everyone's guide to
DISTANCE
RUNNING

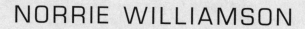

NORRIE WILLIAMSON

THE LYONS PRESS

Guilford, Connecticut

An imprint of The Globe Pequot Press

The Lyons Press is an imprint of The Globe Pequot Press.

10   9   8   7   6   5   4   3   2   1

Printed in the United States of America

Senior Designer: Petal Palmer
Designer and illustrator: Sean Robertson

ISBN 1-59228-438-8

For more information on Norrie Williamson's programs. visit www.coachnorrie.co.za

Author's statement: No sexism is intended in the text when references are made in the male gender only – it is purely to simplify text flow.

Photographic credits:
© photographs – Norrie Williamson with the exception of the following:
Pages 6, 8, 22–23, 46–47, 77, 99, 153 (all), 160, 164, 172–173, 180, 214–215, 220, 223, 241 centre & right, 249, 251, 253, 258 top, 268, 281, 289, 290, 294, 296, 300, 303, 318, 331, 334–335, 336, 338, 341, 351, 352, 354, 356, 386, 391, 396, 409, 412, back cover (top & bottom) – Ryno/Struik Image Library. **Pages** 38 & 48 – Shaen Adey/Struik Image Library. **Pages** 141, 147, 197, 276 – Gerhard Dreyer/Struik Image Library Page 151 – Nick Aldridge/Struik Image Library. **Pages** 216, 236, 258 centre & bottom, 329 – Craig Frase/Struik Image Library. **Page** 227 – Jacques Marais/Struik Image Library Page 241 left – Dirk Pieters/Struik Image Library. **Page** 288 – Anthony Johnson/Struik Image Library. **Page** 299 – Kelly Walsh/Struik Image Library
Log onto our photographic website **www.imagesofafrica** for an African experience

Library of Congress Cataloging-in-Publication data available on file.

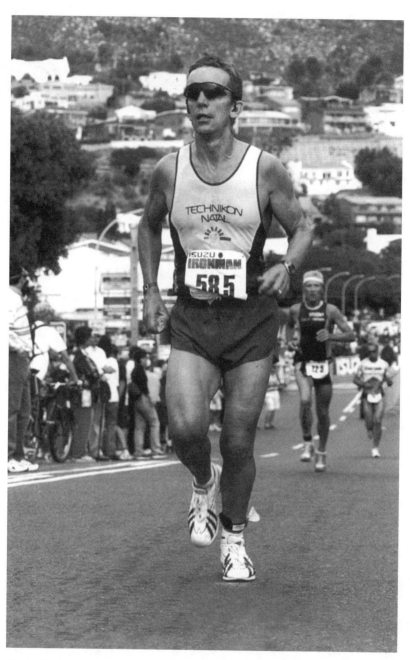

Norrie Williamson in the final 42 km of the SA Ironman, Gordon's Bay 2001

CONTENTS

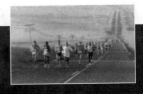

FOREWORDS

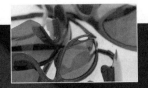

BY BRUCE FORDYCE

Rugby's loss was long-distance running's gain when Norrie Williamson left Scotland and emigrated to South Africa. Like many thousands of runners, Norrie was bitten by the long-distance running bug, which seems to be particularly addictive in South Africa. Thus started a running career that, although rich with major achievements, has been richer still for what Norrie has put back into the sport.

Having met Norrie back in the early 1980s, I've known him to be an outstanding and ferociously competitive runner. He is also a courageous one, venturing into the 'lunatic fringe' of running where he has explored mega-distance running and multi-day events – from 200-km races to JOGLES (John o' Groats to Land's End). Norrie has also excelled at triathlons and duathlons.

Not content to be just a good runner, Norrie has also been a team manager, an administrator and even a hard-working second, running with bucket and sponge.

His combined experience and knowledge has been distilled into this wonderful contribution, *Everyone's Guide to Distance Running*. Even those of us who think we are experienced runners will find that we are mere pupils when we discover the vast knowledge that Norrie has accumulated and successfully captured in his book. Running enthusiasts will find information on every topic, from how to achieve the correct nutritional balance to peaking for the big race. It is all there and no serious runner should be without a copy of this book. I found the personal anecdotes particularly interesting, but perhaps that is because I have been fortunate enough to share moments with Norrie on the road to Paris, or in the pine-covered valleys of Square Valley.

What shines through each page of this book is Norrie's undying enthusiasm for the sport, which can only inspire the reader as much as it has the author.

BY PROFESSOR TIM NOAKES

I first came to know Norrie Williamson during 1984 when he single-handedly organised, managed, coached and even participated as a member of the winning team, in the inaugural London to Paris Triathlon. I learned then that Norrie not only has superior athletic ability, but also a real talent for organisation, a tireless enthusiasm for work and an attention to detail, as well as an unquenchable desire for knowledge. On that trip, nothing escaped his attention. The team's ultimate success was largely due to his personal efforts both as an athlete and as the organising force necessary to cope with the very major logistical problems posed by that unique event.

Although he began principally as an ultra-distance runner, Norrie's proficiency at, and experience in, cycling, swimming and canoeing have allowed him to compete at high levels in both swimming and canoeing triathlons. It is this broad, possibly unique, competitive experience that forms the basis for his sporting wisdom. When that experience is combined with his other special personal characteristics, most especially his genuine enthusiasm for his sports, his inquisitiveness and his desire to communicate his knowledge, it is natural that something unusual should result. The reward of that concentrated effort is this book, which must be required reading for all who have even the most modest competitive running goals.

Everyone's Guide to Distance Running is written for all runners of whatever ability. It highlights the real problems and the important decisions that each runner must make at some stage in his running career. It has been said that already there are too many running books. Why, then, do we need another? The answer is that too often these books convey knowledge but no wisdom. It takes something extra to write a book of wisdom which will materially influence its readers. This is one such book. Norrie Williamson has condensed a lifetime of running experience into a meaningful and valuable message. Runners will do well to consider the wisdom that he has imparted.

INTRODUCTION

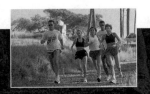

In 1986 I wrote a series of articles for the Durban-based newspaper, *The Daily News*, as a guide to training for the Comrades Marathon. Many clinics had been held and articles written on the subject prior to this, but my series was aimed specifically at the *average runner*.

Any athlete who has ever donned a pair of running shoes in South Africa has undoubtedly dreamed of winning the 90-km Comrades Marathon, but this is a privilege reserved for, and an ambition realised by, a select few. Scientists never fail to remind us that the main attributes required for winning Comrades are dependent on inherited talent.

Such is the conviction of the accuracy of this theory that a calculation by Professor Tim Noakes is frequently quoted to show that even if nine-times Comrades winner, Bruce Fordyce, stayed in bed from January to May, without training, he could probably run the 90 km in under seven hours and still collect a silver medal!

However, in order to win the Comrades Marathon, or for that matter any top-class distance race from 800 m to the longest 'ultra', Bruce as well as other top competitors must indulge in very heavy training and their total commitment to the race is essential if they are to perform to the best of their ability on the day. So great is their dedication that many of them make great sacrifices in their work, family and social lives. For months before a race their top priority is the preparation to peak at that chosen event – all else takes second place.

Immediately, we see that it is not only inherent talent that is involved. A number of other aspects play a part in determining the outcome of an event. It should be a major motivating factor to the reader – regardless of the starting level – to realise that the most talented sportsperson is not always the winner. There are many examples of less talented people beating their more talented counterparts. So how does this happen?

Talented sportspeople don't always win

The less talented person may have a greater focus on the 'goal' and be less likely to be sidetracked by other, less meaningful opportunities. He or she may also have superior control in training as well as during an event, and may have a greater desire to 'win'. It is no coincidence that the majority of the world's boxers, past and present, are from tough backgrounds, or that during the 1990s the great achievers in Comrades came from Russia. They weren't necessarily the best in the field, but achieving a top position represented a major difference in lifestyle. This was best described in a post-match interview by the coach of a rugby team after losing a match to a much lesser team, 'Simply – they wanted it more than us.'

Perhaps only 50 runners in the Comrades have the potential to take home a gold medal, but this does not mean that the other 12 000 plus competitors cannot succeed in the race.

Whilst the majority of runners are not in the position to, nor do they wish to, put Comrades at such a high priority in their lifestyles, there is no reason why they should not be 'winners' in terms of their individual talent, time and lifestyle restrictions, or 'be the best they can be!'.

Everyone may adopt an approach, an attitude and a plan to stretch themselves to achieve what was initially thought to be unobtainable. Even in the best of training conditions they may be unable to compete with the Fordyces or Grishins in Comrades, Tegla Laroupe in the marathon or Paula Radcliff in the World Cross-Country, but they can climb the step-by-step ladder to their own potential.

The same principle applies to any of the major city marathons or other prestige events. In each case there are a few elite, highly talented athletes, in search of the spoils. But there are thousands of others in the field who run without any aspirations of climbing onto the winners' podium and simply want to 'win' within the limitations and targets they have set themselves. A focused, determined attitude can deliver surprising results, and when coupled with the lackadaisical approach taken by some, more talented competitors, even the average runner can reach remarkable levels.

Most Comrades' entrants are unable to squeeze in more than 90 km of running per week, and that is often only for a few weeks during peak training. For many, a last minute, lengthy business lunch or meeting, or a family commitment that can't be broken destroys even these good intentions. This does not mean that you cannot complete the Comrades or any other race to the best of your ability within the limitations of your lifestyle. That is the purpose of this book. It puts into perspective the achievable goals, the training, planning and psychological approach that creates 'winners', and allows you, as a runner, to achieve your ambitions.

The principles apply from 800 m to 1 000 km!

Although my own preference has been towards longer events, this book is not only about marathons, Comrades, 100-km or longer multiday events. The principles, training and advice relate as much to improving at 5 km, 10 km, cross-country, and all other intermediate distances. A popular South African attitude (in athletic circles) is to 'pigeonhole' people and concepts. To do that with the advice in this book is to miss out on a key principles, viz. the faster you are over the shorter distance, the faster you will be over the longer distance.

Even the most dedicated Comrades' enthusiast will do more to improve their potential in their next Comrades by spending a 'season' running only 5-km and 10-km events. Top-notch marathoners and 100-km runners will benefit from sessions that include three sets of 5 x 100 m.

Incredible as that may seem, the truth is there to be seen. It is no coincidence that US athlete Alberto Salazar, a 2:9-marathoner, left the field in tatters in his first-ever ultramarathon, or that Bruce Fordyce could run a 30-minute, 30-second 10 000-m race, and a 2:17 marathon, or that the top Comrades finishers now need to be capable of a 2:10 marathon. In exactly the same way, in order to run a sub-4-minute mile (4 laps of the track each in under 60 seconds), you need to be able to run one lap in less than 56 seconds.

Speed is relative. It is not necessary to have achieved a particular speed before reading this book. What is important is to understand that simply improving your speed over a short distance (whether you started at three minutes per km, or eight minutes per km) enhances your potential at a longer distance.

Naturally, there will come a time when age and training will no longer be able to deliver faster times, but the principle never changes. Instead, the objective then is to maintain your current speed for as long as you can and 'if you don't use it, you lose it!'. So again, speed training remains a key aspect in any schedule.

The two athletic challenges – time or distance

Ideally, it is only as we become slower that we should move up in competitive distance. That was a mistake I made early on. My first race was a marathon, then a 56-km ultra, then Comrades, then a 100-miler, then 1 000 km and ultratriathlons. It was my introduction to Professor Tim Noakes that kindled an understanding of speed and resulted in a 2:35 marathon, 6:07 marathon and 13-hour 100-mile time. Regrets? Only a curiosity as to what might have been achieved if I had first trained to be as fast as possible at 5 km or 10 km before undertaking the marathon or longer.

Not everyone is fast, so the ability to challenge a particular time is limited. Thankfully, those who aren't fast tend to have an ability to go that bit further, which provides another challenge – distance. I take heart from the saying, 'The race is not always to the fleet of foot, but to he who goes the distance.' In running there are two challenges: covering a set distance in the shortest time and testing the body and will against the challenge of distance. A few runners tackle both, but most can only set themselves targets in one or the other.

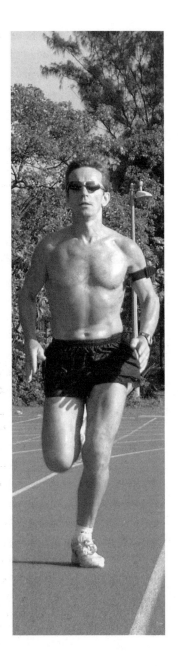

RIGHT *Track training – to be fast over the long distance, you need to train fast over the short distance*

Reinventing the wheel is unnecessary

For you to have confidence in my approach, it is perhaps useful to outline the background to my own experience in sport.

My first sporting love was rugby, a game I still hold in high esteem, and to which I was introduced at the tender age of ten at the Royal High School, Edinburgh, in my home country of Scotland. As was the norm at that age, the forwards were 'selected' purely on size, and since I led the table in the bulk stakes, I was put in the hooking berth. I became noted for my ability to flatten any loose scrum – the only problem was waiting long enough for me to arrive! I vividly remember spending entire matches chasing the game around the field, glad of set scrums and lineouts as opportunities to rejoin the game with the other 29 players.

I had a three-year break from rugby from the age of 16 to 19, after which I returned to play in the former pupils club. In 1973 many of the Royal High F.P. 1st XV decided to pull out of the annual New Year's day fixture against Gala Rugby Club. This was not only because of the Scots' flair for New Year celebrations, but also because Gala was the top club in the country, providing about seven of the Scotland XV, whereas Royal High had experienced a disastrous start to the season.

Although I could identify with the first reason, I always enjoyed the challenge of the game and felt that those players who dropped out made it harder for their team-mates. As a result of this opportunity I was given a chance to play in the 2nd XV and, more through naivety than skill, I had a blinder of a game that ensured my 1st XV selection for the rest of the season. My rapid promotion from 5th XV to 1st XV must have caused some to suspect that it was part of a business deal resembling the cricket match fixing of 2000!

I really enjoyed playing top-league club rugby and in that off season I realised that to retain my place, fitness was essential. Although my hooking ability was good, I carried an 'energy belt' of puppy fat around the field with me. Until then, I had been a safe bet for the last place in any race or training sprints. That, I decided, would change, and my first step was to kick my 30 cigarettes a day smoking habit.

This was probably also when I first started running but my long runs in those days were all of 2–3 km. On one of the early runs I managed to 'conquer' a hill by running to the top but cigarette-induced windlessness prevented even a walk down the other side.

From then until 21 February 1981 I was committed to rugby. By keeping fitter than many of my more talented competitors, I consistently played 1st XV rugby and even made North and Midlands District XV and the Scottish Colleges XV. By training for five days a week as opposed to the usual two – coincidently a strategy used around the same time by Scotland and British Lions hooker, Colin Deans – I became a more mobile hooker. This gave me the edge – certainly it wasn't talent.

The date of 21 February was important because that was the day I flew to South Africa, but such was my love for the game that I wouldn't leave until after the Scotland vs. England international at Twickenham. We played the British Army team on the Saturday morning, watched the international the same afternoon and left a snow-covered Heathrow Airport the following day.

Although my rugby training running seldom exceeded 15 km, I did enter one marathon in the UK, just for the challenge. In that 1980 Birmingham Peoples' Marathon I recorded a time of 2:58:50, which was the winning time for the first Olympic Marathon in 1896 and proved that I was already 84 years behind the times!

The only other races I entered were a Highland gathering at the local rugby ground where I placed well down the field, and an event called the Seven Hills of Edinburgh, which was a cross between a road race and orienteering. Some of the top competitors' lack of local knowledge and a few legal shortcuts by yours truly ensured me a third place and £5 prize money! In truth though, these were very low-key events, and anyone who had previously broken three hours for a marathon was not allowed to enter the Birmingham race!

It was during the flight to sunny South Africa that my change to running was instigated, and a certain English journalist, Bob Holmes, was a major factor in that decision. I had picked up a copy of the UK *Jogging* magazine, (this became *Running* and is now *Runner's World*). He had written an article on a '55-mile race from Durban to Pietermaritzburg'. At that stage I didn't know where the latter city was but I knew that I was going to Durban and Bob's writing certainly motivated me to take up the challenge!

Without the distraction of rugby, since it was the 'off season', combined with the attraction of the sunny days, I was soon running every morning. Coffee and lunchtime chats at work often turned to the subject of the Comrades race and I found further encouragement from my new colleagues.

By March I had joined Savages Athletic Club and ran my qualifying marathon. It was during this first race that I met a runner who, in later years, was to become a very good friend and running companion. We had run together for a few kilometres from around the 22-km mark, when we started chatting. After I mentioned that I was trying to qualify for the Comrades Marathon the following May, my companion commented, 'You'll have no problem if you can run like this.' Here was a chance to talk to someone who had run the race before, so I wanted to know more. I asked him how many times he had run it and his reply became a conversation stopper – 22 times. I spent the next few kilometres puzzling how this apparent 30–35-year-old had managed to run Comrades so many times. In awe at this achievement I forgot his name as we shook hands on the run, but I did remember that his father was of Scots ancestry.

We split up with about another 3 km to go and I couldn't find him at the end of the race (I never looked in the pub!), but in 1983 I got to know Kenny Craig much better when we schemed how we would tackle the Star Mazda 1 000-km race (10 days x 100 km).

Ken's opinion that I would have no problem with Comrades motivated me through the next few months and his words often bolstered me during some of the morning runs when I began to doubt my ability. After all he was an expert – 22 times and so young! It was only later that I discovered his youthful looks belied his 48 years.

Comrades went well for me, with a time of 7:09 and a much-coveted Silver medal and very sore legs to show for it. Despite this I was on an emotional high and even ran the club's time trial the following night! Some senior club members commented how relaxed I had appeared when entering the Jan Smuts stadium in Pietermaritzburg. Already I was being guided towards ultra-events. After all, I knew I didn't have any speed.

I started searching for more distance challenges and in 1982 I entered the track 100 miler. My intention was only to complete the distance but two weeks prior to the event, Tony and Yvonne Sumner suggested that I should attempt a top placing! I was sceptical as Derek Kay, who had been the first man to break 12 hours for 100 miles, was in the field. Derek, however, was going for the 24-hour record and on the day had a bad run in the extreme heat, which gave me the opportunity of a surprise win.

That confirmed it for me and I made the decision to become an ultrarunner, the longer the better. Without testing my speed potential, I had been channelled into the longer events. From then onwards my calendar would centre on the 1 000-km race, and 100 milers. Even the advent of triathlons in 1983 appeared to be tailor-made for the Williamsons of this world. The Leppin Ironman, (21 km-canoe, 100-km cycle and 42.2-km run) and the Carling (5-km surf-swim, 100-km cycle and 42.2-km run) both presented the necessary 'distance' challenge.

I also seemed to recover quickly after these events and started to cram as many as possible into each year and it was only by 1984 that the full impact of my mistakes became apparent.

The year began with the three-day Duzi Canoe Marathon, followed by the Leppin Ironman, the Carling Triathlon, and the Comrades, all of which was training for the London to Paris Triathlon! The latter was a relay for teams of four, running from London to Dover, swimming the Channel, and cycling from Calais to Paris. Having won gold in both the Leppin Ironman and the Carling, 'jogged' Comrades for a silver and captained the Leppin Team to a win in the London to Paris, the emotional wave that carried me forward gave me a sense of invincibility.

It was during the London to Paris that I was exposed to the experience and knowledge of two of the world's sporting gurus, Bruce Fordyce and Professor Tim Noakes, and was introduced to the idea of peaking and the danger of overtraining! However I had already planned an attack on the John o' Groats to Land's End record with Ken Craig, and the full impact of my mistake had not yet taken its toll.

One of the most exciting aspects of this record attempt was to be my return to Edinburgh and I looked forward to displaying my new-found running ability, which in view of my schooldays' experience would startle many friends. In fact, running had also streamlined my figure from an 83-kg hooker's frame to a slender 63 kg. This alone would raise a few eyebrows. After four days I learnt a bitter lesson – what I consider one of the biggest disappointments of my life. I was forced to quit the run as result of a stress fracture to my left leg. What made it even harder to bear was that it happened after only about 400 km, just before Edinburgh, so my planned smooth run through my home city was not to be. Instead I hobbled through to Peebles, a distance of about 160 km, before returning to Edinburgh to borrow my brother's heavy 5-speed bicycle to complete the journey.

However, it was a great privilege to accompany Kenny on the rest of his record-breaking run and he, realising how much the race meant to me, agreed to second me if the chance ever arises to complete that unfinished business. Kenny's record stood for many years, defying attempts from numerous better-known runners. Don Ritchie, a world record-holder at distances from 50 miles to 24 hours, eventually broke it, but only on his second attempt and despite his local knowledge.

The stress fracture meant no running for five weeks and with only six weeks until the Hawaii Ironman, I was cutting it close and digging myself into a bigger hole. It should not have been a surprise that I didn't perform as well in Hawaii as I had hoped. My marathon was of course the biggest disappointment, 3:42 for the 42 km. My only saving grace was that I became the highest placed South African finisher, which motivated me to tackle the 100-mile track race in Durban two weeks later! Thankfully, I finally learnt my lesson, though it had been a hard and disappointing one. With more advice from Professor Noakes and Bruce, I planned my calendar with more intelligence and developed a better understanding of my body's capabilities.

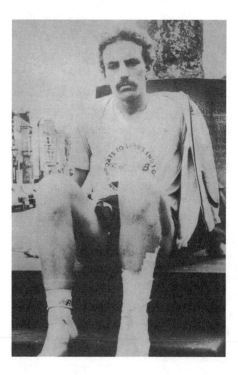

LEFT *'We need to learn from good and bad' – a dejected author in 1984 with a stress fracture after covering 160 km during the John o' Groats to Land's End*

It's never to late too change

Earlier, I made the comment that I wonder what might have been if I had focused on short distances before moving up to the marathon and ultras. Of course we will never know, but it is perhaps some testament to the benefits of more judicious training that in 2001, some 17 years later, I returned to do my second Hawaii Ironman (3.8-km swim, 180-km cycle and 42,2-km run). My time in that race, despite a howling wind that literally stopped runners in their stride, was comparable to that of 1984. In training for the 2001 event, and the subsequent World Championship for which I was selected to represent South Africa, I never ran further than 28 km, swam further than 3 km or cycled further than 120 km. But I did do sprints and intervals in all three disciplines, and plenty of them.

Training methods continue to evolve in the world of sport; there are always new ideas and concepts to be considered and they often arise from a fresh outlook. An example of this is the advice of coach and biokineticist Richard Turnbull. He finally laid to rest my long-held belief that I was the slowest thing on two legs by showing me that I do indeed have speed potential. By accepting this fact I found new inspiration and enjoyment in my running.

Richard Turnbull's inspiration then led me to undertake a training programme that in its own way led me, step by step, to the self-belief that even I could be fast. That produced the desired results, which, in turn, further drove me in search of higher achievements.

To say that I made some monumental mistakes is an understatement. My greatest frustration is that they were not new mistakes but the same ones made by many runners in the past and which others continue to make; the message seldom seems to be passed on sufficiently. Thanks to my exposure to the wisdom of experts I consider myself lucky that the errors of my ways were shown to me early in my running career. Even after 20 years of running I still look forward to the future and view new challenges positively.

The rules apply to us all

To say that I always remember those early lessons would be untrue. Often my enthusiasm or relative success in an event sees me planning another full calendar. A glimpse at the photograph of the dejected runner (pictured opposite), sitting with a plastered, stress-fractured leg on the monument in Peebles, helps to detach myself from the enthusiasm and remember the practicalities. None of us may sidestep the overtraining and overracing rules – we are not invincible.

I cannot state often enough just how good running and sport have been for me. I have certainly had opportunities that I could never have dreamed of when I boarded that plane from Heathrow in 1981.

What makes it all the more fulfilling is that the lessons learned in training and planning for a competition may be applied to all aspects of life and we become richer and more capable as a result.

There are many books on the market that advise the runner on how to become a top-class athlete. These are often written by the world's best runners. And there are others that address the absolute beginner. The problem is that the latter seldom concern themselves with distance events and even if they do, most are written on the assumption that a runner's first priorities are running and winning. In my experience this is not the case for the majority of runners.

The objective of *Everyone's Guide to Distance Running* is to assist the average distance and ultrarunner, so that you may derive as much pleasure from the sport as possible, without repeating old mistakes. That does not mean I will pretend to give you a finite answer in your quest for a perfect training plan, but I aim to put to rest some of the prevailing myths on distance and ultrarunning and to provide you with a good base from which to develop a specialised and individual training programme.

Moreover, coaching manuals often refer to scientific concepts developed by sports medicine sages and scientists and are couched in language incomprehensible to the average runner. This book presents the ideas and principles that guide effective training in an accessible and practical manner.

South Africans are privileged to have in their midst one of the world's top sports medicine gurus, Professor Tim Noakes. He has spent years compiling a book entitled *Lore of Running* (OUP). Many of his concepts are explained here in a very basic fashion with the recommendation that you further your comprehension of these by reference to Tim's book.

Losers let it happen – winners make it happen

If there is one lesson I learnt from sport, it is that 'losers let it happen – winners make it happen'. But sport is merely a microcosm of life, and that simple phrase is as true in business, family and social life as it is in sport.

The principles of the approach proposed in this book, to training, race preparation and race strategies, are the same as those applied elsewhere. There are only a few questions you need to answer. The first is, **'What do you want to do?'** – not the passing whim, but what you really want to do.

If you want something to happen with all your heart,
You will find ways to make it happen:
If you do not really want it with all your heart,
You will find an excuse to explain why it didn't happen!

Steve Waugh, Australian cricketer

We are all capable of far more than we think we are, but thinking, planning and 'wanting' is precisely that, which makes the difference between achieving the goal or not. And the good news is, you are not limited to a single desire, it's an escalating pattern. The more you achieve, the more you realise that you can achieve as your confidence grows. Even the measure of 'winning and losing' changes; it is no longer a simple black and white issue, but rather degrees of success.

Targets are initially set in definitive terms, in a way that implies that achievement is the end, but I now see that achievements are more like mountains. A close friend, Sharonne Emmerick, who also does motivational speaking, has a bookmark that says, 'Climb life's mountains.' This is an excellent concept and you realise that these 'mountain-top goals' become false summits because every time you reach what looked like a peak, is only a change of direction or slope, and ahead lies yet another challenge.

You can, of course, sit on the first ridge and admire the view, but curiosity to see how much better the view is from the higher peak becomes irresistible and another challenge is mounted. Truly, there is no finish line and the more challenges you tackle, the more the opportunities that arise.

As you manage to climb one mountain, you realise that it is not a single peak, but rather a range with many peaks, and the same skills are required to climb a peak on a different mountain – all you have to do is cross the ridges joining the peaks. There is no need to go to the bottom and start anew – all or most of the height you have gained already, may be used on the new mountain with a simple walk across the ridge.

Sometimes you do have to descend slightly before you can climb again, but such descents tend to be small compared to the altitudes you have already climbed. Then it's up again to the next challenge, next peak, next 'exhilarating and giddy' view and the realisation that there are still more opportunities.

At times the slopes are easy and your ascent is speedy, sometimes sheer rock-faces require the assistance of ropes, crampons, and even friends. Progress can be slow. There are even times when you will start on a route only to realise that you are running out of foot- and fingerholds. If you are wise, you will adjust to the path and still reach the summit.

Winners know that achievements are like climbing life's mountains, and the views along the way can be spectacular and rewarding, but the world is full of mountains, each with a different view, and each rewarding in its own right.

There is no specific order that must be followed to climb the mountains and it is unlikely that you will be able to climb them all, but climb those peaks that you think will give you the most appealing view. Beauty is in the eye of the beholder, so what appeals to you and the thrill of your achievement may not evoke a similar reaction from others. Sometimes you may be surprised with the view on the other side, it may not be what you expected, but you will still have climbed to a greater height and that is an achievement in itself.

As you climb, you will find that the number of people towards the top of each mountain decreases. There will nearly always be some ahead of you, but the number below you will increase the longer you climb. Not only do you see more from higher up, but the view is also different. Even one additional step changes the view, and a different view affords you a different perspective.

The more successful you become in achieving your goals, the more mountains you climb, the greater the views you enjoy, and the more perspectives you gain. Do not restrict yourself. We can all achieve much more than we initially have the confidence to believe. This book may delve into the detail of running and coaching, but when you've gained your first running goal, take time to consider the view and decide what mountain to climb next.

Whether it's running for speed, running for distance, or climbing one of life's mountains, the reward can be tremendous, matched only by the **passion required to reach such an achievement:**

To venture into the unknown,
To search for your maximum potential,
To achieve the impossible or highly improbable is life's greatest satisfaction.
It takes intense preparation,
total dedication
and the risk of failure.
If you have paid the price and give 100%, you're a WINNER.

Bob Gries, NFL owner, businessman and ultramarathoner

Earlier I stated that our measure of success and failure changes. Bob Gries hit the nail on the head – if you have tested and challenged your perceptions of your limits, if you honour yourself by extending yourself, if you have focused on a goal and given it your best, then there is no such thing as failure, there is simply another opportunity to go further up the mountain the next time. Better still, you have the experience and knowledge that you gained from the previous attempt!

PART 1:

RUNNING –
A LIFESTYLE F

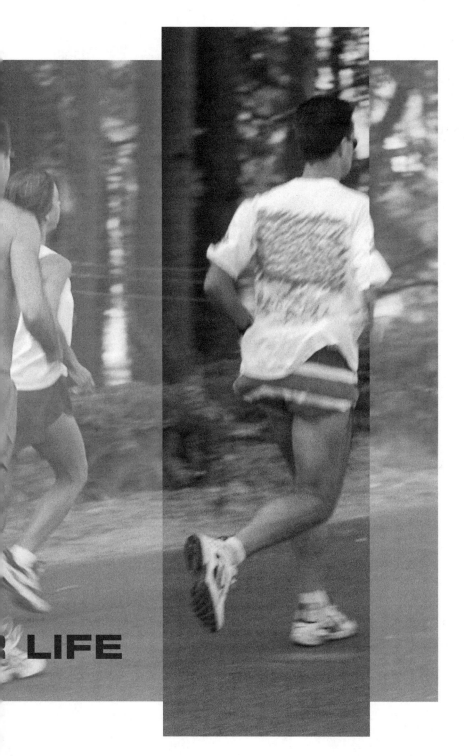

00:00:01
THERE IS NO FINISH LINE!

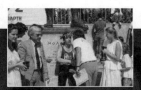

Two phrases dominate the general attraction of, and participation in, running: 'there is no finish line' (also used by Nike sportswear company) and 'the race is not always to the fleet of foot, but to he who goes the distance'. Although they appear to be contradictory, both have long-term messages for runners. To the competitive runner the first may imply that no matter how well you race, there is always more to be achieved. People thought a four-minute mile impossible, but Roger Bannister proved it possible. Within a few months many others followed suit and over the years, the mile record has been systematically whittled down. There is no finish line.

An alternative interpretation is Sebastian Coe's comment that 'there is no such thing as a perfect race'. No matter how well we do, as runners we always look back and wonder if we lost a vital second by rounding a corner too wide in a road race, or an essential fraction of a second in a 400 m by not leaving the blocks slightly faster. Even when everything goes according to plan, the first thing we do is analyse our performance to ensure a better result next time. There is no finish line.

This is the same approach used by Carl Lewis, and one that many runners might adopt when pressurised by the presence of other competitors. By concentrating on striving for your own 'perfect' performance, your focus is redirected from other runners to your own race. Lewis relates how his coach apparently chastised him after he won his first Olympic gold medal with the comment, 'You never left the blocks properly!' It wasn't a derogatory remark, quite the opposite. It was a way of saying there is still more to come, still a better performance. There is no finish line.

However, I feel there is another way of viewing running, one that I often think is overlooked. My future in running will be a combination of these two phrases.

One of the most commonly asked questions of any runner is, 'Why do you run?' It is always hard to come up with an answer that is meaningful to the non-runner, especially if it is asked on the spur of the moment.

Running has many benefits that have been described by medical experts, and there is no doubt that it is one of the easiest sports in which to participate, but I do not run now for either of these reasons. Given my family's poor medical history, exercise was certainly a motivation for my initial introduction to sport, but it has gone much further. Runners encounter various attitudes towards their sport, yet remain committed to some form of participation. It has even been suggested that running is an 'addiction', without which the runner suffers a cold turkey reaction. I am not qualified to comment on the medical validity of that, but I acknowledge that the thought of not running for an extended period is unpleasant. So am I doomed to a life of competition, in constant search of a 'win', initially in the sub-veterans, then veterans, masters and so on?

I sometimes wonder what I will be doing in running, ten years from now, but the question as to whether I will be running doesn't even enter into the discussion. I fully intend to run until I die, and if I die while running, so much the better because, the chances are, I'll die happy! But I honestly don't see myself continuing to, or wanting to be competitive at any distance forever. Not that I would refrain from keeping myself in good condition, as that feeling has become too precious to me, but I would not want to spend the vital extra time required to reach a peak in the years to come.

The great thing about running, which many have come to realise over the years, is that even when there are no prizes to be won or races to be run, there are still challenges to be faced and accomplished... indeed there is no finish line.

At the beginning, the challenge is to run a distance in training so that we can go on to race. Then we challenge ourselves to race faster and beat more people and still later we train to win prizes or categories. This is the progression of a runner. Some runners accept that they will never win any prizes and for them the challenge is to improve their times, or even to complete a race distance and take home a badge or a medal that certifies the fact.

No matter what level of runner you are, there are always new challenges. The lure of a sub-three-hour marathon, completing a Comrades, covering 100 miles in 24 hours, eating up 10 km in 30 minutes, or maybe 50, it's all personal. There can be few other sports where so many different people with varying objectives come together to meet their challenges. Running offers that.

Not all challenges have to be met in formal races and I encourage many runners to consider this aspect of running. The majority of my training as an ultra-distance runner is done alone, not only because it fits in best with my time schedule, but also because I enjoy it. When training for a journey event, or even just for the fun of it, I often plan a 65-km run before work in the middle of the week. I write it into my schedule in advance, but as the time approaches, my excitement mounts, even though it won't necessarily be a fast run.

In order to do the run and be at work on time, I must be on the road just after 03:00. Planning includes leaving a change of clothes and my car at work the night before. I mentally map out a route that is flexible enough to allow me to increase or decrease the challenge, depending on how I feel, but it must take me somewhere specific. Living in Durban, the warm overnight temperatures mean that shorts and vest are adequate clothing. Runs tend to be to and from the town of Umhlanga or Amanzimtoti. The location makes little difference as long as the route is challenging.

I ensure that I have an early night the evening before, and even though it is not a race and there is nothing at stake, the excitement of the 'adventure' keeps me awake and fearful that I might not wake up early enough to do the run.

I head out into the dark only to meet late-night revellers, security guards, policemen or shift workers. At that time of the night we are all defenceless, irrespective of our backgrounds or purpose, and greetings are exchanged. The world seems quiet and perfect and in this pleasant atmosphere I enjoy my run all the more. Four hours later the sun is up, a constant trail of traffic races its way into the city as I return towards work, my goal nearly complete. Despite the distance I still feel a spring in my stride from the success of meeting the challenge and from the knowledge that I have cheated a few extra hours out of the day. It is a wonderful feeling, yet there is no measure of time, no position to log, no competitors against whom to compare my effort, no exact distance to record... just a sense of achievement and personal satisfaction.

The euphoria of the long run wears off towards the end of the day as the early rise takes its toll. I am aware of my need to recover for a couple of days and to restore my rest quota, but that aside, it is a session that holds much attraction for me, one I always enjoy. I see this as something I will do much more of in the non-competitive years.

Running and exploring the high altitude contour paths of KwaZulu-Natal's Drakensberg is another run that has little comparison. Armed with a Walkman or even an MP3 player, some relaxing music, a source of water and an easy-fold rain suit, the world becomes an idyllic place. The initial climb to the contour is taxing as you battle the thinner air, and this too controls the speed at which you can run along the path. But none of that matters as you head off towards the horizon, seeing birds float in the updraught. The mountains seemingly go on forever and a point that appears close is only reached after kilometres of winding paths. The music can make you feel at one with the birds, no other sound is around. Pace and distance mean nothing; there are no kilometre marks, no car can measure the route afterwards, the terrain forbids an even or steady progression and becomes an enforced fartlek session of run, walk and climb. The direction of the run is also unimportant, provided some landmark is taken as the point of return. There is no quantifying this type of run, yet it can become extremely satisfying.

Some argue that it is the effect of the South African climate that makes these ventures enjoyable, but that is not the case. Between 1995 and 1998 I spent a sojourn in Edinburgh, Scotland, which is undoubtedly one of the most beautiful cities in the world. It combines rural and urban splendour and boasts sufficient paths, parks and trails to allow even the fittest distance runner to train off the roads for over three hours without venturing beyond the city boundary.

My first winter of 1996 saw reported temperatures dropping to -20 °C. With clothing layered and hidden under the bulk of a Gore-Tex suit and balaclava, I commenced my scheduled long run. The snow layered the paths and crunched underfoot. From where I lived on the hill, I could survey the Forth bridges, the Pentland hills and the entire western part of the city. This particular run would take me out to the southwestern side and on to paths on the side of the Pentlands. As I commenced my descent from the house, I could see my target turn-around point in the distance. The frost had resulted in a clear, cloudless sky, and combined with the early sun to provide picture-postcard views.

Time would not be an issue, distance would be impossible to measure; it was only about enjoyment and an exploration of the challenge of the conditions. I soon warmed to the conditions as a microclimate built up under the Gore-Tex suit. My stride length varied to meet the needs of different depths of snow, or grip on ice.

There was peacefulness as the city wrapped itself up indoors, giving runners greater freedom and dominance of the roads, paths and tracks. Three-and-a-half hours later, I commenced the climb back up the roads to my house. Now almost midday, a few children were out walking down the road towards me and shouting, 'Hey mister, your balaclava's got ice on it.' With only my eyes, mouth and nose visible, I had been oblivious of my own appearance. The layers of clothing and effort of running had kept me as warm as if I had been indoors. I ran my gloved hand up to my head and brushed off a thin smattering of frost; the heat and perspiration from my head had become frozen on the balaclava. My curiosity aroused, back at home a look into the mirror revealed other winter additions, including ice on my eyebrows! This only added to the pleasure and satisfaction of the run. It was another way of conquering the challenge.

Three different runs, three different challenges and three different experiences – these were not about time, speed, winning or losing; they were about taking and living the challenge of the moment. Failure had no threat, they were merely self-imposed, self-desired challenges. 'The race is not to the fleet of foot, but to he who goes the distance.'

My only desire for my running years from now on is that I will remain fit enough to enjoy these types of runs; these are the challenges and targets for which I will train. Running has something to offer everyone because there is always the challenge, there is always the need to be fit for the challenge within the priorities that you set yourself. There is no finish line!

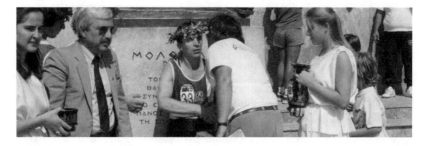

ABOVE *The author is congratulated for his 6th place in the 250-km Athens to Sparta Race in 1992*

00:00:02
THE MAGIC OF DISTANCE

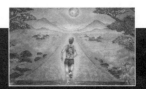

**'The race is not always to the fleet of foot,
but to he who goes the distance.'**

Because my own preferred racing distance is for 90 km and beyond, I am often perceived as someone who is interested only in ultramarathon running. Nothing could be further from the truth. In this chapter, however, I hope to share the magic of the ultramarathon with you, in the hope that, when the time is right, you will explore this aspect of the sport.

Ultramarathons became the focal point of the South African road-running calendar during the years of sporting isolation. Although this isolation was responsible for the initial growth of road running and its boom over the past 30 years, the TV and media coverage that focuses on the most popular races such as Comrades, City-to-City and Two Oceans, has been the catalyst for this growth. Many runners have entered the sport because of the 'accessibility' of the challenge. It is possible that had South Africa not been isolated, national interest may have followed the northern hemisphere trend towards the marathon distance instead.

In London, for instance, some 80 000 people apply to run the London Marathon, and although only 35 000 are accepted, thousands of 'armchair athletes' who see friends and acquaintances in the race, become motivated to take up running and then find themselves motivated to take on the challenge, not of speed, but of the marathon distance. They have no ambitions to win trophies, but simply to test themselves against the distance.

It is the media support and hype of the New York, London, Boston, Hawaii, Berlin and Rotterdam marathons that promotes this interest in the marathon distance to the rest of the world. In South Africa, the lynch pin of the race calendar is the 90-km Comrades challenge, which initiated the same process. Comrades has brought both good and bad fortune to road running; good in that it has attracted thousands into the sport, but bad because it annually tempts runners to move up a distance – often at a young age – rather than down to shorter events, which is the trend in Britain, Europe and the rest of the northern hemisphere. The faster you are at a short distance, the faster and greater your potential at longer distances, therefore you should only move up once you have explored your full potential at the shorter distances.

Another irony of the South African situation is that it is the 90-km distance at which most runners both start and stop, and yet this is only the 'baby' of ultramarathoning. Most international runners consider this to be a mere stroll into the magical land of distance challenge, and think that 56 km is something only for marathoners. Certainly, this view is vindicated by the performances of elite marathoners Thompson Magawana (2:11 marathon best) and Frith van der Merwe (2:27), whose low-flying flight over the 35-mile Two Oceans course set world bests at 30 miles and 50 km that have stood since the mid '80s. Such performances result in many people – runners, administrators and spectators alike – being unable to understand the motivation, athletic endeavour and performances of runners at longer distances. The apparent lack of consistency in the longer distances adds fuel to these observers' fires and it is only when the facts are considered that the magnitude of the problems facing the true ultrarunner may be established.

Internationally, ultras begin with 100 km. For over ten years there has been an Intercontinental Cup, based on a number of events spread over five continents. Athletes' best performances are then compared. There is also the International Association of Ultrarunners (IAU)'s World Cup 100 km, recognised by the International Association of Athletics Federations (IAAF), which became a full-blown world championship in 1993 in Belgium.

Many South Africans initially felt this distance to be comparable with Comrades, and to some extent this is true, but just as there is a 'wall' to be encountered at 32 km in a marathon and at 64 km in Comrades, there is another at 85 km (just when Comrades is finishing) in a 100-km event. If you doubt this, look back at the early performances of top South African Comrades runners' times over the last 15 km of a 100-km race. The final 15 km in the sanction-busting International 100 km in Stellenbosch in 1989 saw Bruce Fordyce's pace drop from a rhythmical three-minute, 45-second pace, to a hard-fought slog, barely under five minutes per kilometre. In 1994, Comrades winner Shaun Meiklejohn led the World 100 km in Japan, only to grind to a halt, surrender the lead and finish fourth in 6:26:58.

In moving up, there is the 100-mile challenge, and many more 'walls' along the way. World records at this distance stand for many years. South African Wally Hayward's record of 12:20:08, set on the Bath road to London in 1953, is still in the top ten best-ever on the road! Don Ritchie's 11:30:51, still the world track record, was set at Crystal Palace on 15 October 1977 and his 6:10:20 record for 100 km on the track, set in 1978, still heads the list. It was only in June 1990, that Ritchie ran his next fastest 100-km track time, 6:46:10, to take the world's best 45–49 age group for the distance. It took even Ritchie, who many consider to be the world's best ultrarunner, until 1991 to match the World & Veteran 24-hour record set by 45-year-old Hayward at Motspur, London, in 1953. Hayward, who won Comrades five times and ran in the 1952 Olympic marathon, returned to Comrades in 1988 to run the 90 km in under 9:30, and in 1989 at the age of 80, he became the oldest finisher ever.

Typically, races over 100 km overseas are won in times between 6:20 and 6:50 with only a few runners achieving under 7:00. Even with a top-class international field in a world championship, 20 or less runners will break seven hours. In an entire year, approximately only 50 runners dip under 6:58 on measured courses. Most 100-mile races are won in times well over 13 hours.

Moving up again, to 24 hours, there are more 'walls' as well as the battle against fatigue. In this category the Greek wonder Yiannis Kouros came into his own and he holds both the road and track records for 12 and 24 hours. He first set a road 24-hour best of 284.853 km in 1984 and improved it to the current 286.463 the following year. In between these, he secured the 24-hour track record with 283.6 km and subsequently moved it up to an awe-inspiring 303 km in 1997. This is the equivalent of running seven non-stop marathons each in 3:20! Kouros holds the eight top 24-hour track performances, with Russian Anatoliy Kruglikov his nearest contender with a 1995 run of 275.982 km. In 45 years, only 20 people have bettered Hayward's 1953 mark.

The Europa Cup for 24 hours has been introduced and athletes may compete in a choice of six races between May and November. A runner's two best performances determine his or her ranking.

Ultra-competitions are, however, gradually getting more international recognition and in 1990 the IAU held an International 24-hour Indoor Championship and awarded the first international vests to competitors. In 1989, one runner surpassed 260 km, four runners over 250 km, and another two over 240 km, with the following six just over 235 km on the track. A similar situation exists on the road. The top-placed runner went to 256.5 km followed by 251.02, then only four over 240 km and three over 235 km. Since then, European teams compete annually in a championship race, and a World 24-hour Championship by 2010 is in the offing. Notwithstanding the increase in prestige and interest, only Kouros, and Russian Ivan Bogdanov were able to place above the 250-km mark on the track, and only seven runners topped 250 km on the road.

Ultras don't stop there of course: there are 48-hour, six-day, 1 000-km and 1 000-mile events, and more, in the search for the ultimate ultra-challenge. Events are held in every conceivable condition including trail, road, mountain and snow and someone has accepted the challenge. Why then such apparently poor performances? Are not enough people trying the longer races? They certainly are. In 2000, teams from over 40 countries competed in the men's World 100-km race and 14 competed for the women's team title. In considering only events longer than 70 km, there are well over 1 000 events in more than 50 countries.

In truth, ultras by their nature require a delicate balance of conditions. The longer an event, the less likely it is that a new record will be set or an existing one matched because, the longer an event, the more there is to go wrong! For success, an athlete must be at his or her peak and the course must be suitable for a record, which means that it should be measured accurately with acceptable amounts of fall (fall is the drop in altitude between the start and finish). Added to this is the major variable, the weather. Ideal ultra-conditions are cool and windless. In a 24-hour race this has to be maintained for a full day! It is interesting to note that all of Don Ritchie's records mentioned above were run in light rain, which doubtlessly cooled the runners. Similar conditions prevailed when Wally Hayward competed in his record-breaking races in the UK in 1953.

Heavy rain on the other hand is a disadvantage. Heat is the ultrarunner's greatest enemy. It has been estimated that a marathoner will slow down by 7% in hot conditions, which turns a 2:30 into a 2:35 in hot weather. Hot may only mean raising the mercury to 20 °C and 68% humidity. Using the same percentage, which is likely to be conservative, would turn a 12:00 100-miler, into a 13:30. This might explain why, in the past 25 years, the 11:56:56 set by South Africa's Derrick Kay has only been beaten twice.

Too cold, too windy or too wet and the times will drop too. So if, as you run your 10-km, 21-km, marathon or 56-km event, your legs feel weary or your muscles ache under the jarring downhill, think of the ultrarunners who have yet another 44 km, 105 km, 20 hours, five days or even longer, to their finish line. Theirs is not the pain of intense speed of marathons or shorter races, but rather the slow, concentrated pain of distance. It is something that takes as much in guts, courage, skill and ability as their speedier counterparts. The emphasis on each aspect is different.

It is difficult to pin down the exact attraction of the challenge of longer events, but the battle to conquer pain and the mind are certainly two aspects – made even harder where the incentive is limited to personal challenge. Without close competition it is not easy to maintain a record-breaking pace when faced with a further 50 km, 100 km or more. This also explains the long life of records. There are few ways to describe the 'pain' of a long run, but one incident during a 1 000-km race in 1983 will give non-ultrarunners some idea. Kenny Craig and I had been running 100 km for six days, and had just completed a 16-hour session, hampered by injuries. As we undressed for a warm bath at the overnight stop, our second, George Thompson, inquired about Kenny's groans, 'Where does it hurt Kenny?' 'Listen laddie,' came the reply, 'I'm so sore that even my blood aches!'

That is ultrarunning, but when you have finished, when you have beaten the pain, the distance and the challenge, the feeling is exhilarating, and all you can think about is the next one.

There is one other aspect to consider about the long-ultrarunners. It is no coincidence that Wally Hayward, Arthur Newton, Don Ritchie and Jackie Mekler have been some of the greatest 'advisers' in road running. When you have experienced these 'extreme' distances, you realise that many of the mistakes made at shorter distances are expanded manyfold. Such mistakes have a magnified effect on the result and you quickly learn lessons that are not so obvious in the shorter events. You only have to read Arthur Newton's three books on running (written in 1924) to realise that he knew many of the 'coaching' secrets of today. He may not have known why his advice worked or the science behind it, but much of it is there. I consider the ten days in 1983 when I ran 1 000 km from Johannesburg to Durban, via Pretoria, to be one of my first real lessons in coaching, and with each of the succeeding ultra experiences, I learned more: the need for pacing, the role of nutrition (not just energy replacement), how the body adapts after three days and the 'pendulum' principle that governs almost all aspects of training. Good books to read are *Just Call Me Wally* (Wally Hayward's biography), Penprint Durban, 1999, or other books by long-ultramarathoners; they nearly all have gems of useful advice.

A new development in sport is the introduction of adventure racing, a multisport event combining a wide variety of activities in an endurance event and normally run in teams, covering anything from about eight hours to a multiday event. (There are some very short events designed as an introduction to the sport, but these really are considered to be 'taster' sessions.) Typical sport combinations include running, cycling, canoeing, hiking, climbing and horse riding. The distances in each event seem quite achievable but the combination is a real test of character, both for the team as a whole and the individuals. The advice in this book may easily be adapted for adventure racing as the principles in the triathlon training section can be used to establish a training programme and the nutritional section will be of particular interest to those competing in ultra-endurance events.

I hope that once you have explored the world of 'speed' where your focus is to see how fast you can cover a set distance, you will consider the ultramarathon option. When your racing seems to be losing its attraction as you finish down the field, or if you feel the need for another type of challenge, consider a move up in distance. Don't be too concerned about the difference in training, as you will discover that most ultrarunners train like a marathoner, with some additional long runs. Ultras have much to offer and are available to all. Why do I like ultras? In those old mountaineering words... probably just because they are there!

00:00:03
UNDERSTANDING THE LIFE
OF A DISTANCE RUNNER

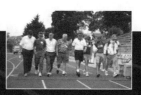

In Boston, Rotterdam and London, it's April. In Berlin and Oslo, it's September. In Amsterdam and New York, it's November, and in South Africa, it's 16 June. All are cities or countries engrossed in marathon fever. All share the same rituals.

For South Africans it doesn't matter where you live – 16 June is the day you become involved somewhere, somehow and at some time in the Comrades Marathon, even if it only means being caught in the traffic jam between Pietermaritzburg and Durban!

Around the world runners are inspired to enter their local mass-participation event. In the vast majority of cases the greatest distance is 42 km. The long years of sporting isolation in South Africa caused the spotlight to fall on an event over twice the length of a marathon and it became the central feature of the national sporting calendar. Each year more than 15 000 people run, and a record 24 000 participated in the year 2000 because the time limit was extended to 12 hours. Had the Comrades not existed, the focus might perhaps have centred on a marathon, but exist it did and a nation deprived of outside sport took the 1970s running boom to 90 km. It is interesting to speculate whether a similar restriction might have taken Britain's runners to the London to Brighton 55-miler (also 90 km).

What is clear is that it is the same level of average runner in New York, Boston, Rotterdam, Berlin and London, who is capable of the Comrades. For this reason, let us consider the role of the runner and the impact his challenge has on the other aspects and people in his life.

In the weeks and months before Comrades, those 15 000 runners will have 'pounded pavements' in their quest for a medal, and each runner's objective and motivation will vary. For the public, it is a tremendous spectacle on the day, but few who are not related to one of those 'mad runners' understand what it takes to make the Comrades' starting line-up. There are stories of runners subjected to challenges in the bar and then, seemingly without training, complete the race in order to win a few cases of their favourite tipple. There are the odd occasions when runners claim not to have trained for the event at all, other than the mandatory qualifying 42-km marathon between October and 2 May. Generally, those few exceptions participate in other sports and draw on that fitness to carry them through.

These anomalies aside, a runner aiming only for a finish needs to complete between 800 km and 1 100 km during the five-month build-up and will average 50–60 km per week in April and May. These figures don't seem all that frightening in comparison to the immense distances covered by the top athletes, but it must be remembered that back runners also train at a slower pace and will have to put in about six hours of running to cover this distance. Add in travelling and changing times and it is almost ten hours per week that a runner must find.

In order to complete the Comrades, a runner must have the speed to finish a standard marathon in under 4:30. Such efforts can be compared over many distances. For example, this would equate to a 57-minute 10-km, or a 45-minute 8-km time trial. In fact, the finish time for most runners can be determined long before the start on 16 June. Pure statistics of their best times over shorter distances and the distance at which they have trained between January and May, show that to achieve an 8-hour finish, a runner needs a 3:20 marathon and around 1 300 km in training. This means a weekly distance of just under 90 km. Silver medallists must be capable of a 3:07 marathon and should cover about 100 km per week, amounting to 1 600 km in the five-month build-up.

When it comes to gold or a win, there are many other factors. On the day, there are probably 50 athletes capable of making the top ten positions, but it all depends on who has a good day and who a bad one. Then there is the planning. Really top runners plan the race like a military operation. They know exactly where their seconds (helpers to provide momentary assistance along the route) will be, what and when they will need to drink, and who the opposition is likely to be. It is such planning and mental preparation that put nine-times winner Bruce Fordyce head and shoulders above the rest of the field. It is, of course, also true that he has inherited the right 'genes' from his parents to make him a world-class runner, but then so have a few others. Fordyce, however, knows how to make the most of them.

To be in with a chance for gold, a runner must be able to run about a 2:25 marathon and train an average of 120 km per week. His total for the five months would be approximately 2 100 km. To win, that should be extended to a sub-2:15 marathon and 2 300 km.

Simply running such distances alone will not ensure a runner a better time; the speed must also be there. Ironically, if a runner overdoes the distance relevant to his speed, he is more likely to finish with a slower time, as he has not allowed himself enough recovery for his standard of training. With the correct training, a runner's time is virtually a foregone conclusion if he paces himself throughout the race. Thereafter, only the positions need to be sorted out and, apart from the top 50, most runners are unconcerned about that. These types of statistics may be applied to any marathon or distance race, and a balance can be determined between the training distance, the current speed of the runner and the desired finish time. If the balance is right, the finish is predictable.

Therefore, on 'marathon day', be that the local 10 km, marathon or Comrades, when you see the TV coverage of the race, you don't have to feel any anguish for the runners, or sympathise with their pain. If they have done their training, the race is a mere formality of proving statistics and can be one of the most enjoyable runs of the year. It is this enjoyment that will motivate them to train for next year's event or the next challenge.

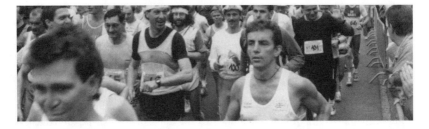

ABOVE *Earning my first GB vest in 1993 at the European 24-Hour Championships in Switzerland*

00:00:04
DISTANCE RUNNING –
YOUR LONG-TERM PROSPECTS

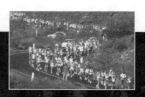

'In order to maintain – continue to train!'

One of South Africa's most popular and remarkable athletes was Willie Mavuma. At the 'tender' age of 67 he was capable of leaving over 95% of the field in his wake, whether he competed in a 10-km race or a marathon. During my first 15 years in South Africa, Willie, who ran for my former club, Savages, never seemed to age and, indeed, appeared only to have slowed down marginally over that period. If it was not for an unfortunate accident, he would no doubt still be alive and running today.

Willie was typical of a growing breed of older runners such as John Walker of New Zealand who aimed to be the first 40-year-old athlete to run a sub-4-minute mile, and John Campbell who at 41 ran a 2:11:04 marathon at Boston, indicating that some runners are able to 'cheat' the ravages of time.

A compilation of recent research on the effects of age (or the process of ageing) on running will give runners of all ages some hope, and perhaps some guidance in this regard. Ageing is a subject that affects everyone, be it now or a few years down the line. No matter what, we all grow old but that doesn't automatically mean that we will become substantially slower. It has long been believed that, as we age, our ability to maintain our previous levels of performance drops off, and that all those long training hours cannot combat the inevitable drop in times. This appears to be substantiated by the fact that most top-level sportsmen and -women retire in their late 20s or early 30s. By 40, it is time to have more respect for the 'fragile' body and to approach exercise more gently. At best, this steers us towards a sedate training pace; at worst it is regression towards the status of 'professional adviser' – a role undertaken by the mass of 'TV experts' on couches throughout the world!

Research has confirmed this belief and shown that even with the adoption of a 'long, slow distance' approach to training, we can expect a drop off of around 9% in aerobic capacity for each passing decade.

In South Africa the modern biathlon comprises a 1-km run and a 100-m swim. Twelve bonus points are awarded to those over 27 years of age on the basis of a 1-second slow-down in both the swim and the run per year. Personally, I think this is slightly excessive but it does acknowledge the problem.

A study that included 14 Olympic competitors ratified that, even at the highest level, a 10–15% reduction of aerobic capacity should be the expectation for a decade of no training. Reduction in VO_2 Max, and Maximum Heart Rate, are two symptoms that are accompanied by an increase in mass. If 'the writing is on the wall', why continue your training regimen? After all, a mere 1% benefit in aerobic capacity is poor return for ten years of continuous training. Could these hours not be used to better effect?

In real terms, the effects of 'age' can be quite devastating and a drop in VO_2 Max of 1 ml/kg/min per year would result in a 2:40 marathoner requiring 3:25 to run the same distance years later. Add to this the weight we gain as we age, which tends to manifest itself in an 'energy belt' around our waists. Such mass increase is of no use and a mere 1 kg increase in weight can cause an immediate five-minute penalty to a 2:40 marathoner, and a further 3% drop in VO_2 Max.

Thankfully, the research that confirmed our worst fears also provided an insight into how many of these seemingly ageless veteran athletes maintain their performance level into their autumn years. What sort of genes, miracle potion or elixir have they discovered that allows them to run times that many 20 or 30 years their junior are still striving to achieve? The phenomenon is most obvious in track and field athletes, and this may be a clue.

Consider the case of 68-year-old Canadian Earl Fee, who entered the 1996 World Veteran Championships in South Africa with 13 World Age Group records on his CV. His specialities are 300-m- and 400-m-high hurdles, 400 m, 800 m, 1 500 m, and mile distances. He attributes his success to exercise of some form every day. Unbelievably, Fee stopped running for 33 years due to injury, but successfully returned to the track in 1982. A daily regimen of press-ups, tennis and skiing on water or snow formed the basis of his exercise during his 33-year racing sabbatical.

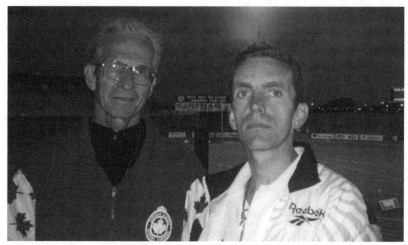

ABOVE *The author with Earl Fee in Durban in 1996 during the World Veteran Championships*

Fee is by no means a freak of nature. A trio of octogenarians from Japan also competed in the 1996 World Veteran Championships in Durban, with Kizo Kimura, the oldest at 87, participating in 13 events, mixing pole vault, javelin and hammer with runs including 400-m to 80-m hurdles. His range of events required speed, strength and flexibility. However, he was disappointed to have left his 91-year-old training partner, Kumazo Kashiwada, at home in Japan! Athletics aficionados will also remember the exploits of New Zealand's Derek Turnbull. Now in his 70s, he still produces competitive times of 2:28:37 for 800 m and 18:34:61 for 5 000 m giving him World Age Group bests.

And it is not only the men who can produce outstanding performances. Which 50-year-old (or should that be young?) wouldn't be pleased to complete 100 m in 12.65 seconds, 200 m in 25.72 seconds, 80-m hurdles in 12.86 seconds and catapult 5.27 m in the long jump? These are the four new World Age Group records American Phil Raschker added to her haul in her 50–54 (years of age) category. This youthful-looking dynamo also bagged seven golds, including the heptathlon. These examples are just a few of the thousands of veteran athletes who have seemingly drunk from the fountain of youth. So where is this Holy Grail?

The benefits of moderate exercise, which include an increase in high-density lipoprotein (HDL) or 'good' cholesterol and a reduced risk of coronary heart disease were highlighted in the Harvard Alumni Study of 17 000 men over a 20–26 year period. This landmark research, which began in 1962, found that each hour of moderate exercise could add roughly two hours to your life! There are limits however, which prevent us from buying back to 'eternity'. The two-year addition is applicable with approximately 25 km of weekly jogging, and the upper limit would appear to be around 50 km per week. In kilocalorie (or kilojoule) terms this converts to about 2 000 (8 400 kj) to 4 000 (16 800 kj) per week. This need not be 'vigorous' exercise, as the research relates to an intensity of about 75% maximum heart rate (about 65% VO_2 Max or six or seven minutes per kilometre jogging for a good club runner – obviously the actual speed will reduce relative to your own ability). Given the added known benefits of reduced blood pressure, reduced risk of insulin-dependent diabetes and reduced risk of osteoporosis (particularly in women), it would appear that we have the essence of our goal in basic exercise. However, there remains the issue of 'quality' as well as 'quantity'.

Research undertaken in Finland made a comparison between endurance sports (running, cycling, swimming), team sports (football, rugby, hockey) and power sports (weightlifting, sprinting). It determined that endurance athletes could add six years to their life in comparison to a couch potato, whereas team sport players only added four years and 'power' people a relatively miserly two years. As a rider to the outcome, the researchers noted that power and team players enjoyed a higher social status, which possibly accounted for their particular increase in life expectancy, taking into consideration their improved nutrition and health care – all of which might result in those who undergo a relatively minimal amount of aerobic exercise becoming septuagenarians. However, to most runners this extension of 'years' is a mere formality, as their lifelong commitment to such miserly amounts of low-intensity work is already grafted in stone. The overriding quest is to maintain a level of excellence.

The Harvard research indicated a link between low-intensity jogging and swimming with longer life, but found that gardening, housework and walking (all often promoted by fitness gurus) did not provide the same results. So the initial link to intensity is evident.

More recently, research on distance runners was undertaken at Ball State University in the USA that included such notable athletes as Frank Shorter, Jeff Galloway and Derek Clayton among the 37 elite athletes first tested in 1970. Repeat tests were undertaken in 1992. In the intervening years, eight had taken to the couch, 18 had continued casual training at a low intensity and 11 had kept to a routine of regular, vigorous training.

As expected, the 'retired' eight had experienced a drop of 12 beats per minute in Maximum Heart Rate and a 10–15% aerobic capacity fall off, and the casual trainers had a marginal advantage with a 9% drop. However, those who had maintained an aggressive approach to their training with higher intensity work had maintained their VO_2 Max, and Max Heart Rate, while their fall-off in aerobic capacity was a mere 2% per decade. One miler's time of 4:05 at the age of 25 had dropped by a mere eight seconds to 4:13 at 45.

Swedish researchers think they might have the explanation. They have proved that, from the age of 40, the nerves that control the fast twitch muscles begin to deteriorate. That the basic premise of intense exercise is a prerequisite for maintaining performance was confirmed by testing 26 elite athletes (including 14 Olympians) by American coach Jack Daniels. Using less elite, but motivated 'average' runners, researchers in Milwaukee, USA, could prove that regular, intense exercise allowed 52-year-olds to maintain their VO_2 Max for a ten-year period (i.e. until they were 62).

So, in practical terms where is the fountain of youthful performance? The secret appears to lie, not with regular endurance exercise, but rather with regular intense exercise. Endurance work will certainly provide an extension to life and a reduction in ill health, but performance is guided by the rule of 'use it or lose it!'.

If you think of your heart as a 'rev counter', your youthful range may be from a resting rate of below 50 to a maximum of above 200. Theoreticians tell us that our maximum may be calculated from 220. Therefore a 50-year-old has a theoretical maximum of 170, which many use to guide all their training. This is merely a rule of thumb, however, as many training athletes find that they are capable of going well beyond this. In our early years of training we grind out high-intensity work with little care for how high our heart rates go. Our intensity is limited more by pride and an 'eye-balls out' creed than a heart-rate monitor. As we age, we tend towards the conservatism of a watchful eye on the upper limit and give more credence to those promoting intensity restrictions, but we still fail to use part of the 'heart-rate capacity' that we have developed. Like a weightlifter, if we only ever lift 60 kg in training, how will we ever lift 80 kg in a competition? Unsurprisingly, this does not mean that we have to make use of maximum revs at every outing, but rather that the limiting factor to our performance should to some extent be self-imposed.

A study to determine the best way of training for a 10-km race was undertaken at the University of Texas by Peter Snell (a sub-four-minute miler in his own right) with ten club-level runners. After an initial base training of six weeks, they were split into two groups, one group had two 29-minute sessions of lactate threshold training, while the other group used two-weekly interval sessions over 200 m and 400 m. Each of the interval sessions was run at a pace between 10-km and 5-km race pace or slightly faster, and the total distance per session was about 5 km. By comparison, the threshold group was to cover around 8 km of continuous running at 12–15 seconds per mile slower than 10-km race pace. The remaining training sessions of both groups were identical.

On completion of the study, the 'interval' group improved not only their 800-m race time (by over 11 seconds on average), but also reduced their 10-km times by an average of over two minutes. In comparison, the threshold runners, who were effectively only training below their race pace and heart rate, improved their 800-m times by only 6.6 seconds and their 10-km by one minute. There are many reasons for this, but most can be encapsulated in the concept of 'using it or losing it'. This is not only restricted to heart rate, but also running efficiency, co-ordination and the ability of the nerves to 'fire' the muscles at the required rate for leg speed.

Even during injury it has been shown that undertaking one session of 5 x 400 m (or 5 x 1–1.5 minutes effort in other endurance sports) per week is sufficient to maintain basic fitness for approximately ten weeks. This is primarily related to the reduction in total body blood volume when exercise is stopped suddenly.

To maintain performance, it seems you need only incorporate one or two sessions per week, which will tax you to the higher end of your capacity. These should be slightly faster but significantly shorter than the event for which you are training, and ties in with the prime training of those world veteran athletes identified at the beginning of the chapter.

These same principles may be adapted for any endurance sport. Given the intensity required, the interval work should be over one minute but probably be no longer than 6–10 minutes. Recovery between efforts will obviously vary depending on the speed of the effort. **As a general guide, start with the following:**

LENGTH OF EFFORT	RECOVERY
30 seconds	40–60 seconds
60 seconds	2 minutes reducing to 60 seconds
3 minutes	3 minutes reducing to 90 seconds
6 minutes	5 minutes reducing to 3 minutes
10 minutes	around 3 minutes

Returning to the 'power and team players' of the Finnish study, it may be that in order to maintain their peak performance, they need to do some 'over distance' work. By their very nature, football, rugby and other team games tend to involve only short high-intensity runs down the wing or midfield, with fairly long periods of low-intensity 'recovery'. This is probably of insufficient duration to elicit the benefits of interval training (a 30-second run would take the player over the full length of a rugby pitch!). Biweekly 'quality' sessions could provide the added boost an older player needs to keep ahead of his younger rivals.

An aspect common to all ageing sportspeople is the natural decline in muscle strength. Muscle density and elasticity decrease with age and to slow down the rate, it is necessary to include a cross-training programme. An older runner or cyclist should spend more time on upper-body strength and a regimen of basic plyometric jumps (hops, stair-skipping, etc) and an older swimmer needs to focus more on the lower body.

The final ingredient to continued performance is motivation. For the elite athlete, this is perhaps the most difficult. After focusing on an Olympic or world medal for 8–12 years, how do you maintain the drive? After all, you can only move sideways in the same sport by defending your title. Given the dedication and sacrifices required by the cream of sportspeople and the lack of reward for those who just fail to make the grade, it is no surprise that they retire 'early'. Their decision may be more to do with lack of desire or burnout than it is with a fall-off in performance (although the two are often interlinked).

Perhaps the future will see more elite sportspeople adopt Andy Ripley's approach. The England and British Lions backrow rugby player of the 1970s made the final squad for selection to the Oxford-Cambridge boat race in the late 1990s at the age of 50! The change of sport had provided him with the motivation to maintain a high level of exercise. And this is where the average sportsperson is at an advantage. Unfamiliar with the 'role of winning' their move into veteran categories will often promote them, closer to the victory platform. In some sports there are even points added for each year of age, or other methods of handicapping, to equate performances. Understandably, there is limited incentive for a previous Olympic athlete to win an age group veteran title, but for the less talented, or late starter, the desire for a world or national ranking in veteran competitions can provide the necessary drive to put in those vigorous training sessions.

With athletes such as Merlene Ottey and Linford Christie competing at Olympic level in their mid-30s, Steve Redgrave winning his fourth Olympic gold medal in rowing, 40-year-olds breaking the four-minute mile barrier, and Carlos Lopes not only running a 10 km in 27 plus minutes but winning the 1994 Olympic marathon one year later at the age of 38, it is time to stop thinking of such career extensions as applicable only to 'freaks'. Although we may not reach the same level of performance, developing the same passion for high-intensity work will assist us to maintain our own peak levels longer.

Our way forward seems to have prompted a new ethos: 'Train to maintain, use some speed to succeed.'

PART 2:

THE BASIC PRIN
OF TRAINING

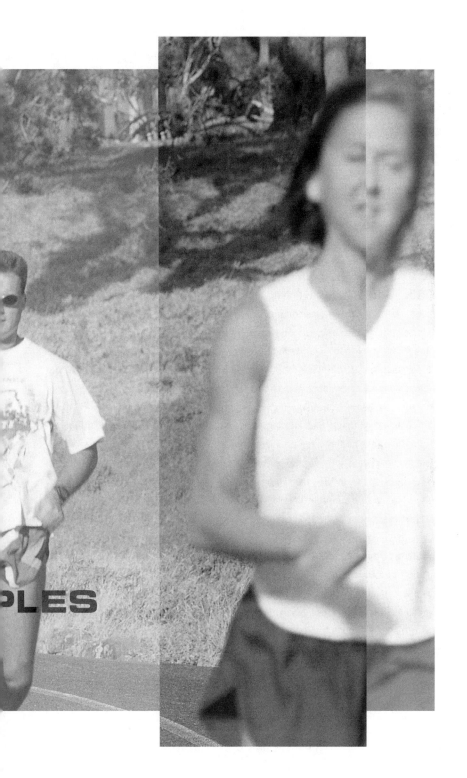

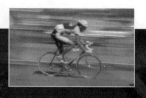

Stress and adaptation

The purpose of training is to bring your body to a state of readiness that will allow you to meet a specific challenge. Training is a process of stress and adaptation whereby the body is subjected to a stress or more exercise than it normally experiences. It adapts by becoming fitter and the stress is increased at regular intervals. This should be carried out over an extended period of time and, as long as the stress is not too great, benefits will continue to be felt up to a certain limit.

Unfortunately, most athletes at some stage in their career, adopt more of a 'do or die' approach to training and expect miracles overnight, or believe they have superhuman qualities that allow them to defy the basic principles.

The concept of stress and adaptation is not restricted to running, or indeed to training for sport, as the same principle applies to many aspects of life. In fact, the scientific belief in the evolution of man is based on the principle that species survive by adapting to the stresses of their environment. If man truly evolved from the ape, we can be sure that it wasn't simply a case of running around on all fours one day and a week later all the apes deciding to walk on two legs. This process took many, many years.

Looking at the different climatic conditions in which man survives, we can clearly see another area where stress and adaptation occurred. How are some people able to live a normal life at altitudes of 3 500–4 500 m, and yet others have problems doing the most basic tasks when they visit these areas? However, if the visitors remain there for a sufficient period of time, they become more productive as their bodies adapt to the stress of the lower availability of oxygen.

These are two simple examples, but they highlight the fact that adaptation takes time. Later it will be seen that it is the very period of inactivity, rest, or light recovery that results in an increase in muscle strength or size. In other words, training is only the catalyst, while benefits are actually gained during the recovery. It is true that enthusiasm is necessary for training, but enthusiasm cannot replace the natural time-scale of adaptation and recovery. What is exciting though, is that because training and adaptation are long-term processes, so too can the improvement be in your performance. This leads directly to the concept of short- and long-term goals.

We are frequently motivated by short- rather than long-term goals. This is particularly true of novices in a sport, who tend to see dramatic improvements in performance for very little effort. For this reason we often bite off more than we can chew and so fail to achieve our potential. With restraint, planning and a more realistic approach, there is a greater likelihood that we will fare much better.

Another benefit of setting short- and long-term goals is that it can supply on-going motivation and direction for us over the years. It is surprising how soon long-term goals become short term, only to be replaced by more long-term goals. The only drawback lies in the scientific belief that our inherited genes largely govern our maximum potential. Nevertheless, one of the great assets of the sport of running is that our goals may so easily be set in comparison to our own previous achievements. There is always room for ambition and improvement.

It is true that physiological variations make a specific runner more suited to a particular event or distance. Nor can it be denied that there has to be a limit to the normal physical ability of an athlete. However, I can't help believing that this 'depressing' concept omits to take into account a number of points. Firstly, if we accept that adaptation is a long and ongoing process, why should it 'peak' at a particular point? Certainly, I can accept that the rewards and improvements may decrease with time, and that there is a point of diminishing return, but I have difficulty in accepting that there is some point beyond which each athlete cannot go. Recent studies in, and results from, veteran athletes also suggest that there is opportunity for greater improvement than previously thought.

Secondly, this concept of absolute limits makes no allowance for the psychological aspects of the sport. Without doubt the longer the distance, the bigger the role the mind plays in keeping the runner fixed on his goal. It is the area of mental control and training that offers the greatest opportunity for future sporting improvement. Though I have nothing but admiration for the mental strength that Olympic sprinters exhibit as they cope with the suffocating and intense pain of running a 200-m race, it must be compared with the mental anguish that multiday competitors experience in trying to combat the constant lower-intensity pain of muscle, bone and joint while striving to cover long distances. This latter experience was best described by Kenny Craig in the Star Mazda 1 000-km race in 1983, when after six days into the ten-day event he said he was so sore, even his blood hurt!

Without doubt, the mind can play a great role in a performance and this is discussed in more detail later. What we do in our everyday training is not only physiological, but to a large extent also determines our mental attitude towards the coming race. Although everyone has a different potential and much of the physical side of that has been determined by our choice of parents, our ability to reach goals is a product of our own mental drive, determination and enthusiasm, factors over which we have more control. Remember, there is no finish line.

I honestly believe that I can improve my running by combining sensible training, motivation and a willingness to learn both from personal experience and from others. This very basic, but important concept is addressed later in the discussion on the role of coaches and coaching. It is most unfortunate that many of us first have to reinvent the wheel before realising the truth of training and adaptation, by which time we can be past our prime.

Lifestyle limitations

If training, and therefore performance, is related to a series of stress and adaptation sessions, then athletes who concentrate most on alternating these two phases of training will show the biggest improvement in performance. This certainly seems to be true of most of the world's top runners, who alter their lifestyles such that they can concentrate on their running, and recovery from it. Other aspects of their lives seem to take a lesser place.

Even though Sebastian Coe was undoubtedly one of the world's greatest middle-distance runners of his time and Bruce Fordyce one of the world's greatest runners over the 50-mile distance in the 1980s and '90s, we can only speculate as to how well they would have fared had they been forced to cope with the added responsibility of full-time careers, married life, night school, children, or many of the other things often faced by the average runner on a day-to-day basis. This is in no way meant to detract from what Seb or Bruce achieved. On the contrary, I respect their determination and motivation to be the best there is, and to reach their full potential. However, it does highlight the fact that different people have different priorities in life.

Moreover, people who direct their ambitions in other fields, have less energy, mental drive and time to give to running and they must accept that they will not reach their full potential as runners. They can, however, make maximum use of the time they do spend in this field to achieve their full potential within the limits they have determined.

It has been said that the only time we are free of stress is when we are dead. The next least stressful time is when we are asleep, which is the 'recovery' period from the stress of day-to-day living. If we miss a few nights' sleep, we quickly adopt a 'Jekyll and Hyde' personality, becoming irritable and unable to cope with mundane situations. We all have our own capacity to deal with stress. Once that capacity has been filled, however, we start on a downward trend physically and mentally. Most people never come close to using their full stress capacity on a day-to-day basis.

Psychologists have estimated that only 10% of people actually make the most of this capacity to achieve their goals. Of course there are those who become workaholics or live in other stressful situations that eventually almost become a way of life. Gradually, the stress leads to a decline in health and attitude until they seem to be constantly in a state of disrepair. The problem is that such changes are not dramatic, but rather a slow, imperceptible decline. One of the best ways to explain this concept is to imagine your capacity to cope with stress as a fruit pie – no matter what you do, you cannot cram so many apples into the pie that you burst open the pastry topping. What you can do, though, is to fill the pie completely without bursting it.

This means that, as athletes wanting to achieve our best, we can use whatever space is left, after we have coped with the other stresses in our lives, to cope with the stress of training. The contents of the pie – and the proportion of our training stress – will therefore be decided by the priority we give to our running. Obviously, the amount of stress available for training changes from day to day, as the stress from items of higher priority, such as career and personal commitments, changes from day to day. When children are ill or we experience changes at work, the stress associated with these events will fill more of the pie; hence the stress of training must be reduced if the pie is not to burst.

It would obviously be wrong to live to maximum stress capacity indefinitely, and would be similar to driving a car at top speed all the time; although it would better cope with this than with over-revving as the car would eventually break down. We must accept that there are periods when we need to cut back on the total stress in our lives so that we can recover from this condition. In fact, such recovery may also benefit us again through adaptation to the stress by improving our overall stress capacity. Perhaps this is one reason we tend to require less sleep as we age.

Gradual adaptation

Following the argument so far, the obvious thing to do is to make full use of the stress capacity left by other commitments, for running training. However, this clashes with another important principle – that of gradual adaptation.

Gradual adaptation fits in well with long- and short-term goals, but is often at odds with our enthusiasm and motivational drive. At the beginning of any training programme, traditional wisdom has always advised a gentle start and a gradual build-up. This is easy to follow because of the breathlessness and hard work that are intrinsic to the first two or three months of regular running. After that, enthusiasm for our new-found fitness often leads us to chase our goals by becoming overambitious in our training. Such an approach frequently results in injury and takes us back to a point where we could end up even less fit than we were originally.

As with most training concepts, gradual adaptation can be illustrated by a simple physical example. Compare the increase in training load to a brick attached to the end of an elastic band. If one end of the band is held and the brick is dropped, the brick plummets towards the ground, building up speed and momentum. When it reaches the full extension of the elastic band, there is enough momentum to break through the resistance of the band, which snaps and the brick hits the floor. The elastic band must first be repaired before the experiment can be repeated.

If, however, the brick is lowered gradually, in such a manner that the elastic band is given time to adapt to its stretching limit, the brick can be lowered until it hangs in delicate balance at the bottom of the elastic band, which is at full stretch. This method maximises the strength of the elastic band instead of destroying it. This is the objective for which we must strive in setting our training programme.

From this analogy we see that in the second case it takes longer to stretch the elastic band to its full capacity, but the rewards are correspondingly greater.

As will be explained in a later chapter, this is also the basis for stretching. In fact, when stretching is applied in this gradual manner – stretch, reduce force, stretch more – the muscle adapts and stretches further than it would otherwise do. This again indicates the rule for correctly controlled stress, rest and adaptation.

Rest

Thus far, we have only discussed stress and adaptation, but the key to training is rest. Training is a process based on the principle of stressing a system to a point just beyond that of which it was previously capable, and then backing off to allow it to recover and rebuild. In this rebuilding, it becomes stronger and can cope with a slightly greater load.

We are all used to this type of progression. In fact, when we first start running we experience it in the most obvious form. The first day out on the road, we battle to make the end of the street, or a lap around the block and we return home flushed, sweaty and breathless. Several months later we would not bother to change into running gear if we were going to run only that distance. In the beginning we are forced into this system of stress and rest but later we seem to forget the early lessons because we are better able to cope with the stress.

The key process in adaptation is rebuilding and strengthening, which occurs during periods of rest. Even in the higher-intensity track and speed training, the benefit is achieved not during the run but in the recovery periods between the runs.

We often hear runners say they would like to be full-time athletes and have all day to train, but this is misguided. The key to the success of full-time athletes is not in having all day to train, but in having all day to rest so that they can put maximum effort into each workout and still recover before their next session.

This was best described by Wally Hayward, perhaps the best ultrarunner the world has seen, who said, 'Being a full-time athlete doesn't mean having more time to train, but means having more time to rest.'

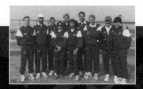

This chapter covers the planning required for eventual success, often an extremely subjective area. Runners who are looking for a 'magic formula' will be disappointed.

It is impossible to write a schedule that will suit your specific needs, as it not only depends on the distance race for which you intend peaking, but also your current level of training, how you react to a hard track session, when the race is, what 'season' of training you are in, among others. The purpose here is to provide some basic principles that will allow you to plan your individual 'ladder to success'.

Setting the goal

Before you can begin a journey, you need to know your destination and your goal. You must have a goal, or rather a series of goals that you want to achieve. Set a target and aim to make steady progress towards it. Once you have reached the goal there is an immediate sense of achievement, followed by an empty feeling as you wonder what to aim for next. The advantage of setting a series of short-, medium- and long-term goals is that you have immediate direction, but remember the necessity of allowing yourself a recovery break before subjecting yourself to the rigours of additional training. When you have achieved your major goal of the year, take an extended recovery period.

During this time you should do your initial planning for the next challenge, which could be anything from a 10 km to a marathon, from a local race to an international championship. In South Africa the goal may very well be the Comrades Marathon on 16 June. The Comrades atmosphere generates its own psychological stimulus.

Before planning, it is important to bear in mind that each goal is not an end in itself. The goal of training should be a continued progression – week on week, month on month, year on year and goal to goal. That is why top athletes often work in four-year cycles, aiming for the Olympics. Planning in autumn 1996 was geared towards a performance in Sydney in 2000, and from there the focus shifted towards Athens in 2004 and beyond. For a first Olympic appearance, the goal may simply be to make the team. Four years later, the focus should change to make the final, or possibly to win a medal. During each four-year period, there are the national championships and trials, continental championships, Commonwealth Games and world championships, each of which provides a focus and measure of an intermediate goal. You may not be seeking such high-profile successes, but the principles you need to adopt are the same.

Returning to the Comrades Marathon, let us consider a single year commencing from the day after Comrades (17 June) and let us assume that your objective is to reduce your PB (personal best) for the distance over the following 2–3 years, with a view to winning a silver medal for a sub-7:30 finish.

If you are a club member you may have some commitments to cross-country leagues, road leagues or other events, which score points for the club and which will need to be factored into your planning. But if you are truly going to reach your potential, there may also be key times when involvement in such an event may not suit your training requirements, and this will have to be explained to the club. In such cases, both parties must remember what they want from the sport and the goals of an individual athlete should take precedence. Remember, life is not a dress rehearsal, you only have one chance of taking on a challenge that is important to you; the key is to know what your priority is and to work towards that.

THE YEAR'S PLANNING COULD LOOK LIKE THIS, STARTING 16 JUNE:

1.   **Race** the Comrades Marathon (previous goal and now the new starting point).
2.   **Active rest** for two to three weeks (to early/mid July) – easy, short runs after two weeks.
3.   Two to three weeks building back to approximately 50% of the pre-Comrades weekly distance but with emphasis on **increasing quality** sessions e.g. short hills and fartlek. (beginning August).

4. Two to three weeks with reduced distance, but including **intervals and tempo sessions**. During this period include a few 10-km, cross-country or other low-key events as quality runs (beginning September).

5. Gradually **increase the distance** of the long run on alternate weeks, of which one session every ten days is to be run at marathon pace beginning at 6 km and increasing to 20 km. This will ideally end with a two-week taper and a marathon in late October/early November. (The objective of steps 3. to 5. is to improve your marathon speed and to qualify you for the following Comrades.)

6. **Active recovery** from marathon for two weeks.

7. Keep weekly distance low and **focus on quality** (short races/relay events/track events from 1 500 m up to 10 km maximum). This is the summer period and although you may not be competitive at these events, improving your basic speed here will help in your goal of Comrades (eight to ten weeks to mid February).

8. **Active recovery** from quality for two to three weeks (end February).

9. **Commence build-up to Comrades** – maintaining two quality sessions (one about 5-km pace and one around 10-km pace) each week. Any long races (30–50 km) entered are to be run at goal Comrades pace, and not more than one run longer than 45 km and two runs of 42 km by last week of May.

10. Ensure a two to three-week taper period, **dropping distance but maintaining quality** with virtually no running in final week.

11. **Race** the Comrades Marathon.

12. Return to 1. and **set new goals.**

It must be stressed that this planner has been suggested on the basis that a runner will compete in Comrades each year. However, in an ideal situation a runner would only compete in Comrades every second year, with alternate years focused on the marathon. That would allow for a greater recovery and a full focus on improving a 10-km time by the following February (end of the South African summer). The autumn and winter should see an even greater improvement in marathon time (the faster you are in 10 km, the faster you will be in the marathon), then back to quality for the next summer (commence again at step 7. above) and into a full attack on Comrades armed with better short distance times and greater potential in Comrades. It may be that instead of a marathon on alternate years, a runner opts to focus on Two Oceans or one of the other 56-km ultras in such years.

At the end of the book are two charts showing possible training plans for Comrades and Two Oceans or a marathon; the principles are the same as the above description. These indicate some events that could be used as second-level goals and stepping stones to the major peak. It is possible to follow one plan the first year (including Two Oceans) and the second the following year, following the suggestion of running Comrades on alternate years. If so, an even better approach might be to omit Two Oceans in the first year and to focus instead on the 21-km race in April, after an extended focus on track, 10-km and 15-km events. Remember, the faster you are at short events, the better your performance at Comrades.

The concept of improving times over a short distance to improve a long distance result is worth more than a second thought. It is more fully explained in chapter 17, but the principle is that your performance at all distances from 5 000 m to 100 km is predictable, based on a relatively simple formula. If the training is done and all else is equal, the fastest 5 000-m athlete will also be the fastest marathoner, and the fastest marathoner will probably run the fastest Comrades and the fastest 100-km race. It is no coincidence that the then World Marathon record holder, Tegla Loroupe, ran in the 10 000-m at the 2001 World Championships in Edmonton, Canada. Although she had little chance of winning a medal, she used the opportunity to sharpen up for her next marathon attempt.

Quality sessions in the summer can improve your physiological indicators, such as VO_2 Max, lactate threshold and efficiency, which will allow you to 'cruise' at a higher speed in your longer endurance training and provide the necessary improvements in the qualities you require for your marathon training. Furthermore, the faster your true 'cruising' speed, the more distance you can cover in the 10–12 hours of weekly training, and therefore the greater the training load you can withstand while still recovering sufficiently.

From the above plan you will, hopefully, see how each year is built around a few 'peaks', each of which is followed by a short period of recovery. Each 'peak' provides a measure to evaluate the effectiveness of the training in the preceding period. However, for such a runner the intermediate 'peaks' may not have the same significance as the major focal point, which is to improve in the following year's Comrades Marathon.

When not competing in Comrades or Two Oceans

The second year plan shown gives an indication of what a year might look like for runners who do not want to consider Two Oceans or Comrades, and is in many ways similar to the programme followed by top international runners. It also helps to illustrate just how difficult the South African fixture list has become as a result of these two great events. Now that South Africa is back in full international competition, it would be a better option for Comrades to be scheduled for October or November. A past Comrades chairman even suggested the date of 11 November (Remembrance Day for soldiers who fought in the two World Wars, and others), as it matched the original reason Comrades was run in 1921. Because of the impact that Comrades and Two Oceans have on prize money (and hence elite athletes), sponsorship, media and other disciplines in the sport, such a move could open up a new fixture list that would create new opportunities for all runners from track and field, to ultra-distance. Ultimately, it would probably attract even more top and average international athletes to the event.

Graduate only when you can go no faster

It should be a logical conclusion that if short distances dictate potential at longer distances, runners should only move up to longer distances when they have achieved the most they can at shorter events. They will then have developed their full potential for all distances. It should apply to all runners, but those who stand to benefit most from this approach are younger runners and novices, irrespective of age, who have been running for two or less years. The greatest improvements come in the first four or five years of running, so focusing on short distances at this stage makes sense. I believe that to be the biggest drawback of Comrades, as it has 'pulled' runners up in distance too soon. It was certainly a mistake I made and one I hope to discourage you from making. It is one of the few 'what ifs' of my running career. As pop star Rod Stewart sings, 'If I knew then what I know now...'

An alternative plan therefore, could be to build around the shorter events for a year, perhaps with races no longer than 15 km. The focus may then go from base and strength training, into the cross-country league season (e.g. 4–8 km), on to the track (1 500–10 000 m), and finally to road races from 10 km up to 15 km. The year would then repeat. Again, remember that some of the intermediate steps may not be 'key' issues to the runner but they would all lead to the goal, which might be to reach the best possible 10-km road time. Then it is not necessary to have a chance of winning the 3 000-m track race, nor does it matter if you come last. What matters is that you are running at a high intensity and improving your speed over the shorter distances. In the late 1980s I competed in a few track events as well as modern biathlons, which included 1 000-m races, and frequently came in well down the field (the challenge was not to be lapped!). Despite coming last, I was disqualified by the referee in one 1 500-m race because my number was said to be the incorrect size! Thankfully, officials today seem to be more open to the participation of non-elite runners in track events.

An important point to keep in mind when planning is that there is a limit to the total distance you can race in a year. Top international runners will only compete in two or three marathons a year, further highlighted by Professor Tim Noakes, who advises restricting the total racing distance per year to 100 km. A runner would then run two marathons and two 10-km events, or ten 10-km races, or three half-marathons and four 10-km events. Again, this substantiates the idea of racing Comrades on alternate years if you really want to achieve your own 'greatness'.

In a previous edition of this book, I used the example of South African David Tsebe. In the early 1990s, people argued against a limited racing approach by pointing to him as an example of how it was possible to race every week of the year. He would put in a world-class 61:03 for the half-marathon one week, and a 2:12 marathon the next, but that was in the restricted racing isolation of South Africa. He knew exactly whom he was up against, their strengths and weaknesses, as well as likely race tactics.

But what happened to Tsebe in 1991? How many races did he win then? Why was he incurring so many injuries? Even compared to his 1989 marathon time, as a relative newcomer, he was two minutes slower in 1990. I was sure he was capable of approximately 2:08, or better.

Shortly thereafter, South Africa returned to full international competition and many top South Africans soon learnt that even though they could dominate the smaller local pool with weekly racing, to be a big fish in the worldwide pool they needed to be more selective. This has paid off handsomely for them. Tsebe went on to win a number of international marathons, including Berlin, and South Africa won the 1996 Olympic marathon gold through Josiah Thugwane, who reduced the 1984 SA record to below 2:07:28 a year later. Top local runners no longer race each week. In fact, the South African racing situation has changed so much that those who run in marathons locally do not achieve times much better than 2:10 and regularly race for small money (in world terms), whereas those who focus on limited turnouts, receive appearance fees and US dollar or sterling payouts for good performances. In the 1980s the SA Marathon Championships participants' winning times were 2:08, with large incentive prizes but no hope of international competition. In 2002 we seldom see anything under 2:11 locally.

If you want to reach your potential, you must select your races, particularly your long races, very carefully. In addition, you will see that it is important to plan your year ahead so that you can focus on these major points.

Goal setting in sport is no different to running a business – the principles are the same. The direction and goals are set for one year and five years, then policies and strategies are adopted to reach those goals. This is necessary to generate profits for shareholders, and it works, i.e. a professional approach is used for professional results. Try the same with your running and you will enjoy your 'share' payout of the benefits.

Assessing your realistic potential

We have discussed the advantages of setting your sights on goals throughout the year, as well as the fact that by improving your times in short events, you will improve your performance in the following year's longer event or marathon.

To construct the ladder, it is important to have a guideline on your own potential and what improvements you can expect to make. The goal-setting system will only work when you are dealing with realistic goals. There are a number of ways to select realistic targets. **The following rules of thumb are an easy way of determining what is realistic for you:**

For the marathon distance:

▸ Take your best half-marathon time, double it, then add seven to ten minutes.

▸ Multiply your 10-km time by 4.65 to get your potential marathon time. So a sub-39-minute 10 km gives a time of three hours, a 45-minute 10 km gives approximately three hours 30 minutes, and to run a 4:15-marathon you need to be able to run 10 km in 54 minutes.

▸ For 8-km race times of 30 minutes, 35 minutes and 43 minutes, you can expect marathons times of 3:00, 3:30 and 4:15 respectively.

From this you should develop some feel for the interplay between 8-, 10-, and 42.2-km performances. The Comrades Marathon (90 km) relates to your marathon time by a factor of 2.42. A marathon of 4:00 will give you a 9:45 Comrades, and a 5:41 finish in the Two Oceans (a factor of 1.42).

In 1986 I developed these marathon factors of 2.42 for Comrades, 1.42 for Two Oceans, and 1.712 for a 56-km race to Comrades, based on the actual finishing results of runners. Because they are based on the statistics of 'real results', as opposed to theoretical results, they have proved to be a good rule of thumb, but are not specific to each individual athlete. That is where a more specific prediction can also be calculated using a computer program (for details see website **www.coachnorrie.co.za**). It is also useful in determining efforts of runs and potential performances, in addition to race predictions.

This program has proved to be very successful and has predicted performances such as Frith van der Merwe's South African marathon record in 1990 of 2:27:36 (predicted as 2:27:35), New York Marathon winner Willie Mtolo's half-marathon sub-65 minutes to within ten seconds, Elana Meyer's South African 10-km record to within two seconds and the finishing times of numerous Comrades runners, including the top South African women's finisher, Carol Mercer, on the 2001 down run. The program will also help you to answer questions such as, what is an 80% effort?, or how fast should you run a recovery run, or a fast continuous run?, etc.

A final point to note on your potential is that it is progressive. If, initially, the above calculations lead you to train to set a personal best of a three-hour marathon, once you have achieved this you will find that your potential also increases at other distances. You may then set a 38-minute 10-km target, which when reached may possibly lead you to a 2:55 marathon. However, as you reach closer to your 'physiological potential', the improvements become smaller and smaller. The final limitation may be the ravages of time as you age each year.

Training time

The next stage in developing your programme is to determine how much time you have to train per week. The object of the programme is to make the most efficient use of the limited time available.

Alberto Salazar once said that in working out a schedule, you should calculate how much time you have and then reduce it by 20%. I believe this to be an excellent proposal as it re-emphasises the importance of rest and recovery. Instead of 'training time', we should more correctly speak of a 'training time – recovery time' balance, each as important as the other. It is no use planning for 4 a.m. rises and 11 p.m. nights if you need a full seven or eight hours' sleep to recover. Of all the points in training, a realistic assessment of your capabilities is essential and this starts with the training load you can handle.

Just because a top runner runs 160 km per week, doesn't mean that is what you require. Such a philosophy doesn't take into account variations in genetic talent or emotional stress from work or family. Certain forms of emotional or psychological stress can have a greater detrimental effect than physical stress. In fact, physical training is often a release for emotional stress.

The laws of training

In developing a training programme, it is important to take cognisance of the 'laws of training' that have evolved over the years. Strangely enough, many were 'discovered' at the turn of the 20th century and although subject to minor modification, remain valid today. At various stages, runners have become slaves to some of these principles, such as the obsession with long, slow distance in the 1970s, but the key is the combination and an awareness of all of them.

Once more I have no better reference for those seeking further information than Professor Tim Noakes' *Lore of Running*, (OUP). He has searched old bookstores around the world and found training references for numerous sports. His subsequent analysis, compilation and summary has provided a list of 15 laws, which I can do no better than to repeat. The author of each concept appears in brackets.

THE FIFTEEN LAWS OF TRAINING:

1. **Train frequently** all year round (Arthur Newton's first law).
2. **Start gradually** and train gently (Newton's second law).
3. Train **first for distance** and only **later for speed** (Newton's third law) – (Note: this changes for ultras).
4. **Don't set yourself a daily schedule,** listen to your body (Newton's fourth law).
5. **Alternate** hard and easy days (Bowerman and Dellinger's law).
6. At first, **try to achieve** as much as you can with a minimum of training (Tim Noakes).
7. **Don't race in training** and run time trials and races only infrequently (Newton's fifth law).
8. Train specifically – **specialise** (Newton's sixth law).
9. Incorporate **base training** and **peaking** – sharpening (Forbes Carlisle/Arthur Lydiard rule).
10. **Don't overtrain** – listen to your body again! (Newton's seventh law).
11. Train under a **coach.**
12. Train the **mind** (Newton's eighth law).
13. **Rest up** before a big race (Newton's ninth law).
14. Keep a **detailed logbook.**
15. Understand the **holism of training.**

It's worth noting just how many of these 'laws' were identified by Newton, an ultrarunner who undoubtedly realised their importance from his exploits at extreme distances (see chapter 2). In 1984 I was captain of a four-man triathlon team to the

London to Paris Triathlon. One of the legs involved a relay swim across the English Channel – the most feared leg of all – and we were indeed lucky that the sponsors, Leppin, had the foresight to appoint Tim Noakes as our manager.

Two days before the event, while walking around London's bookshops, Tim came across a swimming book that detailed Captain Barclay's historic Channel swim. After our evening meal we all retired, only to be met the following morning by a very tired but excited Tim who proclaimed that we were definitely going to win because he knew how to tackle the channel.

He had our complete confidence and had devised a plan and list of necessities for the swim. We did win and, in fact, we even won the swim leg, beating a team of British long-distance Channel and international-class swimmers into the bargain. Such was the power of Tim's research and a good race plan!

00:00:07
THE COMPONENTS OF
A TRAINING PROGRAMME

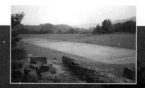

When you first start running everything seems simple, all you do is go outside and run round the block or over a predetermined route. Just completing the route is enough, although you often find yourself forced to slow down or indulge in walk breaks in order to go the distance. These are included for two reasons: firstly, your pace judgement to enable you to go the full distance is not good, as you frequently run too fast, and secondly, you are not fit enough to cover the programmed distance. Eventually, however, both factors improve until you can handle the full run and even greater distances.

At this point, most runners continue to use this 'one pace' running in all subsequent training; the only variations are in the distance, the route, and running partners. So even at this early stage of progression you tend to lose sight of one of the most beneficial yet basic ways of improving your running: speed variation.

In South Africa, particularly KwaZulu-Natal and Gauteng, the main motivation in the sport of running is the annual Comrades Marathon, which has become a major focal point of the athletics calendar. English runner John Tarrant commented that the Comrades was to South Africa what the FA Cup Final is to England – and that was back in the 1970s before Comrades attracted fields of 15 000 runners.

The obsession with Comrades has been exceptionally good in that it has brought a vast number of people, who might have been lost to the sport, into it. On the other hand, Comrades is also responsible for the tendency of so many runners to become long, slow distance runners, irrespective of their natural potential and has created a belief that speed work (or quality sessions) has no place in training for long-distance events. Further side effects of the Comrades tradition are the hand-me-down training schedules and 'old runners tales' about various heroes who ran incredible distances in training. As with most urban legends or stories that are passed on by word-of-mouth over the years, most of these training accounts are exaggerated, such as the hero of the story who not only ran 60 km twice a week, but also ran to and from work. This promotes the runner's total distance to an enormous figure that most runners could never attain.

On hearing such a story, most runners decide that they are doing too little and buckle down to increase their distance with the result that their ability to vary their training pace decreases. Soon they are running all their runs at one speed only, just pacing themselves from one session to the next. It is ironic that the best illustration of the foolhardiness of such training comes from the novice.

The novice's example

New Year tends to signal a new beginning in our lives. We try to keep to the resolutions we made in the final week of the previous year; resolutions to improve in some way. For a number of people this includes some form of commitment to a healthier approach to life, such as a decision to start running.

Although most of the people who contact me about my articles are experienced runners, it is worthwhile to assess the process adopted by beginners. In fact, one can learn from the 'novice' runner.

Take my case for instance. I never started running until I emigrated to South Africa in 1981, but as a 30-a-day smoker and 83-kg rugby hooker, I resolved to improve my fitness with jogging in 1973. The desire to keep my place in the 1st XV and to make a bid for the provincial side persuaded me to don a set of 'not too glamorous' shorts, 'tackies', long socks and an old rugby jersey, and to run the perceived gauntlet of peering neighbours and commence my jog.

I thought, 'If Ron Hill (a leading British marathoner at the time) can run a marathon in under 2:10, surely I can cover a mile or so in 12–15 minutes.' So off I went as a 'fit' rugby player! Perhaps it was the suspicion that people were staring at me, but after 300 m, this 'running' was no fun, and I faced a 'mountain'. In truth, its gradient was similar to that of a freeway off ramp and it was only 150 m long! As a beginner, fighting for every gulp of oxygen in lungs pumping faster than my heart (which felt as though it was in my mouth), this was a major challenge – one that true Scottish stubbornness (rather than fitness) allowed me to conquer. The price, however, was an enforced stop at the top of the hill and a total inability to even walk down the other side. It was then that my resolution to give up smoking became a reality. After a lengthy recovery I was able to 'jog', at a very slow pace downhill and after many similar rests, eventually finished my first two-mile circuit – somewhat slower than the predicted 15 minutes. It wasn't long before I could handle the run non-stop in a reasonable length of time, and the added endurance benefited my rugby. No longer did the other forwards have to use delaying tactics to give me time to reach a loose ruck and flatten it with my large mass.

This story will be similar to the many runners who remember what it was like when they first started. As a sport, running is one of the most difficult in which to make inroads. It is frustrating and even painful for the first three months, but this run-break-run-walk system is the universally successful method of locking us into the sport and results in dramatic improvement. Why then do we immediately throw this method out of our training as soon as we are able to go the distance? Why do we slow our pace to concentrate on slogging out the kilometres?

Traditionally, the New Year sees South African runners commence their annual slog of distance in preparation for the Comrades Marathon. It is almost instinctive. Throughout the following five months a seemingly uncontrollable 'guilt' drives them to grind out a daily diet of even-paced kilometre after kilometre. The objective is to see how high a figure they can achieve at the end of each week. Each kilometre is well within the capacity of the runner – no more the overambitious, lung-bursting speed of the novice, no more the enforced 'chest-bursting' recovery stop.

The need to vary running speed can be compared to weight-training techniques in which the weight on the bar is increased to 'overload' the muscle so that it will increase its strength during a period of rest. Is this not the same way you learn to run? Is this principle not the basis for the fast improvement you achieve as beginner and long for as an experienced runner?

Reconsider those first steps. Aren't all the principles of fartlek and track training in that beginner's run? Periods of faster work with periods of recovery. Running in anaerobic zones for short periods followed by aerobic recovery. These are the same principles that have been shown to be most effective and are adopted by top International runners in their training. It is ironic that it's the novice runner who comes in search of advice and yet it's often the more experienced runners who have forgotten, or overlooked, those lessons they learnt in their early development.

This illustrates that the correct way to train, for any distance, is to combine runs of different intensity, difficulty and distance so as to develop a well-balanced schedule that exploits the runner's full potential. If the single-paced runner has one 'gear', then the runner who varies his speeds in training will develop a 'gearbox of speeds' and perhaps even an 'overdrive'.

This may be complemented with other optional exercises and training to fine-tune the runner or eradicate a particular weakness. Since the options and combinations of intensity, difficulty and distance are numerous, let us first classify runs by intensity and then consider some of the possible permutations within each category.

RUNNING INTENSITY

The long, slow run

There is no doubt that there is a place for the long, slow run in any training schedule, but where it slots in and how much is necessary depends to a large extent on what your target is.

In the case of track athletes in middle distances, the long, slow run woud be carried out during the off season as a means of building an endurance base. The distance of this run, even for Olympic athletes, is unlikely to be much greater than 25 km. By comparison, however, the track athlete's 'slow speed' is quite probably race speed for many road runners. At the other end of the scale, six-day runners will use the long, slow run as the backbone of their schedules and their pace will be considerably slower.

I must emphasise that Comrades is not true ultra-distance running, as the length is only around 90 km! Although the definition of ultra-distance is any event longer than a marathon, most countries around the world consider the first rung of the ultra-ladder to be the 100-km and then the 100-mile, 24-hour, 48-hour, 72-hour and six-day races.

This is not to detract from Comrades. It is a great event, possibly the greatest in the world, but it must be put into perspective when considering the amount and type of training required to complete it. It is generally accepted that a top marathon runner will always win a 50-km race and the 50-mile race is purely an extension of this. The same principles that apply to marathon training can also be applied to ultras, but these schedules need to be modified to cater for the specific demands of the ultrarace. In general, the greatest of these is an increase in endurance, which is where the long, slow run comes into its own in building stamina and endurance. The development of an endurance base involves running for extended periods at a comfortable pace. Training is a series of stress and rest sessions that allow us to become stronger, but what many runners fail to realise is that the stress of a long, slow run comes from the length of time and not so much the speed at which it is run. In training for an ultrarace, the pace of a long, slow run should be close to or slower than the predicted race pace of that ultra.

Bruce Fordyce was an expert at perfecting this. Although he had a best 10-km time of 30:30 set on the track (three minutes per km), a best marathon of 2:17 (about 3:15 per km), and could race Comrades at 3:45 per km, he would do his long training runs in marathons and short ultras, just dipping under the silver medal cut-off time (normally 4:15 per km). In the 'disguise' of helping others to achieve silver, which he did so well, he also provided himself with a way of disciplining his pace in training, to slower than his Comrades race pace. Apart from ensuring that his training was aerobic and did not drain him, he also benefited from training his muscles and joints to a pace that he would use in Comrades. As you change speed, you also change running style and hence the muscles you use. The faster you run, the more you move onto your toes; the slower you run, the more you tend towards a heel strike. Unless you train at the projected race pace, the muscles you use on race day will become fatigued before the end of the race, and I believe this to be one of the major causes of cramps suffered by many runners in Comrades.

By comparison, most runners train too hard in long runs. If they were to do a slow-down as Bruce Fordyce did, a three-hour marathoner would need to 'train' through a marathon in 3:40 and a four-hour marathoner would take a training marathon in 5:15! Just how many runners are willing to do this? That is why so many average runners line up at Comrades overtrained and susceptible to cramps.

Runners must recognise that they have a pace, which they are able to maintain for vast distances without becoming breathless. This sort of running is said to be in the AEROBIC range, because the runner takes in as much oxygen as he is using up – about 70% of his VO_2 Max, whereas his marathon pace will be about 82% of VO_2 Max. Running long runs at marathon pace is clearly too hard and will break a runner down, rather than build him up for a race.

When the pace is increased from an aerobic level, a run is dictated both by breathlessness and a tiring of the muscles. This is a shift into the ANAEROBIC speed range in which a runner is unable to take in as much oxygen as the body is using to produce energy.

In truth, life is not that simple and every run is a combination of both aerobic and anaerobic running, but the objective of the long, slow run is to keep as much of the run as possible in the aerobic range. This type of run not only improves cardiovascular endurance, but also improves muscular endurance, to cope with the distance of the target race. (Endurance can also be developed using intervals, which will be discussed with other track training sessions.)

Speed and strength training is specific

It is important to recognise that slow training will only improve your muscles to work at the slow pace – clearly important for Comrades, which needs to be run at low intensity. It also assists in training the muscles and joints to be used at that intensity and gives a runner the mental confidence to complete the distance. However, it is only the latter, mental confidence that actually requires a runner to do long runs, and therefore doing only one or two runs in the 40–56-km category in the full 12 months between Comrades events should be sufficient. This approach is borne out by the fact that the world's greatest ultra-distance runners at 12 hours and upwards, do not run ridiculous, long distances each week, but rather focus on peak performances.

Since it is necessary to train at the specific intensity used in a race, in marathon training it becomes important not simply to run long, but to run long at marathon pace. However, this session has lost its focus in South Africa because of the pre-occupation with short ultra-events such as Comrades. The way to use a long run in the marathon build-up is to restrict most long runs to around 25 km (muscle damage increases exponentially after this distance) and to include a gradually increasing distance at marathon pace in the middle.

For instance, the initial run may be 21 km with a 5-km section run at marathon pace, while the following run, two weeks later, might increase this to 8 km at marathon pace. This would probably continue until one long run is completed over a total of 32 km with 18–21 km at marathon pace. The non-marathon pace sections of the long run are done at a very easy pace, which even Japan's legendary marathoner, So, ran at five minutes per km. If there is one training session that most South African runners have misunderstood, it is the long run.

Steady runs or threshold runs

The next level of running intensity is that of steady-state running – a pace best described as borderline between anaerobic and aerobic. The objective is to keep the pace of the run on the 'threshold' of becoming anaerobic. This pace is faster than the long, slow run and its prime purpose is to improve the upper limit of the aerobic range. Of course, it is very hard to maintain such a finite pace during a run and even the smallest of hills will put a runner into the anaerobic range unless he slows down considerably. Likewise, a dramatic increase in speed is required on the downhill if the threshold intensity is to be maintained.

Given this, a number of 'threshold' sessions use speed variations to constantly cross over this key 'pace', to keep the heart rate at the 'threshold' pace.

Hard runs

Moving up a gear, the third category of intensity is the hard run – used to classify all sessions that are run in the anaerobic range of a runner's speed.

There are different degrees of 'hard' – generally the distance run will determine this. A run over a 3-km course will be slower than a run over a 1-km course, but both can be equally hard or stressful. This is well illustrated in the comparative distance to speed chart (see page 184), and it is possible to compare a race over 5 km with a race over 21 km. (There is also a computer program that can predict and compare your results at one particular distance, based on your previous results at other distances. Alternatively, you can use it to determine how hard you covered a particular distance. It is a useful tool for determining your personal training schedule. Similarly, it is possible to determine what is an 85% effort at a particular distance if you know what an 'all-out' effort is for that distance – see page 61.)

Although runs may be at different speeds, they can be considered 'hard' when they are anaerobic. It is also necessary to include both short-hard and long-hard runs in a training schedule. The words 'short' and 'long' are, however, relative to the distance of the race for which you are training.

Recovery runs

There is one other run intensity that should exist in every training schedule, that of 'recovery' pace. These are runs performed at very low intensity over the shorter distances, and are 100% aerobic. Their purpose is purely to assist in improving circulation throughout the body after a harder session to improve recovery time, as fresh blood (i.e. nutrients) is pumped to the previously stressed areas, which allows the rebuilding and strengthening to commence earlier.

Recovery runs are often the most difficult because they should be undertaken at a very conservative speed. Most runners find it easier to 'test themselves' in training than to ease back at a slow pace. Recovery and long-run paces are two categories in which a runner can benefit significantly from the use of a heart-rate monitor (see chapter 38) – not to keep the pace fast, but rather to ensure a slow enough pace.

Unfortunately, the real benefit of the recovery run only becomes obvious when a runner returns to the next hard session. Only when you have fully recovered are you able to put a good effort into the next 'quality' training session. Think of it as a pendulum: unless the pace is slow on one side, it will not reach the faster limits on the other side of the swing. The better the recovery, the better will be the quality on the other side.

In many ways, recovery is the most important part of a training schedule and your training is only as good as your recovery. There should be more recovery runs in a training schedule than any other single type of training. The importance of recovery is paramount, and a comment by that great ultra-distance runner and Olympic marathoner Wally Hayward hit the nail on the head. In 1952, Wally had the opportunity to be a 'full-time athlete' and was asked how much more training he would be able to fit in. 'Being a full-time athlete doesn't necessarily imply having the time to do more ... it's an opportunity to get more rest,' he answered.

Picture the relationship between recovery runs and hard training on a sinusoidal graph – the easier the recovery sessions, the harder the hard sessions. If you run recovery sessions too fast, expect poor results in hard sessions. Stress and energy are limited. Many local runners, particularly Comrades runners, run everything at their marathon pace: slightly faster on days of short runs, slightly slower on long run days. They should be running significantly slower (as did Bruce Fordyce) on long or easy days, and much harder on quality days (5-km pace or slightly faster).

EVERYONE'S GUIDE TO DISTANCE RUNNING

TYPES OF RUNS WITHIN THE DIFFERENT INTENSITIES

Although the first two intensities are almost self-explanatory, I shall discuss various aspects in more detail, before considering the variety of sessions available for steady and hard runs.

Recovery runs

My faith and belief in recovery runs are obvious. As a training session, recovery runs are, in many ways, the backbone of any training schedule. They are also possibly the most unstructured training sessions because they revolve around minimal perceived effort. The purpose of a recovery run has been discussed, but since the objective is purely one of circulation and movement, neither speed, time nor distance, are of importance. The pressure is off in all respects and enjoyment should become the prime concern.

I have found the recovery run to be an ideal way to accommodate a number of errands into an otherwise tight schedule and frequently use these 5–10 km jaunts to drop off letters, pay bills or buy stamps. Although it requires some understanding from the shopkeeper and other customers, who are faced with a sweaty runner, it is an excellent way of controlling the workout effort. If my pace is a bit too fast, I have to stop at the first port of call, and enjoy a recovery period. These planned interruptions split the run into sections, which make it even easier.

You may prefer to run non-stop. This is fine but allow yourself to float along in an easy fashion so that you do not feel that any effort is required. You should not feel tired after these runs and in many ways you may feel stronger and livelier.

Work hard at making these runs easy; this will allow you to put greater effort into the hard training sessions.

Long, slow run

As indicated, the long, slow run is purely a method of developing muscle endurance and aerobic improvement. It is a steady-state run which, when training for shorter distance events, will tend to exceed the length of the race. For example, if your race distance is 10 km, a long, slow run may be a 15–18-km distance. However, as you move up in distance towards a marathon, your long, slow run will either be the same distance as the race or, particularly for ultras, less than the race distance.

The trend among world-class marathoners is for long runs to be in the 28–35-km range, although a few have gone to 46 km. Similarly, ultrarunners generally do not run epic distances in their training for 100-km or 100-mile races. Instead, they use various marathons and shorter ultra-events to reach a peak for a particular race in the season. For this reason they might appear to be running many more races than the commonly held 'one ultra a year regime' promoted in South Africa. In Europe there are definite seasons and an 'off season' is virtually enforced by the climate between November and February, which promotes greater recovery from a hard racing season. In South Africa and other warmer countries, it is possible to run year-round distance races and there is little incentive for most runners to specialise.

It is generally accepted that cardiovascular endurance is sufficiently developed by the time a runner is capable of completing long runs of 30–32 km. Any additional distance is unlikely to bring significant further improvement, other than muscular endurance, although Professor Tim Noakes has suggested that this will also be on a scale of diminishing returns.

But there is a further benefit to be gained from the long run — the psychological confidence a runner gains from completing the distance. This is hard to measure and the need for it varies from runner to runner, but I am sure many runners would be surprised at the distances they could run if they paced themselves correctly.

At the longer distances, I believe that putting two shorter, long runs back to back with a relatively short recovery break is probably as good a method of training as one very long run. In fact, I doubt that there is the same amount of muscle breakdown in the double as there is in the single.

The double also teaches a runner how to 'run tired', as the second run is begun in a partially depleted state. The ability to run tired is required in truly long events. Interestingly for Comrades runners, in her build-up to the 2001 Comrades, Carol Mercer only ran the 56-km Two Oceans as a run longer than 40 km between January and June. However, for a few days she ran 25 km each in the morning and in the evening, and went on to become the first South African woman home, sprinting past Grace de Oliveira on the finish line, to record a PB of 6:40. Carol had already gained the experience of racing 100 km (for South Africa in the 1999 World 100-km Championships) and had learnt many of her long race lessons. This proves that a runner rarely needs as many long runs as is perceived, particularly for the ultras.

An additional, often-cited benefit of the long run is that it may help to develop a 'fat-burning' energy system. This system, which will be discussed later, is the secondary energy source that predominates once all the muscle glycogen stores are exhausted. It is thought that the long training run improves the efficiency with which this energy is made available. Even if this is true, I don't believe there is any significant disadvantage with my preference for the double training run technique as opposed to a single, long run. There may even be a benefit, in that the break between runs allows a partial replenishment of liver glycogen – a top priority in the body's energy system. Liver glycogen is responsible for brain operation and therefore the double run system allows runners to complete both runs in a good frame of mind.

To summarise, long runs are an essential part of any distance-training programme, and for short-distance races, will slightly exceed race distance. For longer events, runs will tend to be less than race distance, with consideration given to using back-to-back double runs in preference to a single long run. The benefits of the long, slow distance run are an improved cardiovascular system, improved muscular endurance, psychological confidence for completing the race distance, and possible development of the fat-burning energy system.

Steady runs or threshold runs

Steady or threshold runs are run at a pace that borders between aerobic and anaerobic. Theoretically, when a runner runs at a purely aerobic pace, he could go on forever, i.e. the oxygen requirement is matched by an oxygen intake. In anaerobic running the demand exceeds the supply and a 'debt' is incurred. Scientific studies have suggested that there is a limit to the total debt a runner can accumulate and on this basis a runner should ideally build up this debt gradually and evenly between the start and finish of the race. **This introduces two other scientific concepts:**

> ▸ Running efficiency.
> ▸ The total amount of oxygen that a runner is able to take in.

Professor Tim Noakes has described these in detail in his book, *Lore of Running*, (OUP). Anyone wishing a deeper understanding of the scientific basis would be hard pressed to find a better reference. What follows is a layperson's overview of the concepts to assist in the understanding of the training principles.

While exercising, every individual inhales a certain volume of air per minute, which must match the requirements of the body if the exercise is to continue. As running speed increases, the oxygen requirements increase and a debt develops if the body's requirements exceed supply. The supply has a maximum value that depends on the effectiveness of the runner's cardiovascular system. Because this system can be improved through training, it is also true that the maximum oxygen uptake can be developed to some extent, but this is thought to be only in the region of 15–20%.

This maximum oxygen uptake at maximum effort is commonly expressed as millilitres of oxygen per kilogram of body weight per minute. It is known as the VO_2 Max and is often touted as the be-all and end-all of an athlete's potential. However, this is not true, as you must still consider the concept of aerobic/anaerobic threshold, which is regarded as a measure of 'running efficiency'.

Obviously, if one runner (A) could run at 85% of his VO_2 Max without developing an oxygen debt, he would be able to run faster, and hence further, in any given time than another runner (B) with the same VO_2 Max, who could only run at 70% of the same VO_2 Max value. Runner B would develop an oxygen debt if he tried to match runner A's pace, stride for stride. Runner B would eventually reach the limiting value and be forced to slow dramatically, or even stop completely. Theoretically, runner A would be able to carry on because he was matching his oxygen demand with his oxygen intake. The runner with the higher anaerobic threshold will be able to compete at a superior level, hence the importance of trying to push up the anaerobic/aerobic threshold point, which is the main objective of these steady runs.

Often overlooked in this regard, is that a runner with a lower VO_2 Max but a high anaerobic threshold, can perform at a higher level than a runner with a higher VO_2 Max value whose anaerobic threshold is at a lower percentage. **Consider the examples of runners A and B in the following table:**

EVERYONE'S GUIDE TO DISTANCE RUNNING

RUNNER A	RUNNER B
VO$_2$ Max = 80 ml O$_2$/kg/minute	VO$_2$ Max = 72 ml O$_2$/kg/minute
Threshold = 60%	Threshold = 75%
Oxygen uptake at threshold = 48 ml O$_2$/kg/minute	Oxygen uptake at threshold = 54 ml O$_2$/kg/minute

The benefit of the higher threshold level becomes obvious, and running efficiency can, to some extent, be considered a combination of VO2 Max and threshold level.

The term threshold is often linked with lactate. It is mistakenly thought that lactic acid is only generated when we run in anaerobic zones, and that lactic acid is bad. This is not so, and a layman's explanation may help in understanding this concept.

We continually produce lactic acid, even while sitting, but the amount produced is easily metabolised back into useful energy. In fact, lactate is a source of energy at low-intensity exercise. Visualise it as a tap dripping into a bucket with a hole at the bottom of the side wall. At rest, the drip of lactic acid simply runs out of the hole without any effect on the system. In real terms it is metabolised back into energy. As the exercise intensifies, the flow of the lactate into the bucket increases until the amount of lactate entering is equal to the amount flowing out. This balanced state is the 'threshold' for lactate production. If, thereafter, the exercise intensity is increased, the quantity of lactate is too great to metabolise completely and there is a build-up in the bucket, above the level of the hole (an overload). The system can withstand an overload until the level of lactate is so great that it overflows the bucket's rim. In reality, this is what a 400-m athlete feels as he heads down the home straight in a flat-out race. His muscles tighten and his stride shortens because there is too much lactate in his system. The solution is to decrease the pace, allowing the lactate level to reduce or be metabolised.

If the depth of the bucket is increased (teaching the system to withstand greater amounts of lactate) or the size of the hole is increased (increasing the lactate threshold), exercise can be more intense or of longer duration in the anaerobic zones.

These two analogies show why steady, threshold and hard runs have a positive effect on training and should be a key part of any planned schedule.

Steady runs (threshold runs) should be completed either by running continuously for 5–8 km at this pace or, as noted previously, by doing a number of intervals at this pace with short recovery periods in between. Generally, the minimum interval distance should not be less than 1 km or more than 3 km. The total distance run at this pace in any session must be kept to a maximum of 10 km as these are relatively hard sessions and require recovery time afterwards.

It is simple to determine your threshold pace if you have access to a fully equipped laboratory. However, a rule of thumb is that the pace should be about 30 seconds per mile (20 seconds per km) slower than your flat-out 10-km pace.

Hard runs

This classification of intensity covers a wide range and type of training, from fast continuous runs to intervals and fartlek, to hills. One of the most important rules is, the faster the run, the shorter it should be in training, and the longer the recovery period. This not only applies to intervals but also on a day-to-day basis.

Fartlek

This is a method of playing with speed during a training session and can be either informal or more disciplined. The variations of fartlek are as unlimited as the imagination, but the following are some ideas from which to develop your own.

In an informal session, run easily for a kilometre or so to loosen up, then vary the pace over distances from 100 m to 1 km as you feel able and inclined. The pace should vary from almost flat-out to a jog or even a walk for recovery. There is no detailed list of what you must do, but try to cover a complete spectrum of speeds and finish the session pleasantly fatigued.

Informal sessions require some discipline, but I've yet to meet a runner who looks forward to a speed effort immediately before starting. This approach makes the sessions slightly less taxing than the more formal sessions. Slightly less informal is doing this with one or two friends who take it in turn to dictate the pace. However, be careful that it doesn't become too competitive. Runners of the same ability are the best companions for such sessions, provided no-one is intent on winning.

In formal sessions, the routine is determined beforehand. For example, run an easy 2–3 km, repeat a series of one-minute hard runs four times, followed by a three-minute walk/jog/easy run. On completion of the four hard sessions, an easy 2–3 km completes the workout. Terrain variation also plays a part. The first hard section may be on flat road, the next on an uphill, the following downhill, the next back to flat, or even on grass. The beauty of fartlek is that it can be done anywhere.

Exercises may be included in fartlek for strength and endurance training. Running around a trim track with stops at the stations for pull-ups, stomachs or press-ups, combined with pace variation between the stations is another form of fartlek and provides variation for the runner who is bored with running only.

An excellent extension of this is circuit training. For example, 400 m is done at 10-km pace, followed by a set of five different exercises including some upper- and lower-body work, then straight into another 400 m at the same pace. Repeat this between 2–6 times. (See also circuit training in supplementary exercises.)

Even the old rugby training technique of having teams run around the perimeter of the pitch with the back runner sprinting to the front is a form of fartlek. So too is the pyramid run where runners run to the 22-m line, jog back, run twice to the half-way, jog back, run three times to the opposition 22-m line, jog back, then run four times to the opposition goal line, and so on. However, in this exercise beware of the strain on knees caused by the sudden change in direction.

Fartlek is an excellent introduction to the harder, more stressful, track training, and a good way to develop kicks and surges for use in tactical races. Progression in fartlek can be achieved by increasing the intensity of runs, the number of hard sections, reducing the recovery jogs, or a combination of these. The method of progression will depend on the training aspect in focus.

Hills

Hills are a good introduction to track work, developing leg strength and hill technique. Unfortunately, some runners overdo it, particularly those living in hilly areas who run them every day, causing them to become slow hill runners as even recovery days include hills. One of the keys to good training is recovery, and varying the terrain assists in using different muscles and provides stable recovery. Although there are other variations, hills can be broken down into three basic types.

In many respects, the easiest is to go on a run of 10 km and to push the uphills and recover on the flats and downs. This is not a session of which I am particularly fond since it doesn't really make allowance for your state of fitness at that particular time. Some hills may be 100-m long, others 1-km and a bit too long to concentrate on for the full length. What if two long hills are separated by only a 150-m flat section? This type of run is more in keeping with a fartlek session than a good hill workout. Unfortunately, this seems to be the type of hill session that many runners do and I don't believe that they are achieving as much as they would if they tried one of the other types. If you are going to do one of these sessions, select your course before running, to pace yourself properly and push the hills.

In the second type of hill run, the runner finds a hill of the desired incline and length, and after a warm-up and stretch, runs repeats up the hill to the top AND OVER. This should only be done five or six times, but the runner has some measure of effort as each repeat can be timed and is of equal difficulty. In addition, the recovery is also a measured variable over which the runner has control. Some books suggest that recovery is achieved simply by turning round and jogging down, turning round immediately and running back up the next repeat. I don't believe this to be practical, although I suppose it depends on what you are trying to achieve in the training session. My own preference is to use the session to develop strength and hill technique with less emphasis on endurance, which I feel can come from other sessions, so I walk at the end of each repeat as I turn to jog down the hill. I try to obtain about twice the recovery time as it takes to do the hard repeat and a one-minute uphill effort is rewarded with a full two-minute period to go back down and prepare for the next up section.

Variation in hill gradient and length determines the emphasis I want from a session – steeper hills more strength, shallower hills more speed, long hills endurance and rhythm, short hills power, etc. A 2–3 km jog to cool down completes the session.

It is surprising how shallow a hill needs to be to provide this sort of workout, and care should be exercised to ensure that a good running form can be developed on the hill, which is the first thing to be sacrificed if the hill is too steep.

The third type of hill session consists of bounding to build strength. It involves repeats up a hill with downhill recovery, but the action is more one of extending the ankle of one leg as far as possible, while trying to 'blast' the entire body as high as possible into the air. The other leg must be lifted with as high a knee action as possible. Stride length should be short, and because speed up the hill is not the main objective, a shorter, steeper hill is best. A good way of initiating this style is to use a 'scooter' for a good driving action (see plyometrics, page 113).

Downhill running

The movement of running, particularly downhill, requires muscles to contract eccentrically while in a stretched condition. This is usually felt in the muscle soreness known as DOMS (delayed onset of muscle stiffness) following a downhill race. Each time a foot lands, it is required to 'transfer' the force of the body landing on the ground into a propulsion in order to move the body forwards to the next landing point. Although this is aided by momentum, the ability to improve this projection has a direct benefit on running efficiency and speed. Studies have proved that training on downhills can help protect against DOMS in the following six weeks.

Downhill running is worth including in your training schedule, particularly prior to a race that includes large sections of downhill running. The best way to achieve this is to look for a gradual slope over 500–800 m and to complete six to eight downhill repeats, concentrating on driving from your hips so that you 'roll' from forefoot to forefoot. When you have perfected your style, you should not hear your feet touch the ground and you should experience a sensation of speed and wind through your hair.

Fast continuous runs

Fast continuous runs are run over a distance shorter than your race distance but at your race pace. For a marathon, you may run a 15-km race, at your predicted marathon pace. In addition to pace judgement, such runs will train you to concentrate while under pressure. Choose flattish, or slightly undulating courses, where it is easy to maintain a constant pace. Hilly courses require a constant perceived marathon pace effort rather than a constant speed.

In training for a marathon, many runners try to run too far and too often at their goal marathon pace. You need only start with a 5–8-km continuous run, then on alternate weeks increase the distance by about 3 km until you reach 25 km. Such

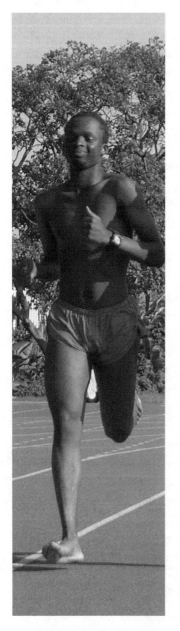

runs must not be confused with the long training runs that are run about 45 seconds to one minute per kilometre slower.

Club time trials are another valuable, but often-abused training session. They can provide an ideal fast, continuous-training opportunity to do a 15-km race in one hour. You would then aim to run the 8-km time trial in 32 minutes and not go for broke as most runners seem compelled to do in club runs. Time trials are training sessions, not races.

Tempo runs

Tempo runs are covered directly after fast continuous runs to highlight the difference between these two sessions. Developed in Russia in a bid to simulate race conditions for runners without the stress of a full-blown race, tempo runs are not to be taken lightly as they are run at a pace about 5–10 seconds slower per kilometre than 10-km race pace.

They are ideal sessions for running in club time trials, but because they are stressful you should prepare well for them. Taper down a few days prior to a run and allow sufficient recovery afterwards. Each time a session is run it should be over the same course so that you can measure your progress using a watch and perceived effort, or a heart-rate monitor.

LEFT *Track work can develop endurance – run a large number of intervals interspersed by short breaks*

NOTE: This is not a flat-out session; if it were, it would be a race. The tempo run is a training method. There is no training method that involves a flat-out race, as that would break an athlete down rather than build him up. Tempo runs should only be done once every 4–6 weeks, and provide vital information on your training progress.

Club time trials

The last two sections lead naturally into a discussion on the appropriate timing of the club time trial. Many runners seem to run their time trials each week in the hope of continually improving their time. This will not happen, as improvement occurs in an irregular fashion with plateaux between. The problem with this approach is that it can become a race, which, as already stated, breaks down rather than builds.

This doesn't mean that runners should not make an appearance at the weekly time trial; quite the opposite, as it can be used in many ways. Two examples have already been discussed. In a six-week period (e.g. between tempo runs), you could use the first week as a tempo run and two other weeks as fast continuous runs. Another two weeks could be used as a formal fartlek session, where, for instance, alternate kilometres are run hard and easy. The final week could be used for a different type of fast continuous run, e.g. run the first 3 km at fast continuous pace, walk and jog the next 2 km, and complete it with a 3-km fast continuous run.

The time trial can also be used as a recovery run, which will give you an accurate measure of how fast you are running and your objective can be to run SLOWER than a set time. This could be an opportunity to run with a friend who is substantially slower than you are. Use your time trials, don't abuse them!

TRACK WORK

Many club road runners only try track work once, before deciding that it doesn't suit them, as a result of adopting the wrong approach. Track work is frequently viewed as something that must be run at the fastest possible pace. THIS IS NOT TRUE.

To emphasise the importance of speed and recovery variance, I shall discuss the whole spectrum of track work, even though the first few types are possibly more closely related to long, slow distance as the primary development is endurance.

Endurance intervals: It is possible to use the track to develop endurance by running a large number of intervals, e.g. 400 m, with very short breaks in between, but these should be run at an easy pace compared with your best 400-m time. Because they are short and there are recovery periods, the intervals are more frequent than if you were to run the same total distance non-stop. Typically, these intervals should be run at 85% or less of your best effort, while the recovery would be in the order of 30 seconds.

Speed and endurance intervals: These intervals are run marginally faster, but there is slightly more recovery time between them and the total distance of a whole session is less. The run intensity is up to 90% effort, depending on the type of race for which you are training. The shorter the race, the higher the percentage effort, but don't run it flat out. Runners who run intervals flat out may as well enter races on their training nights. The distances of these intervals will vary between 200 m and 2 000 m depending on the event for which you are training. The shorter the effort distance and the faster the speed, the longer the rest between them.

Pure speed sessions: Pure speed is developed by running very short distances, such as 60 m or 70 m. They must only be repeated a few times, with long rest periods in between – up to four or five minutes. In general, these sessions are of limited benefit to long-distance road runners, but it is useful to do fairly hard 100-m repeats to improve your basic speed. Such a session almost cuts across the sessions designed for pure speed and power speed repeats. It will be covered in more detail in the following section. However, do remember not to ignore the 100-m distance in intervals simply because you consider it too short.

Power speed repeats/tempo running: The objective of power speed intervals is to develop power, speed and your anaerobic system. They can cause an oxygen debt and fatigue, which must be closely monitored to ensure that you don't overdo the session. Unlike interval sessions, where the benefit of the training is achieved during recovery phases, the benefit of repeats stems from the effort of each run.

Power speed repeats are run somewhat faster than race pace and there should be full recovery between intervals, i.e. your heart rate must return to 100 or below, depending on your fitness level. The distance of the repeats will vary according to the distance of the event for which you are training. Only runners who have already gained some track training experience should attempt this type of session.

Runs at this intensity will also help to develop efficiency in your running style because your foot lands further forward, causing you to raise your hips (and centre of gravity). This action results in a smoother style as it maintains the momentum of movement.

Basically, power speed distances are 200–600 m, but as indicated above, shorter distances can also be useful, particularly a 100-m session. A session could be three sets of five 'sprints' over 100 m, which allows you to focus on leg speed, relaxation and works the short-term energy systems. A 45–60-second recovery time between intervals and 3–5 minutes between sets, allows sufficient recovery to ensure the quality of the work. These 100-m (or 150-m) sprints are not flat out but are of a significantly higher speed than any other quality work, creating 'greater capacity' in aspects of your running. As with all quality work, the measure of intensity is against *your own performance level*, and not that of others. Therefore a session can be used equally by a sub-33-minute 10-km runner and a 50-minute 10-km runner.

One simple sign of improvement tends to show in the very first session. The first set of five for a 45-minute 10-km runner might result in each 100 m being covered in 19 seconds. By the time he starts the third set, his times may drop to 17.5 or 18 seconds for the same effort. This is not a deliberate increase in effort, but a loosening of stride, relaxation of the training and the development of a more efficient running style.

Because each set in this session is short and relatively easy to withstand, there is a danger that you could overdo the number of sets. In fact, the workload is significant and you must be careful not to overdo it. Start with a maximum of three sets of five and don't progress past five sets in any one session.

General considerations in track training
All track work is a product of five variables:

> ▸ The speed of each effort.
> ▸ The distance of each effort.
> ▸ The total number of efforts.
> ▸ The amount of recovery.
> ▸ The way in which recovery is achieved, i.e. running, walking or jogging.

A quick general rule to avoid overdoing a track session is to ensure that the total distance run in any one session, does not exceed the distance of the race pace you are running. For instance, if you are running 1 000-m intervals at 10-km race pace, you should not go beyond ten intervals. Alternatively, if you are running 400 m at 5-km race pace, you would not repeat this more than 12 times. This is a guide for a good club runner; a novice's quality work will probably only represent half that number in the first year of track training.

It is all very well saying that these sessions should be run at set percentage efforts, but deciding what these efforts are in real terms is difficult for most runners to determine, which is probably why many road runners only ever do one track session before reverting to long, slow runs. Most distance runners try to run far too fast when they commence track training, instead of matching their times to the standard of their performances at the longer distances.

The table below compares track speeds and is given as a guide to runners on the possible composition of the different types of sessions:

Best Marathon	Best 10 km	Time Trial 10 km	LSD 10 km	Recovery 10 km	LSD 20 km	LSD 32 km	Track 400-m repeats	Track 1 000-m repeats	90 km
3:00:00	39:15	41:00	45:00	50:25	1:33:10	2:34:30	1:28	3:45	7:15
3:30:00	45:15	47:20	52:00	57:50	1:47:25	2:58:43	1:42	4:20	8:28
4:00:00	51:10	53:25	58:40	65:00	2:01:30	3:23:00	1:46	4:55	9:40
4:30:00	56:50	59:20	65:10	72:00	2:15:10	3:46:45	2:09	5:30	10:54

The main difference between endurance intervals, speed and endurance intervals, pure speed, and power speed repetitions, is the effort with which they are run, and the recovery that is provided between the efforts and the sessions. This is an easy statement, but the trick for the athlete is to be able to identify what this means in terms of time.

Obviously, no hard and fast rules can be applied to what time you must run an endurance interval session, for example. It will vary from week to week depending on various factors, e.g. how the track is affected by wind, how you have recovered from your previous workout, whether you had a hard day at work. However, it is important to have a ballpark figure in mind when you start. Even in a continuous run you must consider the hills and terrain of the route before deciding whether a 42-minute 10-km run is easy or hard. Similarly, you need to consider the aspects that will affect your track effort before determining interval times on the track.

Many runners are intimidated when first trying track or other speed work and can occur on two levels: firstly by the presence of other runners, and secondly by their own perception of how fast they feel they should be going.

Consider the average road runner who goes to the track for the first time to try speed work. After a warm-up and stretch, and with much apprehension, he lines up for his first interval. Unsure of how fast he should run to complete the 400 m in his target time of about 90 seconds, he will normally start off too fast. By the time he reaches 200 m he feels the effort but manages to complete the lap in 86 seconds. Feeling happy with this, and despite knowing that he can slow down, he commences his second interval after the designated rest. This time he is more fluent, both because he has found his stride and because he knows he is up to the task. All of which results in an even faster 83-second lap. Now the 'game is on' and he resets his target to complete all ten laps in under 86 seconds!

The situation is aggravated when he finds children, or others younger than he, matching or passing him during his 400s when they are doing 800-m intervals. Overlooking the fact that they are training for track races and he is looking to peak for a half-marathon, his ego forces him to strive for even faster times. Unfortunately, he doesn't adjust his recovery period as a balance and instead tries to complete the 'new self-revised schedule'.

As discussed previously, each training session targets particular physiological attributes. Changing the pace and recovery time changes the training emphasis and shows how the approach illustrated above can be detrimental to training. The runner ends up racing his training, doesn't enjoy the workout, and may even sustain an injury. At best he finds his recovery from the track slow and he has a decreasing appetite for track and speed work. It becomes a great incentive to revert to the daily long, slow distance runs. Keeping focused on the purpose of each training session is just one reason why every runner needs a coach (see chapter 11).

Each session should develop a specific aspect of running and, as already shown, this is best achieved by varying speed and recovery between intervals. If done correctly, not only will the desired results be achieved, but recovery will also be quicker. Although the effort aspect of such sessions requires discipline and determination, there is a reward that generates enthusiasm for the next track session. Remember the rule of speed training: if you find yourself going too fast, slow down. This mistaken focus on speed by many runners is the reason why I prefer to use the term 'quality'. Your focus must be on running at a particular pace, which will be of a higher quality than the pace of your normal distance, long slow distance, or recovery runs. However, the challenge is not to beat the pace, but to adhere to it.

Another reason why runners don't like track work is that it tends to take substantially longer to cover a distance, and most runners perceive training effect to be based purely on the total distance run in any week.

THE DECEPTIVE FIGURES OF QUALITY WORK

Runners can become obsessed with the figure at the bottom of their training diary. The longer the event, the more the obsession grows. The first 'measure' used by many to assess another runner's fitness is distance. 'How much are you doing per week?' is often answered with an inflated amount to impress the questioner. Moreover, the desire to maximise the weekly number is a prime motivator for omitting 'quality work' from training schedules.

A three-hour marathoner will typically train at an average pace of 4:30 per kilometre and thus covers 13 km per hour. As most runners train between ten and 12 hours per week in peak training, this runner will probably amass around 150 km in peak training and 125–130 km in a 'normal' training week. This means that in a five-month build-up to an event such as Comrades, he can accumulate a magical 2 500 km with ease. However, he would be significantly better off sacrificing some of this distance for quality work to develop a 'gearbox of speeds', instead of a single running pace.

In a simple quality session involving ten repeats of 400 m at 5-km pace with 90 seconds recovery, the three-hour marathoner will run the 400-m repeat around 85–90 seconds. Ten repeats will take 15 minutes, then there will be nine recoveries of 90 seconds giving a total of 13 minutes, plus a slow warm-up of about 3 km and a cool-down of 3 km. These are run very easily, so allow 30 minutes for this and probably a few minutes to change to lighter shoes. Add a few strides and some stretching before and after – another 20 minutes and the total is 78 minutes. Add to this the time spent travelling to a track or similar quality session venue. The total distance covered in this scenario will be 4 km at just faster than 5-km race pace, and 6 km at about five minutes per kilometre, giving a total of 10 km. By comparison a simple 'out the door and run' training session of 78 minutes would reward the runner with 17 km to add to his log.

The benefits of quality sessions, however, do not come purely from distance. They come in many forms as they can increase a wide variety of physiological aspects, including VO_2 Max, lactate tolerance, leg speed, strength and many other elements key to your achieving a new personal best. There are estimates for comparing the effect of quality work to distance training. For instance, 5-km pace training is estimated to be four times the benefit of a run at 'normal' training paces (taken as being 50–75% of VO_2 Max).

Reconsider that 78-minute session. The 4 km at 5-km pace now equates to 16 km, plus an easy 6 km for the warm-up and cool-down results in a total of 22 km – 5 km more than that simple 'out the door and run' session.

Sessions done at 10-km pace are thought to be worth twice as much as the same distance at a leisurely pace, and quality work at 3-km race pace provides eight times the benefit. Of course there are different and important benefits from long, slow training, but undertaking two or three quality sessions can boost your training distance – but it is a 'hidden distance'.

Remember, if you learn to run comfortably at a high speed, even if it is over a shorter distance, you will be even more comfortable at a lower speed, such as a marathon. Progression is achieved in both areas, as the 'gearbox of speeds' is developed. Quality work builds mental tenacity and discipline because it is more challenging to complete a quality session than a long, easy run.

Finally, don't expect miracles overnight. It takes about six weeks of various track work sessions before you see any benefit. You may even feel slightly leg-heavy in the first few weeks as you adapt to this new form of training, but persevere as it is well worth the effort.

WARM-UP AND COOL-DOWN

There is one more intensity of running to be considered. I have deliberately placed it with hard runs even though it is the easiest of all. Of prime importance in any training session is a warm-up and cool-down.

In every book on training, be it running, rugby, football or swimming, there is a section on warming up and cooling down. The physiological benefits of this are well documented and it has been shown that the body performs better when it is 'forewarned of a hard effort', as opposed to being dropped in the deep end. However, many runners find the idea of spending 10–15 minutes warming up and another ten cooling down before a recovery or distance run in the morning rather unpalatable. One reason for this is that they judge their training purely by the total distance run in a week, as opposed to the quality and quantity of their workouts.

I believe there is a way round this for easier, early morning runs. Even though I find the very early morning runs among the most enjoyable, I don't like waking up a minute before it is absolutely necessary. So I set my kit out the night before and after a trip to the bathroom, it's out on the road – total time no longer than 15 minutes from the alarm. Because I don't then feel the impulse to warm up and stretch, instead I purposely take the first kilometre very slowly, and since I inevitably start up a hill, I try to overemphasis my style and take short strides. When I reach a flat, I gradually increase my stride over a few 50-m repeats. This works for me and I fall into a rhythm fairly quickly. Failure to do this tends to lead to bad runs, which I never enjoy.

Any run that includes a few short 'efforts' at a higher intensity early on, always feels that much more enjoyable once the pace has returned to a normal level – surely a clear indication of the effect of a second wind. Such a low key warm-up doesn't work for harder sessions, however, and for these I suggest that you evolve a standard format for a warm-up and cool-down procedure. By standardising, you will build confidence in the success it brought in training and can then use it before races. If it were changed, you will always be anxious that the changes might affect your race performance.

The following is an example of my warm-up that you could use as a starting point from which to develop your own personalised warm-up. Preferring to begin with a jog of about 1.5–2 km, I frequently have to control the speed of my 'jog', as pre-race nerves tend to speed it up. I follow this with six or eight exercises that stretch major muscles and mobilise joints. If necessary, I then change into racing shoes or spikes and am ready to do three strides over 80–100 m, starting with a jog and building to a sprint over 15 m. As recovery, I walk back to the start after each. For longer races, I run a single 400-m distance at the same pace that I do ten repetitions on the track. This helps to calm nerves and 'opens the lungs'. If it is a long race, I do two or three repeats over 200 m at the pace at which I intend starting. This pre-programmes the pace in my mind so that I don't go out too fast. It's really a case of trying to make the 200s *SLOW* enough. A final short jog and a drink, then I'm ready. I try to time my warm-up so as to finish within ten minutes of the start of the event.

A basic rule is to make your warm-ups longer for shorter, more intense races. This may mean slightly more jogging, strides and stretching. For longer events, keep to your basic standard format, but expect it to take between 30 and 45 minutes to complete the above routine.

The weather may force you to modify your warm-up. In cool or cold conditions, do your routine in a rain suit or windproof jacket to create a microclimate within your clothing that will warm you. Conversely, in hot or humid climates, find a shaded area to minimise the effects of dehydration and sunburn. Warm-up is important in both cases; although you may feel warm, the exercise of the warm-up boosts your body's system and helps to prepare you for the task ahead.

The cool-down at the end is somewhat similar with the exception that there are no strides. It is also better for distance runners to do a full stretching session after training. By comparison, track athletes (those who focus on the shorter, explosive distances) spend much more time warming up and stretching before training. One reason for this is that distance runners tend to overstretch their muscles before training because they do not stretch frequently enough. This results in a residual tension in the muscles, which can cause injury when those same muscles are put under pressure from the quality training that follows.

Interestingly, there also appears to be a cultural difference in the act of stretching. At the Honolulu Marathon, researchers have discovered that a high percentage of Caucasian runners injure themselves if they stretch before racing, compared to Asian runners who suffer few ill effects from stretching before the race. This possibly relates to the latter's levels of flexibility and affinity to stretching. In Asian cultures, people tend to spend more time in flexible pastimes and sports, such as sitting on the floor and the use of yoga. From an early age they are more involved in maintaining flexibility.

You must find a routine that suits you. If you suffer badly from pre-race nerves, you may require shorter warm-ups, or possibly to warm up on your own. If, however, you find it difficult to motivate yourself, you may need to be in the company of others to benefit from the atmosphere of the event. Any method is acceptable, provided it prepares you physically for the race or hard session, and brings you to a suitable state of mental readiness. Do not underestimate the importance of this latter aspect, and the use of a Walkman with music, or relaxation tape, can help you to visualise the task ahead or dispel those overanxious thoughts. This will be discussed in greater detail later.

One thing is certain. Not to warm up is to run the danger of injury and will more than likely result in a below-par performance. A warm-up will ensure that you make the most efficient use of your training time.

SUMMARY

From the above you can see that there are different running components that make up a training schedule. By varying the 'mix' you can train for any distance event from 100 m to 100 km and beyond. The task of a training schedule is to tune your physiological system, gradually and progressively, to the event for which you are preparing. However, it is important not to overlook the fact that benefit from training can only be gained if sufficient rest and recovery are provided to allow your muscles to recover between these sessions.

In many cases, the above training exercises may be augmented by additional non-running exercises. These have a place, particularly if a strength or skill is being developed to allow a runner to advance in a particular aspect of running training. A number of these will be discussed in the following chapter. However, it is important to remember that when time is the limiting factor, 'running is the best training for running'. The basis for this is clear if you remember that training inflicts microdamage to the muscles used in a chosen sport, in order to promote the growth of those muscles during recovery.

00:00:08
SUPPLEMENTARY ACTIVITIES
AND CROSS TRAINING

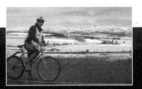

The danger of overtraining is emphasised throughout this book and is, in many ways, the biggest problem faced by the motivated runner. Too often he sees the objective as clocking up as many kilometres as possible. The higher his weekly distance, the fitter he thinks he will be. This is certainly *not true*. Your training can only be as good as your rest and recovery. It is no use piling on distance if your body never has a chance to rebuild the microscopic muscle tears that occur in training; it is the recovery that improves the muscles' performance.

Distance alone only develops one aspect of your performance; a really good performance is the combination of a number of different physical qualities including speed, endurance and power, and this doesn't take into consideration such things as the anticipated weather, psychological preparation and course analysis, to name but a few other variables.

In the search for the perfect performance, there are many benefits to be gained from supplementary exercises. They can be used to vary a training programme. For instance, some long, endurance runs may be substituted by a long cycle because although different leg muscles are used, the cardiovascular system cannot distinguish between running and cycling, it only knows that it is required to supply air! Some supplementary exercises may be used as a means of training through an injury. A number of world-class athletes have run in water when injured and their legs unable to support body weight.

Supplementary exercise such as weight training has been shown to be an efficient way of developing specific muscle strength, and is ideal in the rehabilitation of injuries, or correcting muscle imbalances. (Muscles work in pairs and their strength should be proportional to one another. In addition, left and right muscles must be of comparable strength to ensure a mechanically sound running style.)

The permutations are endless, and in the case of an athlete training to maximum running capacity, these additional exercises can aid progress up the fitness graph to a slightly higher peak. However, such exercises are generally less efficient methods of training for a runner than running itself and, as such, should not be considered as a substitution for running if you really want to reach your potential, and have time limitations on your training.

EFFECTIVE AND EFFICIENT TRAINING

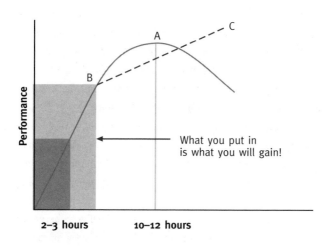

The input/output graph above depicts the correlation between training effort and improvement. Initially, the graph is a straight line showing that up to a certain value, the amount of effort (training) you put in is proportional to the results you can expect. After a certain point (A), the expected return diminishes, i.e. a greater time period yields the same level of improvement. Where that point of diminishing return is, depends on you: the type of training involved, your chronological age, your training age, the amount of rest and other, stress-related factors in your life. The point may even vary at different stages – believed by some scientists to be about 120 km per week for a serious athlete, therefore I think it probably occurs at 80–90 km per week for an average runner with work and family commitments.

If even more time is put into training, performance tends to drop off. This is the overtraining principle – it is a signal and symptom that the body is not recovering enough before the stress of the next training session. Ideally, you need to be at the crest of the graph in time for your peak race. The line reaching beyond the height of the crest is indicative of the role that supplementary exercise can play.

By reducing some of the stress on your muscles or physical aspects that have already been taken to their limit, and training other areas, it is possible to improve your performance to higher levels. It is important to note, though, that the return for time invested in such exercises is never as good as that gained from the running, particularly in the early stages. With this perspective on the role of supplementary exercises, consider the following non-running exercises that are worthy of some of your valuable training time.

THE IMPORTANCE OF A BALANCED STRUCTURE

Have you noticed that every runner has a distinctive style? It is possible to identify runners from some distance by their stride; it's as unique as a fingerprint. I believe that much of this is caused by a runner's mechanical imbalances, which can include inherent 'defects' such as a shorter left or right leg, excessive pronation or supination, toeing in or out of the feet. The list is virtually endless and it is doubtful that any runner has a perfect stride.

However, track runners tend to have a more fluent style than most road runners. Perhaps this is one reason why they compete on the track. On the other hand, a road runner concentrating on longer distances uses a more economic stride than his track colleague, who basically bounds along. The longer the distance, the lower the kickback of the leg as it follows through to start the next stride.

On a visit to Scotland in 1990, I was given IAAF press accreditation to one of the Grand Prix series and witnessed the then new sprint star, Michael Johnson of America. Not only did he run a 19.85 time for the 200 m in Edinburgh, but he also ran 400 m in the relay and clocked 44 seconds. His rigidly disciplined stride in the final straight was impressive; unlike most 400-m runners, there was no evidence of 'tying up'. Closer inspection of his style reveals a very low knee lift action, a vast contrast to a normal sprinter, and one that has obviously come with extensive practice. By 2001 he completely dominated the 200-m and 400-m sprint world.

A number of athletes have tried to adopt a similar low leg lift, recognising its energy-saving qualities. You can and should try it yourself in a series of 100-m intervals. Simply focus on pumping your arms in a greater upward direction; you will be surprised how much faster you can move your arms. That is because the length of the 'pendulum' you are 'swinging' is shorter and moves through a shorter arc. If your arms move faster, your legs can move faster and, combined with a lower leg raise, makes for a very efficient style.

You may question the value of all of this to road runners. As discussed previously, there are times when you must reduce your distance and concentrate on improving speed. Speed is a combination of stride speed (cadence) and stride length. To a limited extent, increasing either will increase your speed but you must take care not to overstride as this causes your centre of gravity to remain behind the point of landing and you have to work against gravity to keep a forward motion.

Your ability to reach your full potential in stride length is directly related to your flexibility, particularly in the hip region. Obviously the more mechanically perfect your style is, the more efficient your running will be and you will either run faster or further at the same speed.

Have you ever considered that your style imperfections may be a result of muscle strength imbalances? Perhaps the tendency of your foot to overpronate is a result of a tight inner set of leg or foot muscles? That is why track athletes spend hours at the track, concentrating on style and flexibility exercises. Whereas distance runners tend to arrive at the track, do a short warm-up, pump out ten or more intervals with short recoveries, cool down and leave, track runners tend to take a more relaxed but longer approach. Their warm-up and stretching can typically be 45 minutes, followed by high-intensity repetitions with long recoveries and more stretching in between, more style or rhythm drills, more stretching and a cool-down. To track runners, poor style can mean the split second difference between first- and fourth-placed finishers.

Better style can result in more efficiency and energy saving, both of which will allow greater speed, and can reduce injuries. Muscles work in pairs; as one contracts, the other extends, and it is the pull by one as the other relaxes that provides the precision control. If you strengthen the antagonistic muscles, they can balance you, and improve your running efficiency. Muscles should also be balanced left to right, but these balances are frequently out of the norm. If you put a mirror down the centre of a photograph of a person, the reflected image will be different to the 'whole' person because we are not perfectly symmetrical. The same applies to most of our muscle groups.

When we run we strengthen the muscles down the back of our bodies, particularly the hamstrings and the lower back, and cause them to shorten. Because the front muscles don't receive the same workout, they don't shorten as much, which explains the tightness that many runners develop, unable to touch their toes, or they may even develop back pain. Part of the answer lies not only in stretching the back muscles, but also in strengthening the front muscles. This is one reason strong 'core muscles' are important to a runner.

To determine precisely which muscle groups need work, consult a biokineticist, who will test you on an Akron or Cibex machine. Basically, pairs of muscles are tested against a moving resistance, and the machine plots not only strength, but also velocity and angles of movement. It can identify raw strength, as well as power and weak points through the range of movement. Of course it also compares the relative strength of the muscle pairings, in addition to one side of the body with the other. After the test you will know which muscle groups need work and can formulate a suitable programme.

It may appear that a weight-training programme is necessary but, as already noted, there is a poor crossover benefit from weights to running because the speed of contraction and relevance of doing sets of weights to the 85–90 cadence of running, is poor. One exception is muscle imbalance, but before opting for a simple weight-training/-lifting programme, discuss your results with a biokineticist. Possibly a programme of skipping, plyometrics or another sport (such as cycling or roller-blading) could be used to strengthen the weak muscles. It is preferable to use an exercise that involves movements at approximately the same speed and that can develop your 'elastic' strength. Training on an Akron or Cibex machine would be ideal but may be financially or logistically impractical.

Track wins are measured in 100ths of a second over short distances. If efficiency is important over short distances, then surely it's even more important over longer distances. Develop a schedule of exercises that you can use in a couple of sessions per week to improve this area.

WEIGHT TRAINING

There is a quite distinct difference between weight training, weightlifting and bodybuilding. Bodybuilding builds muscle bulk, something a distance runner shouldn't have. This is obvious if you recall the earlier explanation of the VO_2 Max i.e. it is in units per kilogram of body weight, hence the lower the body weight, the higher the VO_2 Max.

Weightlifting or power lifting is concerned with the maximum 'one-off' effort and amount that can be lifted in prescribed fashion, whereas running is concerned with a series of movements that are repeated many times per kilometre. As such, weightlifting is of limited interest to runners. On the positive side, because the prime lifts involve large muscle groups and fast, powerful movements, Olympic lifts may be ideal for runners who lack elastic strength. These lifts require special techniques and should be undertaken with assistance from an instructor.

Weight training, on the other hand, concentrates on the development of strength in an endurance mode. The requirements for strength, like all aspects of training, vary with the distance over which you want to compete e.g. sprinting requires greater strength than marathon running. Comparing the physical differences of Michael Johnson and Gert Thys highlights the different requirements. In Johnson we see a highly developed, power-packed, muscular frame, 'designed' to catapult its way off the blocks over 200 m. In Thys, the muscle definition is still there but there is much less bulk. His muscles are trained to do the same exercise many times over; the key is strength endurance. These are extremes in strength training. Obviously, the closer you move to the sprinter, the more 'explosive' strength is required. The longer the competitive distance, the more important strength endurance becomes.

There are many ways of developing strength. Basically, anything that causes muscles to be 'overloaded' will result in strengthening when they recover and rebuild. Overloading can be achieved with hills, running in water, running through sand or rough grass, bounding, or the use of weights or other training machines such as elastic cords and springs. Some of the athletes I coach drag tyres or training partners behind them, to produce the resistance required to improve their strength.

In each case, the runner performs against a resistance, causing the muscles to break down. During the recovery period between training sessions, the muscles repair and strengthen (adapt) to this resistance and can tackle a greater resistance.

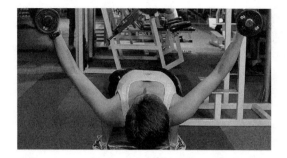

LEFT *Weight training plays a useful role in rehabilitation after injury – it ensures muscle balance, as well as helping to maintain a balanced upper body*

Initially, it appears that the only muscles a runner needs to strengthen are leg muscles, but a stronger upper body is also beneficial to a long-distance runner. For a sprinter or 400-m runner, the arms and shoulders are important for developing, and maintaining, the high-arm drive required. In addition, an all-round, upper-body tone-up assists with correct running style. I believe the need to rehabilitate an injury or achieve muscle 'balance' are key reasons for a weight-training programme.

The objective for a distance runner is not to increase body bulk but rather to develop strength endurance. A schedule that concentrates on a high number of repetitions with relatively light resistance can be beneficial. In the case of weight training, this means doing 12–20 repetitions of an exercise, and performing each set of repetitions three times. A short rest of about 30 seconds is allowed between sets.

The following tables provide **a basic all-round schedule for a distance runner:**

LOWER-BODY SESSION
Warm-up (a 2–3-km easy jog or skipping or cycling on an exercise bike)   Stretching   Bent-leg sit-ups x 20 x 3   Leg extensions x 15 x 3   Leg curls x 15 x 3   Lunges x 15 x 3   Calf raises x 15 x 3

UPPER-BODY SESSION

Warm-up (a 2–3-km easy jog or skipping or cycling on an exercise bike)

Stretching

Bent-arm dumb-bell pullover x 15 x 3

Bench press x 15 x 3

Upright rowing x 15 x 3

Bicep curl x 15 x 3

Incline leg raises x 20 x 3

Stretching

Cool-down (easy jog, etc)

Runners can learn an important lesson from bodybuilders and weightlifters regarding training and recovery. When training, bodybuilders concentrate on one set of muscles at a time, only returning to any muscle group after approximately three days. This allows full recovery (see chapter 5) and maximises the benefit of the training. Doing weight training on the same muscles three times per week will not permit sufficient recovery between sessions and will not produce the best results, as the muscles will not have recovered from the previous training damage when the second and third sessions were undertaken. In fact, this promotes the breakdown of the muscles, which will become smaller (also known as becoming 'catabolic'). To avoid this, ensure that there is sufficient recovery between sessions. Alternating between the upper- and lower-body sessions, with a minimum of two days between any session, will ensure adequate recovery.

Exercises are not described in detail, as you are dealing with weight additional to your body weight, which carries a certain amount of risk and danger of injury. It is very important that these exercises are done correctly and I recommend that you enlist the help of a gym instructor (or biokineticist) the first time you attempt weight training. Initially, you should also select a slightly lighter weight than you think you can handle, as technique is more important than the weight at the start. These sessions, which take about 20 minutes, can be easily accommodated during a lunch break, without having to compromise other running time.

While such exercises may be worth consideration during your base training period, it is important to have the biokinetic assessment, as discussed earlier, and to evolve the weight training appropriate to strengthening your particular weaknesses. Weight training must not be undertaken in the month prior to a major distance race or in the taper period.

ECCENTRIC MOVEMENTS

Many running movements are eccentric, which means that the muscle is put under load while it is already contracted. When the foot is on the ground, the calf muscle is contracted and the Achilles is required to move eccentrically, lowering the heel in a controlled fashion. Running downhill is another example, and explains why runners experience more muscle stiffness (DOMS) after downhill races. It also links into many of the lower leg injuries sustained.

To avoid these problems, focus on some eccentric weight work to strengthen the muscles in these movements. When doing leg curls, most people concentrate on raising (lifting) as big a load as possible, then simply let the weight return to the starting position before commencing the next lift. In eccentric training the concentration is on 'lowering' the weight back to the starting position, in a slow controlled manner. To handle more weight, ask someone to help lift the weight to the top of the lift, then resist the weight by yourself during the lowering.

Eccentric load training may be done for most exercises and should play an important role in post-injury rehabilitation work.

In all weight training (as with all newly introduced training sessions), it is unrealistic to expect dramatic results overnight. It will take a few weeks before your body adapts to this training, but after 6–8 weeks you will reap the benefits.

CIRCUIT TRAINING

Circuit training has already been identified in the previous chapter as an excellent training session. It is also a good transitional phase for runners moving to high-quality track work for middle- and long-distance track racing, or an introduction to strength training as it mostly uses your own body weight. An advantage of circuit training is that it is fairly easy to improvise at the track side and is particularly easy to do in a gym where you have access to a treadmill.

Try the following sequence. Commence with a warm-up and basic muscle stretch as always. Run on a treadmill for 400 m at your 5-km pace (or a lap of the track). Immediately run through the following five exercises: burpess (a standard exercise combining a vertical jump with a squat jump) (6–10), pull-ups/chins (4–6), abdominal crunch (12–20), push-ups (10–15), fast body weight squats (20–30). Continue on the treadmill (or track) for another 400 m (building to 800 m after three weeks), followed by squats and dumbbell press (6–10), elevated feet press-ups (6–10), low-back extensions (12–20), bench or chair dips (10–15) lunges (10–16 per leg). End with the treadmill for another 400 m or 800 m at 5-km pace.

One circuit in the first week, becomes two in the second, goes back to one in the third, but with 800-m intervals. In the fourth week the intervals become 600 m, but the circuit is completed twice, and finally in the fifth week, there are three circuits with 400-m intervals between exercises.

Don't be misled into thinking these are easy sessions. The combination of continuous strength and speed make for a challenging but enjoyable session that combines emotions of love and hate, yet deliver improved performance.

STRETCHING

Stretching is probably the most overlooked exercise by distance runners. They view it as a waste of good training time, or promise themselves to do it while watching TV, but never do. It is, however a vital part of training, but one whose benefit is generally only recognised once they are injured or have many years' running experience.

As already discussed, running strengthens and tightens one set of muscles, leaving the partner muscles out of balance. Running can also tighten complete areas, which in turn restricts flexibility, and all of which results in the impact and driving loads from running being distributed unevenly or onto muscles that have not been conditioned for these loads. This leads to injury.

If there is one area of my preparation that I have neglected over the years, it is stretching and flexibility. Now, with 20 years and thousands upon thousands of kilometres (and more than a few years!) under my belt, I am paying the price with lower limb injuries and a restricted stride length. This is a chain reaction as the running stresses simply continue to search for the weakest link.

I encourage runners to stretch early in their careers and to make it a feature of weekly training. If you have read the track-training section in chapter 7, you know that stretching is emphasised as part of an essential warm-up before training, but it should only be a loosening of major joints, as most distance runners do not warm up long enough for a serious stretching session before track work. Main stretching should be done after a workout, when you are warm and more flexible.

My suggested focus on post-event stretching is supported by research, including a study concerning the Hawaii Marathon. It was found that many of the runners who experienced injury had stretched before training or racing, whereas those stretching afterwards had fewer injuries. Moreover, the results varied according to cultures. Hawaii has a large contingent of Asian runners and it was found that they showed no difference, whether they stretched before or after. Caucasians however had better results from post-event stretching. I think **there are two reasons for this:**

> ▸ Firstly, the Asian lifestyle and culture has a greater orientation towards higher degrees of flexibility than Western sports culture.
>
> ▸ Secondly, if you stretch (or overstretch), the muscle has a reflex reaction that induces an overcontraction, which causes it to shorten (tighten) still further from its original position. If you impose a fast or hard effort on this muscle, it becomes even more susceptible to damage.

Runners are used to trying to persevere through a pain or discomfort barrier, however if this is done with stretching, the risk of injury is increased.

Interestingly, most runners – even novices – instinctively stretch on a minor scale; as they stand around, something 'prompts' them to stretch. Many of these 'natural' stretches cover exactly the areas that runners should include in their core stretching programme. The common ones are to hang forward over the feet, which to some extent stretches the muscles down the back of the body; or to put one foot against a wall or other raised object, which stretches the hamstring area; or even the popular 'push a tree or wall over' exercise that stretches the ankle and calf areas. These appear to be prompted by the body itself and over the years I have learned to respect the cravings and prompting of my body as the very things I need to do.

I cannot encourage you enough to make stretching a regular part of your weekly training. Although you may feel that you aren't making progress, even maintaining your current level of flexibility will pay dividends in the long term. Establish a set time or place each week. A complete stretch session need only involve six or eight stretches and take about 15 minutes, but done regularly, will provide substantial benefit. Either your regular physiotherapist or biokineticist will know the areas on which you need to work.

There are a few basic rules in stretching. NEVER bounce during a stretch. Bouncing can induce the stretch reflex action noted above, causing the muscles to shorten. Subsequent stretching may lead to tears or strains.

POSSIBLE STRETCH SESSION TO USE AS A STARTING POINT

1. **Forward hanging stretch:** Stand feet apart and bend forwards at the stomach until your upper torso hangs over your feet. Keep your legs straight and knees locked. With arms hanging straight, gradually move your hands to one side, then towards each other. Feel the stretch but do not take it past the 'pain' point. This is a good way to warm up for later stretches. If you repeat this stretch at the end of the session, you should be able to stretch further (lower) before hitting the same 'pain' point.

2. **Standing cross-leg stretch:** Cross one leg over the other and keep the heel of the crossed leg off the ground (only the forefoot on the ground). Bend forwards and hang down towards your toes – hold the stretch for a few seconds. Raise your torso and stretch backwards, then repeat the forward stretch. Repeat the procedure with the other leg crossed. The knee of the back leg should remain locked and straight at all times.

3. **Hamstring stretch:** Lie on your back. Pull one knee towards your chest with a bent leg. Raise your head towards your knee. Repeat with the other leg.

4. **Abdominal and upper body stretch:** Lie flat on your stomach with hands shoulder-width apart at chest level. Push up with your arms bent at the lower back. DO NOT pull with your back. Keep your pelvis on the ground.

5. **Quad lunge:** Stand and take one stride forwards until your upper leg or quadriceps or thigh is parallel to the ground. Move forwards to drop the other knee towards the ground in a fencer's lunge, keeping the upper body vertical. The stretch is on the back leg. Repeat, and then repeat with the other leg in the forward position.

6. **Sitting quad:** Kneel on both knees and sit back onto your heels. The stretch will be felt in your quads above the knee. If you are able to sit right down between your heels, take care not to damage the knee joint.

7. **Back stretch:** Lie on your back and SLOWLY bring your legs over your head to touch the ground behind you. Be careful not to jerk your legs over and damage your back. Use your hands to guide and support you.

8. **Calf stretch:** Adopt a pushing position with your hands against a fixed object. Keeping one foot firmly on the ground, bend the supporting knee slowly until you feel the stretch. This can be modified with the use of a wedge of wood, or similar, to assist in improving the flexion of the ankle. Slight variation in movement will move the location of the stretch.

However, during the 2001 New York Marathon I was introduced to a new format of stretching that involves moving through a range of movements, such as knee to chest and running-related movements about eight times. At the extent where the muscle provides resistance, it is held for two seconds before the next repeat. The instructors (all experienced runners) found this to be a better way of warming up and improving flexibility before training because the movements better reflect the speed of running. I was impressed with the results from the couple of sessions I experienced while there.

If you are take the traditional approach, simply take the stretch to the point of 'feeling', hold it there for a few seconds then ease back and apply it again. The second and third stretches will go further and can last 20–30 seconds.

Ease into stretching and don't measure yourself against others. Work within your limitations. Don't stretch when totally cold, at least do a minor warm-up and ideally, stretch again at the end of a training session. Bearing in mind that muscles operate in pairs – one pulls while the other relaxes – it is as important to focus on relaxing the antagonistic muscle, as it is to focus on the muscle being stretched. Muscles cannot 'push'. Strengthening exercises and stretches are required in combination to 'balance' a runner.

AEROBICS

This can be a logical extension of the stretching exercises that will not only improve your suppleness but also your aerobic capacity. Most gyms have aerobic classes but be careful in your choice, as they don't all have suitably qualified instructors.

The benefits of aerobics are fairly obvious and don't require a detailed discussion other than to note that such sessions are also a good method of recovery after a race. Don't be disappointed or embarrassed if you find yourself uncoordinated with some of the movements. Despite appearances, even the best instructors will have experienced that problem when they started.

TREADMILL RUNNING

Treadmills provide an alternative when the weather prohibits training or you are looking for a different session. I have found them particularly useful when away on business as they allow me to put in a 'quality' session even after some late meetings. With treadmill running you have the opportunity to do any or all of the normal running sessions. However, you will not make any friends if you use the local fitness club treadmill for your two-hour long run! Normally, sessions on a club treadmill need to be limited to about 30 minutes to let others complete their training and many gyms limit each session to 20 minutes. This simply requires some planning. Use the stationary cycle for a warm-up or use the first opportunity on the treadmill for an easy 20 minutes, then use the next segment of 20 minutes for your intervals. Set it to your target 200-m, 400-m or 1 000-m track speed, set the incline and lift yourself on and off the belt for each effort and recovery period.

Treadmills offer some benefits; they force you into a leg speed — it's either keep up or be forced off the back. They often have a more cushioned treadboard that reduces the leg pounding caused by tar or the track. This is particularly useful when recovering from an injury, or just for a change. Most treadmills provide an immediate read-out of speed, distance and time – useful for short, speed sessions.

On the negative side it should be noted that treadmill running uses a different stride technique. To compensate for this, set the treadmill gradient at 1% and raise the speed by about 1 km per hour above your target pace, which will provide about the same perceived effort as your target pace.

Although you won't have to push aside any headwind or move air when running on a treadmill, you won't benefit from the air's cooling effect either. Take a cloth or towel with you when treadmill training as your perspiration will not be appreciated by the next user. You will definitely perspire more in a warm indoor climate. Treadmill training requires greater mental tenacity as you are going nowhere and you'll be surprised how long a single minute can seem.

The treadmill offers a good transition session from road to track training as it builds the confidence of handling speed and distance. Doing short, very fast repeats on the treadmill is also a good way of improving leg speed.

Finally, a treadmill provides a good way of measuring training progress, as it is easier to control the wide variety of parameters in running. A simple method is to use the same machine each time, set the same incline and speed, and monitor your heart rate over a 20-minute run. The speed should be around your best 10-km pace. Keep a note of how fast your heart rate drops at one, two and five minutes after you have finished the run. As your training progresses, your running heart rate should drop from test to test, and your post-test heart rate should drop faster in the minutes that follow.

More complicated, but a better test is to warm up at a pace much slower than your marathon pace. Commence on the treadmill at 0.97 km per hour slower than your marathon pace, after two minutes increase the pace by 0.32 km per hour until you cannot maintain the new pace for the full two minutes.

Although it might appear complicated, the following example for a five-hour marathoner will demonstrate how easy it really is. This is not only a good test, but also a good training session. The faster the speed you achieve prior to exhaustion, the greater your racing potential. This test should only be completed every six or eight weeks.

A four-hour marathon pace is 10.55 km per hour, so start the treadmill at 9.58 km per hour (10.55 − 0.97 = 9.58). Each increase should be 0.32 km per hour, **which gives the following progression:**

	PACE – KM/HR	CUMULATIVE TIME (MINUTES)
Ultrarace pace	9.58	2
	9.9	4
	10.22	6
	10.54	8
Marathon pace	10.86	10
	11.18	12
	11.5	14
	11.82	16
10-km pace	12.14	18
5-km pace	12.46	20
	12.78	22

Some fast runners may find that a gym treadmill is not fast enough. The best way to overcome this is to increase the incline. Use 1% increase for each extra kilometre per hour, but remember that you need a 1% basic incline from the start. If your top end speed is to be 23 km per hour and the treadmill only goes to 20 km per hour, you need to set the incline to 4% from the beginning and take 3 km per hour from all the calculated figures as this will be accounted for in the incline. It is not a perfect analogy, but as the test is relative to your own performance, it is accurate enough. It is worth making a note of your race performances following the different test results. Soon you will know how fit you are prior to major events and will be able to set more realistic race targets and strategies.

PLOTTING HEART RATES

As indicated, the comparison of heart rates at different speeds may also hint at the efficiency at different levels of exertion. All runners have a speed at which they are most economical. Such speeds tend to be those at which they are training on a regular basis. It is therefore important for a marathoner to become efficient at marathon target pace. By plotting speed (effort) against heart rate on a graph, it is sometimes possible to pick these up, as there is often a flattening of the curve at these paces. It becomes more pronounced when test graphs are compared.

Testing is a good method to increase motivation when you are training for a race that is a few months away. Each test becomes a small goal on the ladder towards the bigger goal of the race result. A word of warning though, testing by its very nature is a 'difficult' session that requires concentration. Subjecting an athlete to frequent testing can 'dull' his appetite for the test and will have a negative effect on the results.

As with most of these supplementary exercises, the treadmill is a useful tool, but not one to overplay. Remember that the running style is different.

OTHER STRENGTHENING EXERCISES

Strength is a key component of running at speed. Having greater strength allows you to propel a weight (your body weight) through the air. The faster you move a single weight through a distance, the more 'powerful' you are. A sprinter needs enough power to take his body weight from rest in the blocks, through the acceleration zone to his maximum speed, and then to have the ability to hold that speed and momentum. A distance runner needs to accelerate his body weight to a much slower speed, but must have the strength endurance to hold it at that speed for a long time.

Although many consider the use of weights to be the only way of improving strength, this is not the case. The basics of strength training can commence with exercises that involve the athlete's own body weight. This is particularly applicable to young athletes. Any session that causes the muscles to be 'overloaded' will develop an improvement in strength in those muscles, providing, of course, that sufficient recovery is allowed to enable the repair of the muscles.

Since the objective is generally to improve the strength in the muscles used while running, some form of 'overloading' during running is the most efficient. This principle has been tried in many sports, such as using heavier golf clubs or tennis rackets while practising. The main problem is that such methods can change a person's swing or grip, as more and different muscles are brought into play to handle the heavier equipment. Similarly, running with weights can also change your style and is therefore not a good idea. A possible exception to this is to use a container that distributes weight evenly through the centroid of the body, such as a Tripper (see also chapter 27 with regard to drinking during a run) filled with water.

Other possible methods of developing strength without impairing running style, or indeed, that could actually improve running style, include running in calf-deep water e.g. along the beach, sand running and hill running (see the previous chapter). It has become a tradition for the British athletic team, as well as teams from other sports, to do repeats up and down some of the steepest sand dunes in Wales. Take care when running on sand as your feet tend to sink into the sand and greater strain is put onto the Achilles tendon. There is also the problem of the slope of the sand towards the ocean as this can result in knee injuries. When running hard on sand, some people twist their feet and because it is not their natural stride, it can cause problems. A period of adaptation is necessary for all of these reasons.

Dragging car tyres across grass as a means of developing strength and a good driving style is an activity I like to use with athletes. The tyre is 'attached' to the body by means of a harness, which should be worn around the hipbone. This causes the drive to come from the hips and promotes a good driving position. I prefer this to using an upper body harness, which tends to encourage the athlete to lean forward too much. These sessions are preceded by a thorough warm-up and then comprise 3–5 sets of 4 x 80–100-m efforts with sufficient recovery to allow the session to be completed. If you finish the session with a series of three sprints over the same distance without the tyre, it feels as if someone has attached a turbojet to your back!

Stair running can also develop strength. Running up 30 flights of stairs in an office block, stepping on each tread, builds more strength endurance than sprinting up the short but steep grandstand stairs of a rugby stadium, which is more geared to strength. Be sure to move into stair training gradually as the workload on the calf muscles can be quite dramatic.

In 1998 I managed the Great Britain Ultra-team to the World 100 km in Japan. During a stopover we stayed in a 100-storey building and I could not resist the challenge of climbing the emergency stairs, although spent the next two days visiting the team sport masseur. A more gradual introduction would have been better, but there are times when you simply have to accept a challenge, as the opportunity might not present itself again. Luckily for me, my next race was a long time ahead and I was able to fully recover from that effort. Most of the above exercises focus on the development of leg strength, but upper-body strength is also important to the correct carriage of arms and to aid breathing.

A trim track can be used for this purpose; stop at various stations to do pull-ups, dips, sit-ups, press-ups and a host of other exercises against gravity and body weight. Use hand weights to tone up the upper arms, but it is important not to use too heavy a weight as this will alter running style. Weights in the region of 5 kg per hand are ideal.

PLYOMETRICS

Most distance runners have a leg speed of around 90–110 strides per minute. Exercises that require this type of muscle contraction against a resistance slightly greater than that experienced in normal racing will improve a runner's ability. For this reason plyometrics provide the ideal training for distance runners as they develop elastic strength – the ability to transfer weight and power from foot to foot quickly. It is necessary to prepare joints and ligaments for the plyometrics by having an initial strength base developed in weight training.

Plyometrics exercises promote such elasticity. Commence with basic skipping and hopping, and progress to bounding, height and depth jumps. The biggest danger is to do too much too soon and, as with weights, programmes for young athletes should be highly restricted. Even older novices may take months to reach a level that is anything more than basic plyometrics.

Long-distance runners will find the heights and depths they're able to achieve in these exercises significantly less than those of their more powerful sprinting colleagues. The longer a runner has been running long-distance events, the more difficulty he will have in commencing plyometrics as the distance will have reduced his muscle elasticity.

After time, bounding up (and down) steps and even over hurdles becomes a possibility. The importance of elastic strength is perhaps best illustrated by the fact that it can be used as a direct indicator of an athlete's ability. For example, a top-class 800-m runner will bound 25 m in 12–14 bounds, but plyometrics are beneficial to all runners as they improve elastic strength.

Two cases have reinforced my belief in this training. The first was the progress I noted in running style and performance by a group of runners I coached following a ten-week programme of plyometrics; they improved their 10-km half-marathon and marathon times. Of course, plyometrics represented only one aspect of their training, but were used instead of normal weight training.

The second came from an interview in September 1999 with Carl Lewis, arguably the greatest Olympic athlete to date, in which he revealed that he did not subscribe to weight training, but rather to plyometrics for strength training. The reason? They mimicked the requirements of his sprint and long jump events more closely. Now retired from competition, Lewis still 'pulls out the boxes' for a weekly plyometric session as a 'recreational and health runner'.

Sebastian Coe was another Olympic star to believe in plyometrics. He regularly undertook a session of plyometrics that had him bounding over 1 m plus vaulting horses, or jumping astride a 300-mm box. There are pictures of him 'dropping' off a vaulting horse with a 15-kg weight around his waist, then immediately going into a long jump.

Closer to home, many rugby teams now use plyometrics to develop the power of their players. The sight of 100-kg plus Sharks' prop Ollie le Roux jumping more than 1 m from a standing position to land on top of a box is surely sufficient endorsement that this is a useful method of developing elastic strength.

The variety of exercises is limitless; a full session of these may take 20–30 minutes and can improve rhythm, style and coordination, as well as strength. One example is to 'run' a 50-m section while kicking your heels up to your buttocks as many times as possible, progressively increasing the speed of these. Synchronise your arm movements throughout the exercise. Another example is to repeat the same distance with high knee lifts and very short strides. These may seem very simple exercises, but try repeating each exercise four times and you will soon notice how they work muscles that you never knew you had!

A good introduction to plyometrics is simply to hop down a set of stairs. Pick a flight with 10–12 steps and hop down on one leg, climb back to the top and hop down on the other leg. (Use the handrail for safety and confidence if you need it when you begin.) The small eccentric bounding prepares you for some of the more substantial bounding exercises later. Starting with a total of 20 hops, you will soon build up to about 50–80 per leg. To derive maximum benefit from these sorts of exercises, you should aim to do the explosive sections at a running pace (approximately 85 steps per minute). Keep it fast, rhythmical and explosive – you'll soon discover the rewards are great.

SCOOTING

Those gleaming silver scooters that children use to create havoc on the streets can be a useful tool for runners to develop leg drive and as an introduction to plyometric bounding. Like running, the key to good scooter speed is a strong leg drive, something rarely developed in distance training. Consider good 'scooting' technique: the unsupported leg touches the ground slightly ahead of the supported leg, maintaining the momentum of the scooter as you drive the free leg backwards. This drive should be long, smooth and hard, but not overexaggerated, as it will delay the return time for the next 'kick'.

Running at quality speeds is similar. While many runners overstride on their forward swing i.e. allow the foot to touch the ground too far in advance of the body, few distance runners have a really good leg drive as it moves through to the back of their stride. A good drive makes for more efficient running, particularly on hills and at speed.

To benefit from using one of these scooters, ensure that you have the correct positioning. Compensate for the supported leg being 75 mm higher on the platform by keeping the supported leg bent. This will keep the hips level throughout the stride. Maintaining this 'partial squat' position also improves the hip, abdominal and support leg muscles as it is the key to scooter stability. Adjust the handlebar height and angle so you do not lean too far forward. Your torso should be almost vertical with your hips, tilted slightly upwards. While stationary, check your posture in a side mirror. Take note of your foot position on the platform as a point of reference. Moving your foot will change your posture.

Find a relatively gradual 30–40-m hill with a smooth surface, safe from traffic and pedestrians. 'Adopt the position' on the platform and drive your free leg backwards against the tar to propel the scooter uphill. Make these drives as long and powerful as you can, but sufficiently fast to maintain the smooth motion of the scooter. With short strides, the direction and supported body movements become erratic. If the strides are too long, the scooter slows down between 'kicks'. Only use 30–40-m uphill repeats in the early sessions and change legs each time – about ten sets per leg is a good introduction. You will soon feel the difference obtained from various drive lengths and you may find the following surprising: the strength and muscles required to maintain the partial squat position; the difference between leg strengths and styles; and how 'short' your normal running strides have been.

Once you have 'mastered' the initial sessions, try some track 200s or 400s. These are similar to normal track running and aim to improve length and cadence of strides. Keep to 1½ –2 minutes recovery between each repeat and concentrate on style. Alternate the legs and the directions in which you travel. Start with only a few repeats, approximately 5 x 200 per leg.

Such scooting sessions are taxing, particularly to the hamstring muscles, which are required to operate powerfully over a greater range of movement. Listen to the 'tweaks' and niggles of the following day before doing any other quality work. As you become used to it, return to the hills for longer repeats of 100–150 m.

Scooter work is much closer to the muscular and neural speed and actions of running. Although you run about 85–100 strides per minute, in weight training you only push weights around 10–20 repetitions per minute, often in a seated position. The closer your training is to the specific speed and action of running, the more effective it will be. Scooter work is a good introduction and **allows you to concentrate on the action of one leg at a time** (something that normal running doesn't allow) **and can provide:**

▸ Better drive strength and style.
▸ Improved support and core strength.
▸ A good neural workout.
▸ Improved bounding technique.

CYCLING

Cycling has experienced a 'second wind' as a mass sport with the Pick 'n Pay *Argus* 110-km cycle race in Cape Town each March, attracting in excess of 35 000 entries. The value of cycling, in complementing running, received a major boost with the introduction of triathlons and duathlons in the 1980s. More recently, this sporting code was further bolstered by the explosion in mountain biking, either for off-road use, or simply to travel to and from work.

Like running, cycling is basically an aerobic sport, although it can be used to develop all the same aspects as running, viz. endurance, strength and speed; it depends what sort of training session you undertake. There is much debate as to whether there is any carryover between cycling and running. Camps are split, but I certainly believe in the benefits of mixing cycling and running.

The cardiovascular benefits of cycling are similar to running, provided the effort of the cycling is hard enough. Cycling can also improve leg muscle strength as a result of hill repeats.

Similarly, the 'spinning' undertaken by cyclists must surely help in improving the leg cadence of runners. Spinning, or fast, low-gear pedalling, in which legs turn over at a speed in excess of 90 revs per minute have also benefited a number of runners I have coached. In fact, both friends and I have run some very fast sessions immediately after a short cycle. (Such sessions are extremely taxing and must be used with care – see triathlon training, chapter 15.) An average club cyclist spins at around 95 revs per minute, while better cyclists turn over at approximately 100 revs per minute.

What I have proved with runners I have coached is that there is definite benefit to be gained in terms of hill running from cycle training on hills. Cycling teaches the need for gears and how to tackle a long hill with a rhythmic approach, which is an excellent way of teaching a runner how to run up long climbs in races. Too many runners 'charge' hills at the bottom and grind to a halt near the top, whereas cycling teaches them better use of stride length and rhythm.

The benefits of cycling during injury recovery are well illustrated by Gordon Baker, who became 'Mr Lead Bike' in the Comrades until 2002. For many years he was one of the top runners and earned a number of gold medals. However, during one year he was sidelined by an injury for most of the January to May build-up period and took to cycling instead. By Comrades race day, he had very little running under his belt but had trained substantial distances on his bike. That year Gordon still managed a gold medal, which must prove something about cross training.

In terms of time benefit, an American triathlon source suggests that, as we ride at approximately twice the speed of running, it will take an hour of cycling to equate to 30 minutes running. I'm not convinced that this is quite accurate and think it's more likely to be a 3:1 ratio.

The greatest drawback to cycling is the danger, which is not always a rider's fault. No matter how safety conscious you are, the fact that you are sharing the road with high-powered motor vehicles implies substantial risk. Such an accident happened to a very dear friend and team colleague, Dave McCarney, who was hit from behind and killed, by a large truck. Cyclists should take every precaution, from what they wear, to the mirrors and reflectors fitted to their bikes. It may not be fashionable to wear a hard helmet, gloves and bright cycling top, or to fit a handlebar or helmet mirror, or to have a host of reflective material over the bike, but it's better than becoming a statistic. Be bright, be seen and stay alive. A useful tip when cycling past a road junction at which cars are stopped is to watch their wheels rather than the body of the vehicle. Small movements are more easily detected at the wheels.

A training session that is exceptionally hard, yet 100% safe, is the use of indoor wind trainers. The bike is fixed to a rig and a fan (or magnets) and turned by the rear wheel to provide resistance. This is a very taxing session and allows the rider to do various high-intensity repeats. Being indoors, it also tends to become hot and humid, not to mention mentally tiring, as you are always stationary. On the counter side, it is possible to combine this with various testing and monitoring procedures that allow a standardised testing procedure to be undertaken.

Indoor cycling also provides the opportunity to obtain much finite information with the use of small computers on the handlebars. Speed, time, distance, average speed, heart rate and cadence (revs per minute) all help to measure progress or replicate previous conditions. A good test is to warm up with some light spinning, select a relatively high gear that you can maintain for six minutes. Set the resistance of the turbo trainer and cycle as hard as possible for six minutes non-stop, keeping the revs up above 95 or 100 per minute. As you pass five minutes, put in a last ditch sprint to the six-minute finish. Make a note of all information: distance covered, average speed, maximum heart rate, the gear you were wearing (the same gear must be maintained throughout), and the resistance on the turbotrainer. Repeat this session at six- or eight-week intervals to monitor progress.

In addition, use the average speed of the test for some interesting turbo training sessions. For instance, warm up, then cycle 20 x 30 seconds at the same pace, gear and speed as your test. Give yourself a 30-second easy between each set, then cool down. This is a good session and means that you cycle for ten minutes at the same pace that you managed for only six minutes, but your heart rate will be up in the same zone for around 15 of the 20 minutes.

Regular tests in this manner can assess fitness and it is even possible to determine VO_2 Max and threshold levels with the use of a heart monitor. However, this can only be used as a guide because your cycling technique may be slightly better or worse than your running, with a consequent minor variation in the results. The biggest drawback to this cross-training benefit is that cycling does not use exactly the same muscles as running, thus there is no direct relationship.

SWIMMING

Swimming is an excellent sport, and one that tones up just about every part of the body. If you go for a swim, notice how firm your muscles feel when you've completed even a relatively short session. Using both the upper and lower body, swimming makes major demands on your cardiovascular system and, because your breathing has to be controlled with the stroke, it is a good way to regulate your breathing.

You can even use different breathing rhythms as part of your conditioning. Try swimming with bilateral breathing – every three strokes for two lengths, then go to breathing every five strokes, then seven, and finally nine strokes to one breath. You will soon feel how your lungs are taxed. Studies have shown anaerobic capacity to be improved by swimming distances underwater, by limiting the oxygen supply. This ties in with research on runners who performed breathing exercises for six weeks. They practised breathing against resistance both on inhaling and exhaling. This was found to improve their VO_2 Max by a substantial amount, the implication being that learning to breathe correctly and exercising those breathing muscles is an easy way of making some progress.

A swimming session should follow the same format as a track session. A few easy laps provide a warm-up, followed by some repeats of 25 m, 50 m, or 100 m at a faster pace with limited recovery, and then a cool-down. You can use hand paddles to increase the workout on the upper body and flippers or kicking to increase the lower body workout. Simply swimming long, slow distance has limited benefit, but can make for a relaxing session on a rest day. The use of flippers can give an added workout to the leg muscles, particularly if you are suffering from tight or sore leg muscles.

In swimming, your body weight is totally supported by the water, probably making it one of the most useful sports while recovering from an injury. The main problem is that it is a high-technique sport, and if you don't already know how to swim properly, the chances are that it will take you a considerable time to learn the required techniques. Learning to 'kick' bad habits developed in casual swimming often proves to be extremely difficult. The irony with swimming is that the better you are, the better your line and the shorter the distance you need to swim. Conversely, a swimmer with poor style tends to swim further, and usually slower. I know this from my own participation in the annual Midmar Mile (1 600 m), and will soon have completed my twentieth Midmar 2 km.

It is interesting to note that most champion swimmers are relatively young; in fact, even children who participate seriously are subjected to 10 000 m of swimming per day! Obviously, this is far in excess of the swimming that you would use as an alternative or a supplement to run training. In such cases, a session may only involve swimming a total of 1–3 km. Swimming is the least taxing and damaging of the three triathlon sports (running, cycling and swimming) and recovery from a hard swimming session is fast, which is why young swimmers can cope with such long distances.

RUNNING IN WATER

Running in water is more allied to running itself. Many world-class runners have used it as a means of training through major injuries and have recorded much improved performances shortly after resuming running. It is achieved by being supported in the water in a vertical position while simultaneously driving with the arms and legs. This may sound easy but done correctly, a 20–30 minute session can become a heavy workout and should only be undertaken gradually. In such exercises, the resistance is not only on the downward foot drive, but also upwards against the water.

The water session can be tailored to different requirements, using different exercises or adding various boards and floats to provide additional resistance to your movement. In this way you can gradually increase the load on an injured muscle or joint. For most lower limb injuries you should run in deep water so that you cannot touch the bottom, and can gradually apply load to the legs by reducing the depth of water.

A foam back belt can be used to assist you to float in a vertical position, but after a number of sessions it should be possible to do this without any float as you become familiarised with the technique of running in water.

CANOEING

Canoeing is included because it is a popular sport among a number of runners who also participate in canoe triathlons, the Duzi Canoe Marathon and other outdoor activities. Canoeing may be used as an alternative sport, but it is predominately concerned with upper-body movement and the benefit to running is much more limited.

One aspect that does improve with canoeing is basic core strength. Sitting in a canoe requires stability, similar to sitting on one of the 'physio' balls used for developing the stability muscles around the waist and hips. The conclusion therefore is that novice canoeists can develop their ability and stability by doing exercises on a 'physio' ball, while canoeing and surf paddling will be beneficial to anyone wishing to develop core stability muscles.

MASSAGE

Although massage is not a sport or exercise, it certainly has a place in training programmes, and is a very worthwhile 'tool' in training, race preparation and recovery. When I was appointed senior manager for the UK athletics ultra-squad, I requested that a sports masseur be made available to squad members and be given preference over a physiotherapist when the team toured overseas. The reason for this is simple. If an athlete needs physiotherapy before an event, the question must be asked whether he is fit enough to be in the team, but all team members will benefit from massage before and after an event (and during, in the case of the 24-hour championships).

Many forms of massage are advertised, indeed some relate to a 'sport' of a different sort! The first problem for a novice to such treatment is to determine what type of massage is appropriate and what credentials a masseur should have. Massage is an excellent way of improving blood circulation to muscles and joints, improving the alignment of muscle fibres and muscle flexibility, treating minor intrinsic and potential injuries, and has both a stress-reducing and physiological benefit to the athlete. The emphasis on each of these areas may be altered through the use of different types of massage 'strokes'.

A trained masseur can mentally attune an athlete who is lacking in motivation for a competition, using one type of massage. He can also reduce the anxiety level to a desirable status in an athlete who finds himself 'uptight' from apprehension prior to major competitions, through the use of more relaxing strokes. Massage method should vary according to the stage of training being undertaken, and **can be widely classified into three areas:**

> ▸ **preparatory massage**, which deals with the training period. This is used to aid the recovery of an athlete after a heavy session and also to prepare him for the following quality sessions.
>
> ▸ **pre-competition massage**, which is used to bring an athlete to the right state of physical and mental arousal immediately prior to competition. This too will vary, depending on the type of event. If it is a sprint, many short, fast strokes are required, while an endurance event requires longer, deeper massage techniques.
>
> ▸ **recuperation massage**, which is undertaken after a competition to improve an athlete's rate of recovery. Again, the techniques will vary with timing. A deep massage immediately after a marathon is not the most beneficial or pleasant experience. Similarly, a light massage a week later will have little benefit. The massage must be suited to the training.

A masseur must have a thorough understanding not only of the massage techniques, but also the athlete's objectives at any point in his training. This requires a background in physiology and to a lesser extent, psychology. A good masseur is capable of work on minor injuries, as well as assistance in preventative care of potential injuries. For these reasons an athlete and masseur must work together over an extended period to develop the necessary rapport.

Such regular attention only becomes viable for many runners if a friend or family member is suitably trained in such techniques, and to this end, it may be more beneficial to attend a course on massage rather than face the relatively high costs of regular attention. This will depend on the priority a runner places on reaching peak performance.

Much of the scepticism to which massage had been subjected has faded, but some runners still fail to understand its advantages. Unfortunately, their negativity is often reinforced by experiences at less knowledgeable establishments. The practice of mixing massage and training is used by world-class athletes around the world and I have no doubt that, if applied correctly, it will benefit runners at all levels. Your training is only as good as your recovery and anything that improves recovery will allow you to train more effectively.

00:00:09
THE DIFFERENT PHASES
OF TRAINING

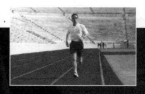

This section should help you to put the 'meat' onto the skeleton of the schedules. Obviously, the type of schedule will vary according to each training season and its objective. It is important to know exactly what you're aiming to achieve every time you cross the threshold of your door for a training session.

You need to know where you are going and precisely how you will accomplish it, if you want to reach a destination or goal. Planning is all important. However, as that great Scottish poet, Robert 'Rabbie' Burns put it, 'The best laid schemes o' mice an' men gang aft a-gley,' (or 'often go astray', in more common parlance), and the fourth law of training (see chapter 6) reminds us that a schedule must be flexible.

If I have a track session planned and for some reason an office commitment means that I would have to train at 4:00 in the morning, I must have the flexibility to change my sessions around, because to try track at that time is more likely to court injury than benefit. Conversely, I must not use flexibility as an excuse to shirk unappealing training sessions.

ACTIVE RECOVERY

The following sample weekly schedule is probably the most flexible as its objective is to allow the body a chance to recover fully from a competition season, while at the same time maintaining a basic standard of fitness and movement. It incorporates a few rest days of total inactivity and also provides an opportunity to make use of some or all of the supplementary and complementary exercises discussed earlier.

DAY	TRAINING
Day 1	Rest
Day 2	Cycle 1 hour
Day 3	Run 8–10 km
Day 4	Rest
Day 5	8 km off-road/cross-country
Day 6	Swim 1 km
Day 7	Run 10–12 km

The permutations are endless and will vary according to your fitness level, but it is important to remember that this is a time of 'no pressure' and if you feel like missing a schedule, you're entitled to do so.

BASE TRAINING

Once you have recovered, you are ready to tackle your next goal. The first step is to re-establish your endurance base. Most of your running during this phase will be of the long, slow type, but not exclusively so. Be careful with this definition. Long may be 10–12 km when focusing on 10-km and shorter events, while slow will also relate to the forthcoming race distance. Runners who have, for instance, already completed Comrades, hardly need to build up an endurance base, but do need to ease their way back into training, perhaps for a forthcoming 21-km event. Your schedule must also introduce things such as strength training after a few weeks; cycling can be used as an alternative way to develop the long run.

One of the easiest places to start when setting up a schedule is to determine which day you want as a rest day. In my early running years I made the mistake of not having at least one day's full rest a week. When I realised my mistake and incorporated a rest day, my running improved immediately as I had a renewed zest the following day. Although I may sometimes run some distance on days that I have set aside as rest days, I still maintain the principle of regular, total rest days, and benefit from the concomitant physiological and psychological renewal.

Some runners may find that they need two rest days per week. This is fine; remember the sixth law of training: try to achieve as much as possible with minimum training. Don't slide into an obsessive training routine, or become a slave to weekly distance. These wheels have been invented and reinvented many times and have always been proven unsuccessful.

The next step is to divide your training runs into one long run, one medium run, one fartlek-type run, and the remainder as short recovery runs. This, in effect, gives you three harder sessions, three easier sessions and a rest day.

As noted, what constitutes 'long' or 'medium' will be decided by the race for which you're training, as well as your current level of fitness. The fartlek is to prevent you from slipping into a one-pace format in this training and may be as simple as speeding up three or four times in the session to 15-km race pace as opposed to training pace. These faster sections may only last a few hundred metres, but will prove invaluable. They should not be used as hard efforts, but rather a change of gear.

Runners who have never done any speed work before tend to train at their marathon pace most of the time. Elite marathon runners, however, train much slower than marathon pace, although their marathon pace is slightly under three minutes per kilometre! Seiko, like many other top Japanese runners, actually trained much of his distance runs at five minutes per kilometre despite being capable of running sub 2:10 marathons. Once average runners begin speed work, they too develop a relatively wide range of training gears and speeds. Remember, long, slow trainers become good long, slow runners.

Bearing in mind the fifth law of training (alternate hard and easy days), it is necessary to apply the alternating principle to weekly, long runs. If your maximum weekly, long run is currently 15 km and you are building to 30 km, try the following scheduling: week one – 15 km, week two – 12 km, week three – 22 km; week four – 14 km, week five – 23 km, week six – 18 km, week seven – 26 km, week eight – 19 km, week nine – 30 km. This may seem slow, but remember the second law of training (start gradually and train gently). This will allow you to recover well and will establish a good base. In general terms, **a weekly base schedule may resemble the following:**

DAY	TRAINING
Day 1	Rest
Day 2	Medium run (about 20% of weekly total)
Day 3	Short run
Day 4	Fartlek (about 12% of weekly total)
Day 5	Short run
Day 6	Long run (not more than 35% of weekly total)
Day 7	Short run

Short runs should be a third of the distance left in the weekly total. If your total is 80 km, a long run would be 21–26 km, a medium run 15 km, fartlek about 10 km, and short runs about 8 km each. This has proved to be a well-rounded schedule. After a few weeks, a couple of strength training sessions may be introduced. Depending on availability of strength training facilities, they could be done on days two and seven, or three and one. But do not mix them with the hard sessions such as six and four. Possibly, day seven's run could be replaced by a cycle of an hour, which would again assist in recovery. The variation prevents mental boredom.

RACE-SPECIFIC TRAINING

After a base has been built, it is possible to include training sessions that deal with the specific needs of the event in which you are competing. Generally, this will be speed-orientated, but in the case of some of the trail races that are becoming popular (in the USA in particular), training may be geared towards running on trails. If the course is very hilly, hill technique may be a predominant aspect.

This period of training needs to focus not only on the speed and physiology of the race, but also on all other factors that impact on how it will be run so that the training specifically adapts a runner to the needs of the competition. This said, the objective is not to become obsessed with these requirements, but rather to develop a balanced programme around them. It is important to note that you cannot do everything at one time. During this period, which may last from 6–12 weeks (as previously discussed), the emphasis may change to cover all the requirements at a gradually increasing degree of difficulty. For example, if your event requires speed, the training period may introduce a couple of fartlek sessions per week, then change to one fartlek and one hill session, to one hill and one track session (relatively easy), and finally to two or even three track sessions per week. Your progress in moving to track will depend on your past experience with quality work. In general, there should not be more than three hard sessions per week; more would not allow for sufficient recovery.

Initial fartlek sessions are introduced in a very easy format in the base training. To a certain extent, there is a carryover effect between these 'training phases'. Hills may be introduced towards the end of the base training. The progression is generally from endurance to strength, to speed, to taper (sharpening and recovery), and finally to competition.

Keeping this in mind, an average runner training for **a half-marathon may well have a schedule similar to that shown below:**

DAY	TRAINING
Day 1	Rest
Day 2	Track (3–4 x 800 m for speed endurance)
Day 3	Recovery run 12 km
Day 4	Track (5 x 200 for speed, 5x 400 at your 5-km race pace)
Day 5	Recovery 8–10 km very easy
Day 6	Cross-country race or fartlek
Day 7	15–18 km slow distance

This will result in a total distance of about 60 km for a week, yet still provides variation. If the hard sessions are truly hard and the easy sessions easy, good results will follow. The above schedule is merely a guide and the content of the track will vary as the training season develops. Notice the reference to a cross-country race, but it is compared to a fartlek session, and that is the approach you must take. Prior to the 'race', you and your coach must decide what time or where you should finish in comparison to your flat-out effort.

Such an approach to races requires supreme discipline and willpower. Perhaps the majority of runners are incapable of this and should possibly refrain from races. What tends to happen is that they see a runner they know they're capable of beating, or a friend that they always 'dice', and then the 'game is on'. The training race becomes a flat-out effort, and instead of developing their fitness with training, they end up drawing on their reserves in a race situation. Remember, **Racing Requires Recovery** – think of it as the three Rs.

On the other hand, as you approach the race for which you are trying to peak, it is essential to sharpen up in a few races. This allows you to experience pre-race anxiety, race tactics and conditions, but these are not necessarily 100% flat-out efforts. Many of the world's top marathon runners use a 10-km race about ten days before a marathon as a result indicator. It is important to note that the race they use is over a shorter distance – often where a club time trial may come in handy; e.g. a 4–5-km time trial may be ideal for a 10-km race, and an 8-km can be a good predictor for a half-marathon.

American runners have a rule of thumb for the recovery period after a flat-out race: to allow one day's recovery for every mile (1.6 km) raced, after which a runner may start building up again. Thus, after a hard 5-km time trial, allow about three easy days. This once again emphasises the problem of 'racing' a club 8-km every week. No sooner have you recovered than you have the next week's club time trial to run, leaving no days for training!

TRAIN HARD – REST JUST AS HARD!
Recovery week during the training build-up
In any build-up to a distance, there are always periods of heavy training. Each of these should be followed by a shorter period of recovery before moving on to the next period of heavy training. The recovery period allows the body to 'repair' and benefit from the 'overload' effect of efficient training. You should enter periods of high distance feeling fresh and eager to train. In the following weeks there may

come times when it seems that there aren't enough hours in a day, as you try to squeeze in the distance. Starting the endurance block with an easy week will allow you the opportunity to complete things that your training may later overshadow.

What makes up a recovery week?

A recovery week doesn't mean doing nothing, nor does it mean simply going for slow runs. The idea is to keep to the basic training principles, but to reduce the workload sufficiently to allow your body to recover fully and be well rested. It also means that it is pointless to reduce your training merely to replace the stress by working all hours of the day and night. It is important to ensure that you continue to use a variety of speeds during the week's training. A single, high-quality session will ensure that you don't lose any of the fitness you have already built.

Taking an entire week off is not as beneficial as the balance of reduced stress and activity, but there is nothing wrong with adding an extra day's total rest to your schedule. If your work allows it, rather move your early morning runs to the early evening, or even lunchtime, in such a week. That will allow you to enjoy an extra hour or so in bed – something you may have to sacrifice in the following weeks! **Your week may look like this:**

DAY	TRAINING
Monday	Rest
Tuesday	8 km easy (marathon pace or slower)
Wednesday	8 km with 5 x 100-m pick-ups at 5-km pace
Thursday	5 km moderate (15 km – half-marathon race pace)
Friday	Rest
Saturday	Track 4 x 400 at five seconds faster than best 5-km pace
Sunday	12–18 km easy

Such a schedule could be used as a recovery week in a marathon or ultra-build-up. The following week, you could move to your new training schedule and then start moving towards your specific training goal.

The difference between a recovery week and active recovery is only minimal. A recovery week maintains a higher level of 'quality' work and is a temporary 'lull' in the build-up to an event, whereas active recovery is more orientated to circulation and ticking over.

TAPER

Every schedule that builds to a peak performance needs a period of tapering. I feel that this is so important that it warrants a chapter in its own right (see chapter 16). The influence of this will also be seen in the section on racing and schedules at the end of the book. Tapering is an essential part of your race preparation.

FINAL WORDS

In all of the sample schedules above, it can be seen that there must be a good balance between effort and recovery, and although implied in many of the 15 laws of training, there is one more that I believe needs to be stated more forcefully: where there is any question or doubt about hard training, choose the conservative option. It is better to go into a race slightly undertrained than overtrained. At worst, you can always improve for the next race, but if you race when overtrained, you will slip further down the spiral and may even be sidelined by injury.

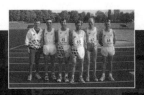

I have always felt that one of the greatest disadvantages to the average South African runner is the lack of defined seasons, as found in the northern hemisphere. The same applies to any country situated around the tropics, particularly those in the southern hemisphere. However, the problem is exacerbated by the focus on Comrades and Two Oceans. In comparison with their European and North American counterparts, local runners really don't have an off season. Even if the mornings are cold, very few places in South Africa prevent training for extended periods of time.

Let us consider the problems associated with such a climate, and how the more extreme seasons of the northern hemisphere can be beneficial to the planning of training and racing.

In South Africa, there are a substantial number of races around the country every month of the year. To some extent, international isolation compounded this, as exceptionally large sponsorships were ploughed into local events, creating a large number of high-profile races. It leaves the average South African runner with a choice that changes the question of 'what to race?' to 'what to leave out?', rather like a child in a sweet shop with unlimited spending money.

Let me state emphatically that I am extremely grateful for the sponsorships that contribute to making the sport of running a multimillion rand industry in this (or any other) country, but a 'cluttered' fixture list of high-profile, highly sponsored events presents most runners with a dilemma in deciding when to choose an off season for recovery and base training. It forces many local runners into the less desirable alternative of doing base training throughout the year, which means that they never truly peak for any particular race, or realise their true potential.

Examine the following typical year for a South African runner. October to February is preoccupied with running a Comrades 'qualifying marathon', followed by March and April when the focus is on the short 50–60-km ultras (e.g. Two Oceans, Korkie,

Loskop, Om Die Dam). Each offers a substantial reward of a gold, silver or bronze medal. In June it is the 90-km Comrades. July sees the start of the provincial championships at the 10-km and 21-km distances and many other high-profile 10–21-km events, all of which attract major sponsors and exciting handouts. August sees the 50-km City-to-City, and it is already predicted that the Durban City Marathon, which was initiated in September 2002, will become a major marathon (similar in status to London or New York). The Soweto Marathon follows in November and the year ends with a mass of festive races.

There are also cross-country options between April and September for those who enjoy a bit of off-road, as well as approximately nine ultraraces for those wanting to do 100-milers, etc. This doesn't even include the weekly races, which have also become more high profile, attracting fields of over 1 500 runners. When does the average South African runner rest?

Clearly, there are some wonderful choices. An immediate problem is that you are only considered to be a runner in South Africa once you have completed the Comrades. A classic example of this is Willie Mtolo, who had twice won the SA Marathon Championship with some of the fastest times in the world (2:08), but remained a relative unknown runner to the general public until he finished second in Comrades. Thereafter he was asked for his autograph everywhere and earned far more in sponsorship than he had from his world ranking as a marathoner. While Comrades is one of the best races in the world, it is sad that it takes so much precedence in athletics, and has undoubtedly forced talented runners to move up in distance too soon.

In 1996 John Disley, the IAAF Measurement Coordinator for Africa, on a visit from the UK, noted that the start of a half-marathon in Johannesburg had to be delayed to allow a club race to clear a section of the half-marathon route. Two races, one day, one area, and over 2 000 runners in each. This public and sponsor interest may seem utopian to some, but it overlooks the benefits of seasonal training.

By comparison, the European seasons are well defined. Winter and cross-country lasts from late October to February, March to October is the road season with most marathons allocated to spring and autumn, and ultras are placed towards the end of summer. The track season starts in late April through to a championship peak in August and leagues finalise in October.

Such a seasonal approach prepares the athletes for a structured race build-up, from active rest to base training, to speed and sharpening, to competition and back to active rest. The incentive and temptation to compete at a high level all year round, in search of elusive medals or cash prizes for the elite runners, simply doesn't exist. Even if it did, the inclement weather would step in to control any such urge. Although northern hemisphere ultrarunners do run a number of ultras in one season, they are forced into a period of recovery or hibernation as the weather turns nasty – more in keeping with the 15 laws (see chapter 6). If you want to reach your true running potential, you must adhere to training seasons.

The next step is to identify your competition season, and then work backwards to allow a taper period, your sharpening (peaking) season, your base season, and your rest/recovery season.

As already noted, rest and recovery don't necessarily mean doing nothing. In fact, to do so would contradict the first law of training – to train frequently all year round. It does, however, mean cutting back on distance and effort and having an active rest. Conversely, there is nothing wrong with doing absolutely nothing for a short period of time, particularly after a hard race or competitive season.

This is emphasised again by the fifth law, which directs you to alternate hard days with easy days. This principle can be extended to the macrosituation where hard periods of training are followed by easy periods. For instance, three heavy weeks' training may be followed by an easy week.

The exact length of a season is difficult to determine, because it generally depends on the individual. Although elite athletes are capable of sustaining 10–12 weeks of heavy training before the symptoms of overtraining start to rear their ugly heads, my experience suggests that an average runner, who is under greater pressure from work and family, can only handle about six or seven weeks of hard training before something 'gives'. Inevitably, the priorities in his life dictate that running is pushed aside.

The length of the taper period, however, is somewhat easier to ascertain, but will also vary, depending on the race distance. A short race may require only an easy couple of days beforehand, while an ultra or marathon taper could be as long as two or three weeks. Another variable in taper length depends on how hard your training build-up has been.

EVERYONE'S GUIDE TO DISTANCE RUNNING

To a limited extent, base training can be handled for extended periods as it is not necessarily that taxing if the distance and the long runs are kept under control, but such training will not produce results that reflect your true potential.

When should your season start?

As the IAAF takes greater cognisance of cross-country, road and ultramarathons, this question will become increasingly confusing. The answer will depend on the event and aspect of the sport in which you wish to make the greatest improvement. For instance, if it's for cross-country, your 'peak' season will be winter. If your interest is in track, the major events are in July and August. Marathon runners typically have their major championships in August, and city events take place in the European spring (March to May) and autumn (September to early November).

World championships in all aspects of athletics have forced elite athletes to specialise more in their training. The opportunity to reach the top in both middle-distance track and cross-country will soon disappear as the calendar becomes more crowded and 'year round'.

Clearly, the real question that local runners must ask themselves is not what races to do or to leave out, but rather what they want to achieve. If you want to find out just how good you could be at a particular distance or event, you need to adopt a focused approach, which requires a 'seasonal' and periodic training outlook. It certainly doesn't mean missing all events, but it does mean becoming very disciplined in what you do.

Apart from coaching some top runners who have gone on to international level, I have had the privilege to coach many back-of-the-pack runners, who have set their sights on achieving a particular goal. These have varied from simply running under 50 minutes for 10 km, or a sub-10:15 Comrades, to aiming for a Bill Rowan (sub-nine-hour) or silver (sub-7:30) Comrades. The point is, they have achieved much more than many dreamed possible simply by focusing on a specific goal and working for it. One of the most rewarding aspects of these achievements is that the same attitude carries over to other aspects of their lives.

When, in 1998, I first met Carol Mercer (the first South African women to finish Comrades in the 2001 race), she was by her own admission an upper-average club runner with a marathon PB of 3:11, and a seven-hour plus time for Comrades. Carol had a sprint background from her schooldays, but had followed the 'normal' road-racing route, running many events each year. She decided to find out exactly what she could achieve. In 1999 she ran a 2:55 marathon, was selected for South Africa in the World 100 km where she finished nineteenth (and ran the most even-paced race of both the men's and women's field), became the first South African women finisher in the All Africa Games marathon over a hilly altitude course in Johannesburg, and won a gold medal in Two Oceans. In addition, she ran a 6:40 Comrades in 2001. Obviously, she had the potential, but only by focusing on what she really wanted to achieve, did these goals become a reality. That meant choosing her races carefully.

Such an approach is open to everyone. You simply need to ask yourself what it is you want to achieve and how badly you want it.

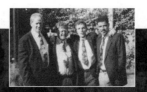

The art of preparing a runner to maximise his running potential is not easy – too little preparation, the wrong mix, or too much training, and the runner will fail to peak. A fine balance between optimum and too little or too much puts the runner on a razor's edge. As if this is not difficult enough, there are still matters of race preparation, planning and confidence boosting.

Some people contend that most of these things are of a personal and individual nature, so who better than the runner to know his body's reactions to the preparation. Certainly, there is a need for the runner to become totally aware of his body and its reaction to situations and conditions, but most runners are not in a position to be objective about themselves. How then do we explain those very successful runners who, it is claimed, coach themselves?

Perhaps in the commonly accepted perception of a 'coach', they do coach themselves, but I am sure that they also use at least one other person as a 'sounding board' for an objective assessment of their programme.

How often have you heard club members chatting about another runner, along the lines of, 'Joe can't expect to do well this week, he's been doing too much distance, and run so many races, he is overtrained' or some similar diagnosis. Runners easily spot the early signs of overtraining in others, but have great difficulty in recognising it in themselves. They tend to have a feeling of invincibility about their own endeavours.

It shows in many runners after a race in which they have done well. Floating on an emotional high the following week, they are motivated to train harder, even to enter an additional race. I do it, yet I can't put my finger on the reason why we fall into this trap. We know it is a mistake, but we are tempted. Because we had a good race means that we have put substantial effort into achieving the result and the logical thing to do is to rest and recover before building up for another challenge.

WHAT WOULD A COACH DO IN THIS SITUATION?

Most people think of a coach as someone who, in conjunction with the runner, sets the training schedule, evaluates the results and progress, assists with the planning and provides mental and physical support. The coach may be at the track timing the intervals, he may be the second on a long run, he may even be the person that you would want to share problems with and may be your closest friend.

The typical image of a coach is embodied in Sam in *Chariots of Fire* who became Harold Abrahams' mentor. The duo was inseparable in its goal to achieve Olympic gold. Such coaches do exist and the Athletics South Africa coaching structures have long been the official 'production line' for the development of coaches, generally admired for their high standards. However, it is unfortunate that there has been a tendency for coaching progression to require a candidate to recruit top-level athletes to their squad, rather than developing a system that promotes assistance to runners of all abilities, be it the novice jogger or the elite national athlete.

I make special mention of this because to my mind there is a great need for runners and administrators to realise that coaching is not the preserve of elite athletes, although this is a commonly held belief, even amongst runners. This belief is so deeply rooted that awards, coaching qualifications and appointments tend to be based on the number of provincial and national athletes to which a coach can lay claim. This, to me, is the wrong way round.

Elite runners certainly need 'coaching', but many of them have enough talent to make it to that level with or without a coach. They also have the motivation to do it by themselves. The role of the coach, therefore, is to take them to their absolute peak, but the chances are that, even if the coach fails, the athlete will still have enough talent to perform at a high-enough standard to assure the coach of the award or qualification. If the award system alone is the coach's goal, it will promote the 'poaching' of athletes and runners. In fact, the conclusion is that a coach must have an elite athlete to be able to meet the requirements of the National Coach Award.

Although coaching is an art and a science, I am not convinced that there should be a differentiation between a coach who uses his knowledge, skill and communication to take an average or back runner to his highest potential, and one who takes a naturally talented runner to the same relative extreme, but who happens to compete at international level. It is not clear to me how the ability or knowledge of the coach is any different in these two cases. Both take athletes to their maximum potential, and should surely enjoy equal recognition.

Consider an alternative where the emphasis is placed on improving the ability of average runners. Such improvement will cause elite runners to be challenged by runners previously considered to be of lesser ability. To stay at the top, elite runners will be forced to work harder, which they will do because they have the motivation. In addition, many so-called 'average' runners might discover a talent for the sport that was not previously exposed because of poor training methods. This will also improve the sport at top level.

I have yet to hear of a successful business whose major effort only developed the upper echelons and ignored the base of the pyramid. Yet this is an inherent part of many athletic (and other sports) structures. The traditional Eastern Bloc countries thrived on a system of early assessment of an athlete's potential, after which he was channelled to maximise his potential. Because the initial emphasis was at grass root-level, champions were spawned as a consequence. The system didn't wait for elite runners to find themselves and then provide them with a coach.

An argument against this is price, but the cost of even mass education (coaching) material e.g. videos, training charts, newsletters, is small in comparison to the numbers it can reach. Do the coaching incentives really have to be based on elite athletes? Surely those coaches who work to bring runners into the sport and develop them to club-class runners are equally serving the sport and the athletes.

A vast number of female runners have been brought into the sport by an event such as the Spar Ladies Series. Many have been coached or encouraged on a one-to-one basis by people at club level, or by existing athletes, others by 'coaches' such as newspaper columnist Dave Spence or Blanche Moila. Few of these runners have yet made provincial or national status but surely the 'coaches' have a place within the sport. Taking a novice to the point where he has reached his maximum potential is surely just as much 'coaching' as taking a naturally talented athlete through to his maximum potential. The difference is purely in the starting and finishing points of the journey!

Many coaches worldwide are only in telephone contact with their 'elite' charges, which begs the question, 'What is a coach?'

The latter coach may well be serving the needs of a national-class runner, in which case he is fulfilling the role of a coach, but whether he deserves higher or special awards simply because his athlete is at elite level, is debatable. The requirements of a coach vary from athlete to athlete. On one hand, an athlete may only require this distant contact and sounding board, another may demand virtually full-time attention from the coach. The amount and extent of the coach's attention and expertise may change as you develop in the sport. There should be no stigma attached to coaching and it should not be reserved for elite runners. It should be accessible to all runners.

It's all very well reading books, listening to lectures, gathering information on training techniques and even knowing how to put a training schedule together, but when it comes down to it, there is no tried and tested formula that applies to everyone. Here, objectivity is required.

Human beings are not naturally objective, and it is therefore worthwhile having someone to appraise or assess what you plan to do or have done, and offer knowledgeable comment. Such comments are often enough to highlight a glaring omission or even a subtle point overlooked in your schedule. I repeat, even a runner with the smallest amount of experience can spot overtraining in another runner. Conversely, a runner with vast experience can overlook the same symptoms and make the same mistake many times!

A sad story that illustrates this point well is that of Dr. Tony Venniker, better known to many South Africans as the 'radio doctor'. Tony had a regular radio slot and helped many people. He was always willing to listen to problems and offer assistance. A very knowledgeable man, he was gifted enough to spot troubles early enough in others to ensure fast and efficient medical treatment. However, by his own admission, it was his failure to diagnose his own illness early on and to do something about it that led to his premature death. Tony was one of the oldest-ever novices to finish Comrades. His real-life story is symptomatic of most runners' inability to coach themselves.

WHAT DOES A RUNNER REQUIRE FROM A COACH?

Probably the most important factor is that you must have confidence and trust in your coach. It is no use looking to someone for advice or encouragement if you doubt their integrity. For this reason, the 'world's best coach', if such a person exists, may not be suited to the world's best athlete. The relationship between coach and athlete, be it runner, golfer, tennis star or any other, is based on a sound relationship and understanding between two people.

The remaining requirements will vary in terms of what you expect from your coach. If it is total control of your sport, look for someone who has plenty of practical experience. If its purely a 'sounding board' for ideas, a fellow runner may be able to help you, as all you really need is 'objectivity' and someone to play devil's advocate. Perhaps, if that is his need as well, you could 'coach' each other.

If you already have the knowledge and know how your body reacts to various conditions, it may be possible to ask your spouse to act as a 'coach'. He or she could well pick up sufficient knowledge from a few books to assist you in questioning what you have done, what you intend doing, where you are going, and whether your planning is correct? For some runners this is enough.

The coach-runner relationship is based on interaction, not demands. A coach works with a runner to develop a training programme; not every runner responds to the same training in the same way. An athlete must be comfortable with his schedule and surroundings, because the one thing more tiring and destructive to an athlete than heavy racing, is emotional stress. For a programme and regimen to be successful, the athlete, not the coach, must be comfortable.

In one case, a national-class runner was instructed to move home to be closer to her coach. Her success until then had been within a family home environment, a place in which she was extremely comfortable. I think it would have been more appropriate for the coach to have moved nearer to the athlete if he felt so strongly that they needed to be closer together, and that he was the only coach for her.

Sometimes, administrators and officials seemingly forget that without the athlete there would be no need for officials and administrators. Without officials I can still run; there wouldn't be the same standardisation or organisation, but I can still run!

An issue that the increasing professionalisation of sport has brought to the fore, is the payment of coaches. The argument is that if an athlete is winning significant amounts of money, shouldn't the coach who is helping him to do so, also be paid? Definitely. Another consideration promoted by one local coach is that if a small, regular monthly fee is charged, athletes will be more committed to coaching sessions. This is a valid point, as many runners seem to think that it is acceptable to contact a coach, have him draw up a training schedule, and then disappear into the distance, with what they consider to be a magic formula. That will never be successful because a coach can only write a suitable training schedule once he knows the runner and his abilities. A runner should also realise that he has no right to demand time of a coach unless he respects him, and affords him the basic common courtesy of letting him know how the training schedule is progressing.

I don't believe that there is a coach in the country who would turn away a runner in need of assistance but unable to pay. Indeed, I and many other coaches have 'athletes' from different sports and backgrounds who have never been asked to pay for the extensive coaching they may have received. Similarly, there are coaches who rely on funding to enable them to live or to be available throughout the day for 'after school' classes. Ultimately, it depends on personal circumstances but I don't think that a coach who charges, should be considered any less or more of a coach, than one who doesn't charge. After all it is his time that he is sacrificing and he is entitled to charge whatever he feels is appropriate.

If you are interested in finding a coach, you could contact the provincial and national athletics bodies, who should be able to refer you to coaches in your area.

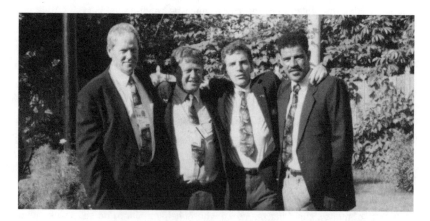

ABOVE   *Ian Harries, Kaai Prellor, Norrie Williamson and Roger Adams – coaches and management to the first Unified SA Student Team to the 1993 World Student Games in Buffalo, USA*

00:00:12
KEEPING TRACK –
LOGGING THE MILES

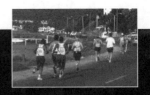

Life is an experience and we grow through our own experiences and those of others. However, the greatest guide as to what works for individual runners, comes from monitoring their bodies' reaction to training and racing experiences. Dr George Sheehan called training 'an experiment of one', which highlights the need to learn from experience, and what works for one person may not be good for another. We must keep a note of what we do, how we feel and how our bodies and running reacts to training. This allows us to look back and tailor our training to the specific requirements of our racing.

Unfortunately, human nature is such that we tend to remember highlights and forget the critical details that are key to analysis. If notes are kept on training sessions at the time they are completed, the exact distance, time and 'feeling' is recorded for posterity and easy reference.

I remember asking Dave Box (the 1970 World 100-mile record holder) how much training he had undertaken when he ran one of his 100-mile track records. At the time of the conversation he told me that his training featured a weekly 60–80-km run at weekends and several fairly long runs during the week. However, he said that he had kept notes and would check them for me. A few weeks later when he passed me his training log, he remarked that he was surprised to see just how little he had done in the build-up to the race. Memories play strange tricks! On inspection, his training prior to his record, was perhaps one of the lowest he had undertaken in years.

WHY LOOK BACK AT YOUR TRAINING?

Frequently, we aim for a specific target and initially have the enthusiasm to complete the 'mission'. Fired with this enthusiasm we plot out our training, building in strength work, track, hills, fartlek and endurance runs. More often than not, this initial schedule is too ambitious. A better approach is to look back to the last occasion you ran a race that you felt was your best performance, and base your plans on the training you did prior to that last success. Such training obviously suited you and therefore should only be modified slightly to suit the new target. Similarly, it is also useful to look back at your bad races to compare your preparation for those. That will reveal the pitfalls.

This is the theory of a training diary, but its use is only as good as the information it contains. Merely recording distance and time is not enough – the more information, the better. Everything that seemed important at the time will still be important when looking back.

HEART RATE

Your pulse immediately after wakening is a good indicator of your body's response to the previous days training, and should be logged daily. Even after a few days, a 'base line' will reveal itself. Any deviation will give an indication as to what intensity you undertake in training that day. As your fitness improves, the 'base-line' reading will reduce, but on a specific day, it may actually rise if you have not fully recovered from the previous day's effort.

For example, I know that at my fittest I have a waking pulse of 38 beats per minute, but in 'tick-over training' this tends to be about 41–42, and if I have done a hard session the night before, it may rise to 44–45. This indicates the need for an easier day and if it is above 46, then a recovery day is required. I have reached the stage where I know when I am ill, or perhaps even about to become ill, because my pulse goes up despite two days of easy training. If I visit the doctor and he tells me that my pulse is 'normal', I'm able to point out that it is in fact up 10 beats a minute, or 25%! After all, a doctor bases his judgement on the average pulse, which is around 60–70 a rest. Clearly, morning pulse is one of the items that is very useful in determining your reaction to training.

Similarly, heart rate monitoring during exercise has the advantage of providing a measure of the intensity of a training session (see chapter 38 for more detail on this). Keep a record of your heart rate. If you compare your heart rate during a specific session with that achieved when the session is repeated, you will gain a good indication of your fitness level. In this manner, if you are commencing training at a lower or higher base fitness, it is possible to modify the required heart rate to match the intensity of a proposed session. The times might differ, but the intensity will be the same.

WEIGHT

Your early morning weight, before eating and after visiting the bathroom, can also be an indicator of training response. Professor Tim Noakes regards a sudden drop in weight as a possible sign of overtraining. While not disagreeing with that, I also believe that runners, particularly in humid climates, may experience a gain in weight as a sign of overtraining. Tim notes that an increase in the amount of fluid taken at night is another indication of overstressing, as is water retention by the body (to assist with 'repair'). Runners who train in humid climates can lose large amounts of water during training. I can 'lose' 1.5 kg during a 10-km run on a summer morning in Durban, before work. This is only water and not true weight loss. If I'm not careful to replace this water on finishing a run, I soon become stressed. My weight 'see-saws' over 2–3 kg in a day and, in fact, my early morning weight tends to go up. This always occurs when I overdo things, so I have learned to watch out for it.

Another symptom that I experienced, which substantiates this, is that my joints and limbs became swollen during long journey runs – also a direct result of water retention. This first happened under the extreme conditions of the Johannesburg to Durban run where I was covering over 100 km each day for a week or more. Thus weight is another useful factor to log.

SLEEP

Throughout this book there is much emphasis on the need for recovery, therefore it makes sense to log the amount of nightly sleep, allowing you to spot any tiredness resulting from the lack of proper sleep.

In this regard, it is not usually the night before the 'day of tiredness' that causes a problem, but rather the 'night before' the night before, i.e. if you feel tired and washed out on Wednesday, it is probably as a result of poor sleep on the Monday night prior. In the same way, in race preparation, an anxious, restless night immediately prior to a race is not as detrimental as a poor night's sleep two nights before. That is the most important rest night.

On one occasion when I ran from Johannesburg to Durban, a sleep laboratory monitored my sleep pattern every night. Interestingly, the first two nights' sleep were totally disturbed by the extreme activities of the day's running, but by the third night I showed signs of adaptation, and although I was still sleeping insufficiently, my normal sleep pattern was returning. A similar three-day adaptation occurs when running multiday events and it is reported that many shift workers have experienced similar patterns when they move from day- to nightshift or vice versa.

TRAINING INFORMATION

For the training itself, you should log the route, the distance and the time, as well as your feelings about the run. Was it a good run? Record your objective. Was it recovery or fast continuous effort, or a long, slow distance run? Alternatively, if it was track or fartlek, the details of the session must be more specific. Again, the more you record, the more 'advice' you will have to fall back on later.

Some runners record items such as the shoes they wore, the weather and their running partners, all of which can be useful. Develop your own personal diary format. Your diary may contain pieces of information that, although not directly associated with the actual training, will have some impact on stress levels or lifestyle. Often, the significance of these will only be seen later, when you look back to see what was good or bad about your training.

Problems with diaries

Just as a diary can be of assistance, it can also be the downfall of a runner, particularly for those who believe quantity is everything. Runners can become obsessed with weekly distance targets as opposed to a balanced quality training week. Similarly, the booking of exact routes and times can cause runners to continually test themselves and improve their times over routes on each outing. Such approaches are doomed to failure.

There will be times when your runs are slower than usual, when the pressure of work exhausts you and takes its toll in an extra few minutes on the road. There are times when you need to go slower, such as a recovery run. There are times when your weekly distance will drop, but the amount of your quality running increases. These all depend on the relevant period of training and what you want to achieve.

One way to overcome distance counting during periods of quality training is to use the basic workload guide, as indicated in the training chapter. Effectively, all distance done at 10-km pace is thought to be worth 'double' the actual distance, i.e. 5-km pace work equates to 'four times' the distance, and 1 500 m per 3 000 m work equals eight times the actual distance. If this format is monitored weekly, it provides a better reflection of the total workload and progression, and reduces the concern of an apparently low distance week.

It is tempting, and dangerous, to become a slave to diary filling; there is nothing as satisfying as recording a full page of good training. Though an empty couple of days may look bad, they often result in a much better performance when it counts – in the race.

Heed a serious warning of one of the biggest and most common pitfalls that runners make: IT IS NOT THE DISTANCE YOU COVER THAT MAKES THE ATHLETE, IT IS HOW THE DISTANCE WAS COVERED. DON'T BECOME A SLAVE TO WEEKLY DISTANCE.

High-tech logs

With the advent of personal computers, it was only a matter of time before a running diary was developed for the PC. Developed in the USA, it has made its way around the world. I have reviewed a number of these, and while they do provide a method of recording your training, most have substantial drawbacks.

In most cases, the amount of space available for recording your training is limited and useful detail has to be omitted. Ironically, this is the very thing you need when 'researching' through them in later months or years. A further drawback is that these programs do not permit formatting for information that you might consider important, such as pulse, weight, time, etc., nor will they allow you to substitute a cycle or swim for the run because you can't log it properly. In comparison to a hand-written log, the flexibility simply isn't there.

However, these computer records are useful for producing graphs, which show weekly or daily distances and personal bests. These can be used to show trends more easily than a book. From this point of view, I believe that a combination of both is probably the best, but I am sure that there is a market opportunity for a well-written, highly flexible program that will allow runners to log their training in a personalised format.

Possibly the best way to create your own diary is to design a suitable spreadsheet; I have progressed to this method for myself and for the athletes I coach, particularly those I work with via e-mail. I store various pieces of information, yet only send them the proposed training for the following 7–10 days. The record can include goals, personal bests and test-session results.

For my own use, I not only record training information, but also allocate space to record anything that suits me, such as cycling, running, swimming and weights, as well as how I feel, my pulse rate, weight, hours of sleep and eating habits, without having to draw up new sections or cramp my writing into a set space.

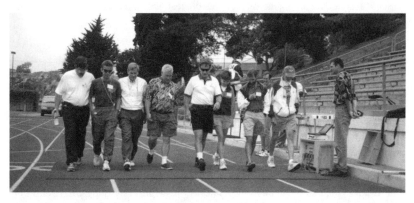

ABOVE *Evaluating the new 'chip' timing system as an invited guest to the USA Track & Field Technical Conference, Santa Barbara, USA, 1994*

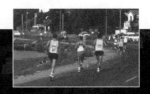

LESS CAN BE MORE

Sometimes, less is more. This is an important, but difficult lesson for all runners to learn, but particularly those who run marathon and longer races.

By this stage, you will know my opinion on the apparent obsession that many runners have with distance. It's certainly a trap that I fell into, particularly in the first few years of my running. There were times when the driving force behind my training was to maintain a 'set' target mileage per week, in the mistaken belief that this alone would ensure success. In 1983/1984, for instance, my weekly average was over 145 km for the full 52 weeks, and that included periods of illness or injury. During that year I ran over 1 600 miles in races and competed in many triathlons that also required cycling and swimming training.

This meant that the vast majority of my training was undertaken at one pace. It had to be because I had no energy left for quality work. By Thursday I would find myself totting up the distance run since Monday, and planning how to reach the magical 100 miles (161 km) by the end of the week. Come hell or high water, I wouldn't be truly satisfied unless I did. Luckily, by this time I had selected the long ultras such as 100 miles as my races of choice, and to a limited extent this type of training suited that 'diversity'.

However, and this is important, had I known then what I know now, I would not have chosen that direction, and I can only ponder at how much better I may have been in some events had I adopted a different approach. (The frustration to any 'coach' is to see athletes reinventing the wheel. This concern alone has motivated me to write this book.)

It certainly made me a good one-pace runner, but did nothing for my speed and left me sadly lacking in shorter distance races. Most runners don't share my 'love' for long races and yet it seems as though average runners are automatically drawn to making this 'distance obsession' the backbone of their running.

I am reminded of it each weekend when, even if there are no local, long-distance races, I see hordes of runners on their own training runs. As I venture into town on Saturdays and Sundays, I see a number of runners obviously finishing yet another long, slow distance session, yet a trip to King's Park athletic track often finds the stadium deserted.

Although this can, to some extent, be understood in the build-up to a marathon, the same situation exists at all times of the year, even when there are no marathon races in the offing. Many runners simply don't consider it worthwhile to run short 5–10 km races unless they are on their doorsteps.

Ironically, these shorter distance races can be ideal, quality-training sessions if you don't race them flat out. If you are looking to put in a top-rate performance at such a distance, the longest run you need is about 15–20 km, so the longer run is of little or no benefit.

This again reminds me of my interview with Sebastian Coe. While discussing travelling and running and the fact that some top runners even go for a run around the airport grounds while in transit, Sebastian maintained that he thought it pointless, as the only time he went for a run was when he could do quality training, be it 15 km or a track session. Those 'airport runs' were only worthwhile if they were quality workouts, otherwise they were a waste of valuable energy.

The benefits of the long run are well detailed in other chapters, and it should be clear by now that there is much more to be gained from shorter, more intense work.

The difference in requirements of the shorter races should be mirrored by different approaches to training. When not training for a marathon, dropping distance is a key way to improve performance. This does not necessarily mean that the total weekly training load will be any easier, indeed it may actually seem more stressful, particularly for the first six weeks.

Whereas a marathon is run at a fairly even 'energy' expenditure rate, 5–10-km races require a runner to maintain the 'pressure'. There is no point in running speed work on the track, with long breaks and recovery periods. After all, you can't stop for such breaks during a race.

It is preferable to run a fewer number of times with shorter breaks. A track session of 3–4 x 1 000 m at best 10-km pace with one minute rest, is closer to the requirements of a 10-km race and will improve an average runner quite considerably.

Including a warm-up and cool-down, this will only add 8 km to the training distance, and will take the best part of an hour to complete. The benefits will, however, far outweigh those gained from running a long, slow 12–15 km.

Of course there is room in the training week – in fact, probably three times per week – for a continuous run, which could be over 18 km, 12 km and 8 km. However, the pace of these continuous runs should be slightly faster than the normal pace used in a marathon build-up. There are many theories on how fast such runs should be, and heart-rate monitoring is one of the best guides. Most theories suggest running at approximately 65% of your 'working heart-rate range'. For a 40-year-old, with a resting pulse of 60 and a maximum (estimated from the equation: 220 – your age) of 180, the 'working pulse range' is about (220 – 40) – 60 = 120. This runner should aim for 120 x .65 + 60 = 138, as a minimum pulse during such runs. He should not push it much above 150 for any length of time (i.e. working between 65% and 75%).

When I first began monitoring my heart rate regularly over a three-month period, I found that only after the first 10–12 minutes of a run did my heart rate reach my required range, which, if nothing else, proves the need for a warm-up. If this is the intensity required to benefit from training, it becomes obvious that the benefits of a 20-minute jog or very easy runs, even over long distances, are minimal to those wishing to improve in the shorter races. The role of those short, easy runs is purely one of active recovery.

As noted before, the benefit of working at 10-km (double), 5-km (quadruple) and 1 500 or 3 000-m pace (eight times) is far superior to merely plodding out more distance for the sake of a figure at the end of the week. Therefore, it makes sense to reduce your distance. Put two or three track sessions (or other quality sessions) together per week, add three shorter continuous runs and see how less can be more. It may only add up to 50–60 km per week, but it can have the same energy drain as 100–120 km.

Remember, even if you don't find racing these shorter distances challenging, a period of lower weekly distance with higher quality running, every week, will assist you in the longer events. A variety of training and the reduction in distance will allow your body and mind the recovery required for your next marathon build-up, fresh and eager to take up the challenge.

SPEED AND DISTANCE DON'T MIX

If you have followed my advice thus far, you are probably doing more speed work and quality sessions than before. If you are an experienced runner, you will have noticed the reduction in your weekly distance compared to your previous training. For most of your training for the longer events, you will only be covering about 60–70% of your previous total distance capacity each week.

Although marathons require good endurance, the mistake many top runners make in their attempts to go for 'gold', is to combine the rigours of frequent 'speed sessions or races' per week with a simultaneous increase in their weekly distance. This is impossible. In the early months, the objective is to improve your basic endurance, whereas later in the build-up, the emphasis moves towards speed endurance. However, it is important to note that in training for events longer than 80 km, the reverse is true. Initially, the training is aimed at increasing speed capacity, and later the emphasis will change to improving your endurance.

Unfortunately we tend to think that if a little of something is good for us, then a lot must be much better. This is not the case in running. There must be a balance and the basic training principles must be observed.

As the need to increase distance predominates in training for an ultra, the number of quality sessions should drop from three to two. Even in those two sessions it may be necessary to increase the recovery between intervals slightly, or to reduce the number of intervals, but don't discontinue the sessions entirely. On the other hand, runners who normally only train once a day, may add in an extra session on one or two days during the week. The midweek, long run should be gradually increased by 10–15%, and the weekend run increased on an alternating basis. This will allow your weekly distance to increase by 10–15% so that it will peak at your maximum distance capacity, approximately six weeks before the race. You can hold that distance for three weeks before commencing a taper to your chosen ultra.

If, however, you are training for a marathon or shorter, you will find that the 'endurance' and 'speed' blocks are reversed, allowing you to first build endurance and then improve speed. Endurance is decreased by 10–15% and the number of speed sessions is increased from two to three, and the recovery interval is reduced.

Remember to maintain the same principles regarding recovery or easy weeks between each training segment. Your training is only as good as your recovery.

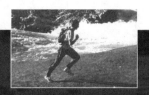

00:00:14
COPING WITH
THE ENVIRONMENT

There can be little doubt that the climate in South Africa is very conducive to training and is vastly different from that of the UK, the country of my birth. Different environments affect our ability and motivation to run. What follows is a short discussion of how I perceive various weather conditions to have affected my running and some recommendations on how to counteract the effect of the weather. Wherever possible, I have made reference to scientific research but, in some cases, there does not seem to be much information available. Although some of the conditions discussed here are not commonly found in South Africa, they have been included, following the move towards ultra and adventure racing, plus an increasing participation by local runners in international events.

HOT WEATHER

High temperatures are the greatest problem faced by runners in South Africa and the need to keep cool is well documented. It is best done by wearing 'airy' clothes such as mesh vests and fabrics that are light in weight and colour. Large muscles are the body's major heat-producing areas, as they are the hardest working and need to be sponged down.

Interestingly, Bruce Fordyce did not like his hair to be wet, even though he acknowledged that much heat dissipates through the top of the head, and to keep it wet seems, to me, to be logical. Perhaps the irritation of wet hair was more of a problem for him. This is ultimately a matter of personal preference.

For the same reason, your choice of hat is important (see chapter 37 on equipment). In my view, it is best to opt either for one of the new 'high-tech' caps or promotional foam peaks that are often handed out at races, or to go without. The need to keep well hydrated is equally important. The importance of drinking enough is covered in chapter 26 on fluid loading.

Whether to wear suntan lotion or not, is controversial. I don't like putting anything on my skin as it may prevent easy sweating and, since this is my prime cooling method, I sacrifice all for that. Rather than use a suntan lotion, I prefer to enter a race having already had some exposure to the sun. Again, I stress that this is based on personal preference rather than proven fact.

In general, my recommendations for hot-weather running are to wear as little as possible and to air your body as much as you can. This is based on the assumption that the running takes place in fair to high humidity. When running in a sunny, hot and dry climate, I have found a pure cotton shirt to be the best protection from the sun, and there is no problem with chafing. However in the Augrabies 250-km six-day marathon where participants also had to carry a backpack, I found the use of a Nike Dri-Fit long-sleeved shirt the best option, as it provided protection from the chafing of backpack movement and also wicked the moisture away.

For a runner who travels to a warmer climate to run, the biggest challenge is to adapt to the heat and humidity. Adaptation to heat generally takes a minimum of ten days. It is a good time to use a heart-rate monitor, as it allows you to put in the same effort for your sessions that you would normally do, but the pace will be slower until you have adapted. Because you are forced to run more slowly, the temptation will be there to keep all your sessions at the same pace, but you should continue to vary the pace of the sessions to the same variation of heart rates that you normally use in training.

As with all adaptation, it must be undertaken gradually and increased gently. Start with 30 minutes and build up to about 90 minutes over the ten days. If you are able to spend more days in the heat prior to the race, so much the better. A temptation is to suntan as soon as you arrive. This can become a problem, so develop it gradually, particularly if you have fair skin. It is worthwhile to increase your consumption of vitamin A when you arrive in sunny conditions from, for instance, a Cape winter, as this will assist with sun protection.

It is probably better to consider humidity as something you 'become used to', rather than something to which you 'adapt'. I do not believe that you ever adapt to humidity and often its effect is confused with that of heat. As the humidity increases, your ability to cool down through sweating decreases, as the air is too moist to dry perspiration. It is the removal of sweat that aids cooling. High humidity, be it during exercise or 'normal' living, is a big drain on the body, and it is essential to increase your fluid intake each day.

Furthermore, humidity tends to reduce the amount of sleep possible and longer recovery may be necessary between sessions. Taking a 'siesta' during the hottest part of the day may help to regain some lost sleep, but staying indoors in air-conditioned rooms all day will not prepare you for the energy-sapping effects of humidity. The keys to dealing with humidity are to acclimatise to its effects and modify your target time, as well as fluid- and energy-replacement strategies. Cities with high humidity often also have high-pollution levels. If you look down at the city from the top of an outlying hill, you will often notice a yellow-brown layer of pollution hovering at skyline level. Take that into consideration in your preparation. By the time the flag was lowered on the 1998 Commonwealth Games in Kuala Lumpur, several UK coaches and managers had drastically changed their preconceived views on how to deal with humidity. Runners who have not experienced the humidity of Durban in February would do well to complete a trial event there before attempting a major race there between November and March.

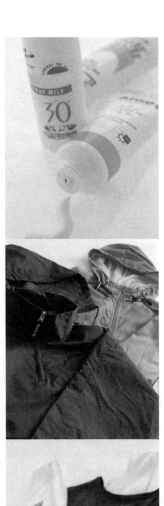

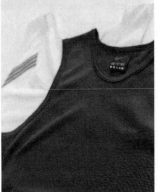

RIGHT *Runners are faced with all-weather conditions – dress appropriately and take the necessary precautions*

COLD WEATHER

The chapter on running gear (chapter 37) deals with the type of clothing suitable for cold weather. Wear the amount of clothing that allows you to feel slightly cold outdoors at the beginning of the run. As you run, the heat generated will soon take you back to a comfortable temperature. If you are warm at the start of a run, you will soon overheat. It is important to consider your extremities in cold weather, i.e. hands and feet. It is worthwhile to make the first part of your training run a short loop that will allow you to return to base to make additions or reductions in the clothing, if necessary.

There is a perception that if you train in a temperate climate, there is no need to drink, as there is limited evidence of a high sweat rate. This is a fallacy. The cooling effect still takes place, but is less noticeable. Furthermore, if the weather is so cold that you need to wear a windproof jacket, you effectively create a microclimate inside the jacket, which can become very humid. There is a definite need to increase your fluid intake under such conditions – both during and after a run.

There is a dearth of information on how the environment affects performance. Although it is recognised that the ideal running conditions are windless and slightly overcast with a temperature of 11–16 °C, there are few references on how other conditions may alter your performance.

It may be helpful to examine extremes such as the 100-mile records. The world records of Derek Kay and Dave Box in Durban between 1969 and 1972 were set in what were considered to be 'bad' conditions, i.e. rain, cold and overcast skies. Likewise, the current world best by Don Ritchie on the track in 1978 – and yet to be bettered – was also set in cool conditions. Even Wally Hayward's 1953 100-mile and 24-hour records still make the top listings, while Derek Kay's remains the fourth best.

The reasons are many. A race such as this requires an athlete to be at a peak for a full 24 hours, as many things can go wrong in such a long event and, most importantly, the weather must be kind for the full length of the race. Twelve hours without strong wind (a gentle breeze can be a bonus), a constant temperature of 11–16 °C, and even light rain, will make for ideal ultra-conditions. Heavy rain requires protective clothing, and presents the danger of a poor foothold on the road. Light rain, however, is cooling and refreshing.

Now consider the running of 100-mile races in South Africa or any other hot climate. Many runners have achieved the same times as Kay or Box for shorter distances, but have never matched them over 100 miles. It is true that they might never have reached the same peak, but you must also look at the conditions. Typically, during the 1980s and early 1990s, 100-mile track races were run in conditions where the heat had reached and even passed 30 °C. The slow times are scoffed at, even by 'knowledgeable' administrators of the sport, because the races were won in 14 or 15 hours.

But is it fair to compare these times with those set under more favourable conditions? The hot-weather results may not be world records, but Dr Stephen Browne, who has done some research on hot-weather running, classifies a 'hot' race as one in which the effective temperature is over 20 °C, and a 'cool' race as one in which the temperature is less than 20 °C. Effective temperature is a combination of both humidity and air temperature, and can also be increased or decreased by the effect of wind. A head wind will obviously have a cooling effect. Racing times in hot conditions, according to Browne, can be expected to be at least 7% slower than times set in cold conditions, and this increases with rises in temperature.

According to an article from *Runner's World*, July 1975, researchers C. Foster and J. Daniels have estimated that for every degree above 7 °C on the dry bulb, the running time in a marathon will be 40 seconds slower. I suspect that since then more has been 'discovered'; I know that Professor Tim Noakes has also researched this problem and will no doubt shed new light on the subject. In other ultras, e.g. the 1988 Komani 200-km race, in which 'bad' conditions (rain and wind) prevailed, good times resulted. When conditions have been hot over the same course, times were worse. Bad spectator conditions can be good running conditions.

This principle suggests a beneficial effect for hot-climate runners who run in European conditions. If runners from hot climates can run 2:10 marathons in hot and humid conditions, imagine what they could achieve in kinder conditions, such as in the London or Boston Marathon. Obviously, 7% at that level means much less in terms of minutes and seconds than at 100 miles, but the principle is the same.

Having run many races in a number of countries, I agree with Browne. A week before the 1985 London to Paris Triathlon, Tim Noakes and I, both on the management team, were given the weekend off and we decided to visit my family in Scotland. With only 48 hours' notice (and no specific training), we ran the Edinburgh Marathon. It was certainly cool and in that regard, ideal. Despite a strong head wind for much of the run, I recorded a 2:36, my personal best by three minutes. Similarly, in 1983 I ran the London Marathon in 2:43, again a personal best, and the next day ran the Boston Marathon in 2:45.

In terms of Browne's formula, anyone running a 2:35 in hot climates can expect to do a sub-2:30 in ideal conditions and vice versa, while someone running around 3:08 in hot conditions could achieve a sub-3:00 in cool conditions.

WIND

Wind is quite possibly the environmental factor most disruptive to running. Winds are never constant. They gust through built-up areas and are prone to tunnelling and eddy effects, all of which disrupt the rhythm of a runner. Even a direct head wind on an out-and-back course results in slow times. More effort is needed to counter the effect of a head wind, than is gained from the effect of a direct tail wind. Don't expect the loss of time when running into a head wind to be gained when you turn. It won't be.

Another problem with winds is that they have a cooling effect. The table on the following page shows how wind can reduce the effective temperature considerably and even lead to hypothermia. This table originates from research done for cycling, which deals with speeds higher than those of running, but the principles for running are the same. A tail wind will cool you down less than a head wind. In addition, because you are not as aware of the sweat you are producing, it has the potential to lead to dehydration because of insufficient fluid intake.

RAIN

I have briefly mentioned running in the rain and how light rain can have a cooling effect. South African runners are lucky that, in general, it does not rain too often. For this reason, many runners do not train in the rain, confident that by the following day the sun will be out again. However, many are actually missing out on some great runs.

The initial period is the hardest part of running in the rain, before you are properly wet. Once you are thoroughly wet, and provided you are warm, the run

HOW WIND SPEED INFLUENCES EFFECTIVE TEMEPERRATURE DROP								
Wind Speed (M.P.H)	Air temperature (degrees fahrenheit)							
	+ 50	+ 40	+ 30	+ 20	+ 10	0	- 10	- 20
5	48	37	27	16	6	-5	- 15	- 26
10	40	28	16	4	- 9	- 24	- 33	- 46
15	36	22	9	- 5	- 18	- 32	- 45	- 58
20	32	18	4	- 10	- 25	- 39	- 53	- 67
25	30	16	0	- 15	- 29	- 44	- 59	- 74
30	28	13	- 2	- 18	- 33	- 48	- 63	- 79
35	27	11	- 4	- 20	- 35	- 51	- 67	- 82
40	26	10	- 6	- 21	- 37	- 53	- 69	- 86
	LITTLE DANGER				INCREASED DANGER			GREAT DANGER

takes on a completely different aspect. I can't explain it, but I always enjoy running in these conditions. Incidentally, I have yet to find a rain suit that keeps me completely dry and allows my body to breathe and rid itself of the internal sweat. No matter what happens, you will be wet, so why not enjoy it?

The most effective item available seems to be the Gore-Tex suit, a product that I believe was designed and manufactured in Scotland. That makes sense, as it was a Scot – one Macintosh – who invented the raincoat! Although even the Gore-Tex suit has its limitations, the benefit of this type of clothing is that it keeps the wind out and helps to maintain body temperature at a comfortable level.

Normally, the most annoying aspect of running in the rain is wet feet, and socks that crawl down into your shoes (to hide from the rain?). The latest sports 'tech' socks, however, actually wick moisture away from the feet, keeping them warm and dry. Buying two pairs of shoes will also pay benefits, as the wet pair can be left to dry out for a day. Wearing shoes while wet will advance the rotting of the stitching.

ALTITUDE

Running at altitude was something completely strange to me until I came to South Africa. My first encounter with it in 1981 convinced me that I should avoid it – I found running very difficult and thought I might suffocate. It felt like starting running from scratch again. There is substantial evidence, however, that it is useful to train at altitude and compete at sea level. The time spent at altitude increases your ability to transfer oxygen through the body, which effectively increases your Vo_2 Max. Tim Noakes, recognising the way in which altitude reduces the ability to train at intensity, suggests that the ideal is to live at altitude, train daily at sea level, and race at sea level. For many this is a theoretical ideal, but it also explains why more consideration should be given to establishing an altitude training camp for sports in the Drakensberg. Not only can you live at an altitude of 2 800 m, but within an hour you could be on the track or road in Pietermartizburg, while a further 45 minutes will take you down to sea level. With thought and planning, this could be an ideal opportunity for both local and international athletes.

The use of altitude training however, has to be considered carefully and, once again, reactions are personal. UK Olympic marathoner Ron Hill relates how the British Olympic team once attended a training camp at altitude for three weeks prior to the 1976 Olympics. The athletes moved 'down' to the Games site one week before their events. Nearly all of them performed poorly. However, a week later, in the traditionally held post-Olympic Coca-Cola International meeting at Meadowbank in Edinburgh, those same athletes recorded personal bests and beat many of the Olympic medallists.

Obviously, adaptation took longer than had been anticipated would be necessary. If you live at sea level and find yourself spending time at altitude for whatever reason, don't expect to do the same amount of work or put in the same amount of effort. Accept the fact that it will take you a while to adapt – possibly as long as two or three months. For me the worst time is the first three days at altitude, after which I gradually improve, but I never reach normal levels, although I have not yet been at altitude for longer than two weeks.

I also prefer to drive up to altitude, as flying means that I have to withstand the cabin pressure of the flight, which can be equivalent to 3 000 m. Because the effect of altitude is based on blood gas pressure, it makes sense to me that a change of altitude should be as gradual as possible. Certainly, I don't find the drive as tiring as the flight. If I am to compete at altitude, I never do any exercise prior to the race once I have arrived there. I prefer to save oxygen for the race. Even at the start of the race, it is important for me to take it easy and gradually adapt to the more 'stressful' environment.

At one stage during the late 1980s and early 1990s, I had reason to travel up to altitude approximately once every two weeks for three days at a time. I experienced something for which I have found no official explanation. After doing this for about two months, I found that I was able to handle the transition from sea level to altitude better and could even run some good track or hill sessions on the first or third days of my trip. I cannot say for sure if this was the effect of adaptation; it may be that I had simply learned how to cope with the changes, but I must admit that I ran well over that period, recording some good times in races. Perhaps regular, short trips to altitude are another form of compensation. Was it co-incidental that it was the same period in which I ran 6:07 in Comrades and had a very good 100-mile run later in the year?

The only athletes who appear to benefit from the move to altitude are short-distance sprinters and field throwers. The reason for this is that the air resistance is less at altitude. As air resistance is based on the square of the area presented to the moving object, it makes sense that thinner air offers far less resistance.

There are gadgets on the American market that are reputed to help you adapt to the effects of altitude. To my knowledge, none have been scientifically proven successful. I have tried two of them and found them to be quite awkward to use, not to mention the fact that you look like a space cadet when wearing them!

Moving from altitude to sea level, is not as much of a problem. I believe that many runners overemphasise the advantage of this without taking care to find out exactly how long they need to ensure maximum benefit. I think Ron Hill's story about the Olympic team's experience highlights this.

This is not a detailed or comprehensive description of all the environmental conditions you may encounter, but I hope it is sufficient to make you aware how conditions can affect performance and what steps you should take to counter adverse conditions.

00:00:15
TRIATHLON TRAINING

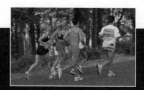

Although triathlons have been part of the world of sport since 1978, my introduction to them came in 1983 when they were first held in South Africa. Even the early events, such as the Computackie Triathlon held in the Free State, and the first *Rand Daily Mail*/Leppin Iron Man (comprising a 21-km canoe, 100-km cycle and marathon run) held at altitude in Gauteng, attracted relatively large numbers of competitors, which augured well for what was to become the boom sport of the 1980s and has since gained Olympic status.

Whereas running and cycling races took many years to progress from the small fields of competitors to today's large and sometimes restricted entries, triathlons have, in a brief period, grown to a stage where fields consistently number a few hundred competitors.

The problem with such rapid growth is that a tried-and-tested recipe for triathlon training has not had time to develop. This, coupled with the fact that triathlons are a combination of three established endurance sports, each with its own requirements for dedication and skill, makes the mere training for such an event a challenge in itself. In addition, the background, as well as the strengths and weaknesses of a triathlete, will also impact on the balance of his training.

There are so many different aspects to multisport training and so many variations in individual needs that it will take many more years before more definitive approaches to training have been determined. What follows are the modifications and pointers I have found to be successful for myself and triathletes I have coached. You will see many of the same principles promoted in the chapters on running, underlying this chapter.

There is perhaps a basic rule, which like many of the other comments made in this book, applies to all sports. In my opinion, we never really feel that we have run the perfect race, we always think that there is something more to come. After each event, we should question the good and the bad, and learn from the answers.

It is, without doubt, better to discuss this with a training partner or colleague, as they recognise the merits and flaws more objectively; we are too involved. Throughout my 21 years of running, I have been surprised at how often a novice will present an idea that was overlooked (or resisted) by seasoned runners, and this reminds me that we are never too smart to learn.

In deciding whether or not an idea has merit, I use the concept that if it sounds logical, it is probably correct. This requires me to view the suggestions objectively and without emotional involvement.

Although much of this chapter may be found elsewhere in the book, I will repeat it here as it will serve as a complete approach to the athlete wanting to set himself a target in the sport of triathlons.

SETTING GOALS

The first step in any training programme is to establish your goals. It would be futile to decide to train for triathlons without any idea of the events, distances or disciplines of the relevant competition. The training for the Hawaii Ironman differs from that for the 1.5-km swim, 40-km cycle and 10-km run format, in the same way that marathon training varies from that required to be successful at 10 km.

Then there is the question of participation in canoeing or swimming triathlons. Up to a point, this debate has been resolved because the number of canoe triathlons have reduced dramatically over years, especially since triathlon has moved through World Championship to Olympic status. However, there are still some canoeing triathlons, and you need to decide whether to focus on the swim or canoe option. Training is specific and it is essential to know what your aim is before you decide how you are going to do it. For this reason you must set a long-term target, along with a number of intermediate goals, which will bring you closer to your planned objective. The long-term target is normally easy – perhaps you want to complete the demanding Iron Man Canoe Triathlon in Vanderbijlpark. The difficulty is often not only to determine intermediate goals, but also to keep them relevant. Intermediate goals may be as simple as learning to balance in a canoe, or as seemingly formidable as completing a half-distance event. The objective is purely to build yourself a ladder to reach your final target, and to keep the ladder as straight as possible.

After two years of running in ignorance, I found myself performing reasonably well in endurance events and concluded that I could tackle anything that required competitors to 'stay upright' for long periods. There were numerous challenges, 100 milers, ultratriathlons, and canoe races, all of which I wanted to combine with the usual weekly, shorter social events. The consequences of this 'Jack of all trades' approach was not only that I was training at base-level intensity all the time, but also that I had no sooner completed one event, than the next one was upon me.

Another problem reared its head; I would break down or injure myself in events that really mattered to me, but survive through those of lesser importance. All the incidentals culminated in fatigue, knocking me back just when I really wanted to do well. My mistakes were brought to my attention by the seconding team for the 1984 London to Paris event, but it took a further three months, much persuasion by Bruce Fordyce and Tim Noakes, and another ruined hope to see it clearly.

I tell this story deliberately because it illustrates not only that we must be specific (and the outcome of failing therein), but also how set in our ways and blind we can be when we are emotionally involved. What concerns me is that I could see the same thing happening to another triathlete in 1986 and, despite similar warnings from three people, my colleague made the same mistake. It appears that many of us only learn by our own mistakes, but those who are truly clever will take heed.

To summarise: set your long-term goal and then plan your intermediate short-term targets so that you stay on the straightest road. Don't become involved in training for the sake of it; it rarely leads to progression and often becomes boring.

TIME MANAGEMENT

There are few better definitions of time management than successfully fitting a well-rounded triathlon-training programme into a normal lifestyle. Triathlons are time-management events.

Firstly, you need to identify all the aspects of your lifestyle and determine the priority of each in relation to achieving your long-term target. (These priorities are often short term and will change after you have attained your goal.) Normally, you need to apportion daily and weekly time to family, career, socialising, sleep and sport. Although sleep and sport are listed separately, later you will see that they are closely linked.

Secondly, you must make the most efficient use of the time you have allocated to each item. In training for a triathlon, I picture my day as a pie chart and try to fill it so that there are no gaps between the sections. An example of this would be to leave your car at work so that you can cycle in the next morning. It may normally take 20 minutes to drive, but will take 40 minutes to cycle. Even if you allow ten minutes for changing (good transition practice!), you've still only used 30 minutes training time. Ask yourself, 'What do I do during lunch? What is the minimum time it takes to leave the house in the morning?' After setting out a proposed programme, ask the final question, 'Is this the most efficient use of my time?'

It is obvious that a professional triathlete or a student has more time and more manoeuvrability within the confines of the 24-hour limit, but good planning can often make for a more successfully trained athlete.

Thirdly, consider which of the three disciplines will give you the most reward for the time spent on it. Again, this is an issue of time efficiency. It may be more pleasant to spend two hours swimming intervals or distance in the pool, surrounded by those scantily clad goddesses of the sun, but for some triathletes more will be achieved in the next event by spinning their way over the hills and valleys of the roads. Once you have determined the proper place for triathlons in your life, identified the times that you can commit to them, and determined the order of priority for each of the three disciplines (run, cycle and canoe or swim), you will be in a position to determine what you are going to do.

CONSISTENCY

The hardest part of any endurance event is correct training and unfortunately for those of us who enjoy ultras, the longer the event, the more important this becomes.

Because triathlons are made up of three events, they are always billed with each of their individual distances, e.g. 1.5-km swim, 40-km cycle and 10-km run. At first glance you sneer at such distances. You may know what it is like to do each of these events separately, but the combination can be a totally different game. If you consider that elite triathletes take approximately one hour and 50 minutes for such an event over an ideal course in ideal conditions, perhaps it could be compared to a road race of 35 km, a cycle of 75 km or an 8-km swim. Suddenly, it becomes more apparent that it is an endurance event.

Success in this sport cannot be achieved with the three-day training week that some sportspeople allocate to prepare for the rigours of rugby or football, or any other single sport. To realise your vision in triathlons, to do more than simply battle your way to the finish line and exhaustion, a more dedicated approach is required.

This more consistent approach to training has physiological reasoning as well. It is better to increase your training load gradually, rather than subject your body to the shock treatment of irregular heavy sessions. For every action there is a reaction, and the reaction to shock treatment can so easily be enforced rest through injury.

If you look at the two running schedules **in the table below**, you will see that it is possible to reach the same overall mileage in each case. Schedule A, however, demands that three large blocks of time be set aside each week for three, relatively

DAY	A (KM)	B (KM)
Monday		6
Tuesday	21	9-km time trial and warm-up
Wednesday		18
Thursday	22	10
Friday		rest
Saturday		10
Sunday	42	32
TOTAL	85	85

large, volumes of running. Such an approach is likely to result in substantial periods of recovery, both after each bout of exercise and after a probable injury. Schedule B, on the other hand, requires only that a small amount of time be 'budgeted' each day and will result in quicker recovery. It also allows more flexibility and opportunity to vary the pace, time or location of the exercise, and keeps it interesting.

EVERYONE'S GUIDE TO DISTANCE RUNNING

Smaller periods of regular training not only appear to be easier to handle, but also permit the development of a routine that makes the training easier and more pleasant. Two words are closely linked to consistency: adaptation and progression.

ADAPTATION – PROGRESSION

As previously indicated, a good simile for the adaptation/progression system is to imagine a weight attached to an elastic band. If the weight is heavy enough and dropped from a resting position, it will plummet earthwards, immediately snapping the band. However, if the same weight is applied gently and lowered in a controlled way, the band is more likely to stretch to its fullest extension. This is what you want to achieve in training – to reach your physical limit without 'snapping the band'.

Before finalising your programme, you must consider the effects of the input/output theory (see diagram on page 94). While initially there may be a direct relationship between the amount of time you put into an exercise and the resulting improvement (line o – A), after a certain point the rate of the improvement diminishes and may also peak out (time B results in a peak at B). Furthermore, additional time spent in similar exercise may well result in reduced benefit and moving beyond the peak training load will lead to overtraining.

In a single sport the object is to train at time B during a heavy period and possibly extending your returns with a supplementary exercise, as indicated by line B – D. However, in triathlons it is unlikely that you will be able to train at that intensity for each sporting code. In fact, you may very well commit competitive suicide if you undertake the training loads required by each of the specialist events in a single week.

Triathlons, particularly the longer events, only require you to be 'capable' in each discipline, not expert. Obviously, the more 'capable' you are in each leg, the more successful you will be. As a result, it is probably better to train each discipline at level and time A on the diagram. However, A and B are only relative to your state of fitness at any given time and your programme must be formatted so that these points will move further and further from the origin.

At the top end of the scale, 'professional triathletes' who are free to train all day, will want to become an expert in each of the sports, and they will have the time for the necessary recovery to allow for that amount of training. Progress at the elite end of triathlons has been such that top athletes, swimmers and cyclists are now forced to choose between events. In the 2000 Sydney Olympics, a Canadian 10 000-m runner first competed in the triathlon, before considering whether to race in the 10 000-m heats the following week.

An advantage of triathlon training is its 'cross-training' effect, i.e. the enhancement of running and swimming fitness as a result of cycling. This appears to be a contradiction of the earlier decision to be specific. On closer examination, however, it may be seen that the cardiovascular system, for instance, is trained by all three disciplines, and, therefore, to gain the same improvement from a single sport, would require much more time in that single sport than is provided during the multidisciplinary training. For a runner who is only committing time A to his sport, it would be inefficient to spend time cycling, but a triathlete compelled by the nature of the sport to train at each of these disciplines can use the effects of cross training to advantage.

As with any stress, it is essential that a recovery break be allowed after the period of stress to permit development and growth. In the case of the elastic band, the weight is lowered in increments, allowing the band time to adapt to the stress of the weight. So too in training it is necessary to factor in recovery, by the use of alternate periods of hard and easy work, and by the occasional rest period.

Ironman requires quality and technique – not distance

In 1986 a new triathlete entered Durban's triathlon scene. She came from a swimming background and very quickly came to terms with the basic principles of hard/easy training and recovery. As the women's winner of the Durban 3.5-km swim, 140-km cycle and 32-km run triathlon, she won a trip to the Hawaii Ironman event. Within a few years Paula Newby-Frazer not only had a string of Ironman wins to her credit, but also dominated the professional triathlon scene in North America. Throughout her career she stuck to the basic principles and proved that limited quality training can far outweigh the benefits of large quantities of low-intensity distance work.

For me the message of low-distance, quality training was reinforced again in 2001, when I made a return to the full Ironman distance. In 1984 I had competed in Hawaii after finishing second in the 1984 Durban swim ultra. In those days, I believed in a diet of distance rather than quality and had finished eighth in my age category and was the top South African male. Seventeen years later I trained for the Isuzu Ironman in Gordon's Bay. Allowing for the exceptionally high winds, which brought both cyclists and runners to complete stops, I completed the event at a similar level to that which I had achieved in Hawaii years before. Certainly, the technological advances in bicycle equipment accounted for some of this, but my training had concentrated on quality. The longest run had been 28 km, the longest swim 3.2 km, and the longest cycle 110 km for an event that covered 3.8 km swimming, 180 km cycling and 42 km running. It was sufficient for selection to represent South Africa at the 2001 World Ultratriathlon in Denmark. Even at elite level, top triathletes restrict their running to around 40 km per week. The secret is in the quality.

Mixing hard and easy across the sports

Not only should the day-by-day progress of your training be based on the hard/easy principle, but also the weekly progress. The determination of what constitutes a hard day and what is an easy session, is best monitored by the body's reaction to the previous day's load. Parameters such as an increase in morning pulse rate, loss of weight and increase in thirst, are the telltale signs of too much, too soon, too often. (Tim Noakes' book, *Lore of Running* (OUP) gives a detailed description of the telltale signs of overtraining.)

With the limited time available and the amount of sessions needed to cram into a week of triathlon training, overtraining is seemingly inevitable; the alternative being that you arrive at an event underprepared. However, with careful planning, it is possible to combine the less stressful items of one discipline with the more stressful items of another. A hard session in running one day is followed by an easy run the next. Within each discipline it is important to mix both the distance and the pace of the training. Although running is not a high-skill sport, time can be well spent in technique sessions in the other two disciplines.

In order to improve, you must increase the stress as you continue to train. In the same way that initial base training is later followed up with speed training when you train for a single sport, so too must you adopt this principle for the three-sport competition.

Once you have written down your programme for each session in a day, plus each day of the week, it should encompass the principles of training for each individual sport, as well as the balance of the three sports, which are determined by the requirements of the event in which you wish to compete. Your programme must not be one of rigid finality, but be flexibile enough to substitute, for instance, the less taxing effect of a cycle for that of a joint-pounding run when your body is telling you to beware.

However, do not mistake flexibility for laziness. I have often been tempted to substitute a cycle for a series of hard swim intervals, but it was my preference for that exercise that was willing me to mount up rather than swim. The greatest determination is often necessary for me to complete swim sessions, while the greatest willpower is required to stop me from overdoing the running. An honest appraisal of your own programme will always reveal preferential faults, and when changed, results in better time management.

The object of this chapter is to assist in the formulation of a suitable training schedule and it would not be complete without an example. The problem with such an exercise is that, as with all training, it should be personally tailored, and specific to the event itself.

However, I have used the skeleton programme given to ten of the country's top triathletes when they were selected for the Leppin London to Paris squad in 1985. They were selected in the May and asked to prepare themselves for a trial in early July that would be of similar format to the event itself. The triathletes were given these guidelines and a 'Possible Peak Week Training' schedule, in the hope that it would assist them to prepare for the rigours of the event.

Those of us familiar with this event know that, despite it being of a relay nature and spread over a three-day period, the +160-km run, 35-km swim and 300-km cycle event requires each of the four team members to be in a condition of peak fitness and to work together like a machine. There were those in our squad who doubted the difficulty of such an event, but who, during stolen moments of recovery in Cape Town during the trials, confided to Professor Tim Noakes and myself that this had indeed been one of the most taxing weekends of their sporting lives.

The following table shows the details of a typical week's training prior to this trial. Distances have intentionally been omitted. Notice that the programme is

DAY	RUN	CYCLE	SWIM
Monday	recovery	fast distance	intervals
Tuesday	track		technique
Wednesday	recovery	slipstream	time trial/ intervals
Thursday	fartlek		distance
Friday		technique	intervals
Saturday	recovery	long cycle	technique (optional)
Sunday	long run		surf swim

biased towards the swim in the same way that the event itself is biased towards the swim. An important feature is the combination of sessions of different exertion levels in one day and throughout a week.

As mentioned earlier, it is important to have intermediate goals, thus progress in training forms the basis of such goals. If you succeed at each of these smaller steps, it gives you the confidence to succeed in your long-term target. Once you have established a plan of attack, have confidence in it and give it the chance to work.

Bricks

'Bricks' are two or more disciplines in a triathlon placed back to back in a training session, e.g. go for a one-hour cycle, change immediately and run a relatively high-intensity run of 5–8 km. The run should be just under the 'red-line' intensity.

These sessions tend to be fairly tough and require good recovery in the following sessions. They are, however, of key importance to the preparation for a triathlon and should be included approximately every 14 days. The cycle-run version should not be considered the only option, however. Swim-to-cycle or -run, or other combinations also offer significant benefits, as well as the opportunity to practise the transition procedure.

Recent research shows that bricks can also be beneficial for specialist runners. A runner will often do a track session, only to find that he is no longer able to maintain the set intensity in yet another interval. At this stage, he could use a bicycle (or a bicycle on a turbo trainer) to knock out another couple of intervals over a similar period of time. In this manner, although the muscular work is slightly different, the training in the same 'energy system' may be extended.

Transitions and punctures

The standards in triathlon continue to improve and the impact of time lost in the transition area is becoming increasingly relevant. In sprint events, most of the 'changing' should be prepared for in the final sections of the previous discipline.

For instance, just before you reach the cycle-to-run transition stage, undo your cycling shoes (some triathletes even remove their feet from their shoes), unfasten any cycling gloves and mentally 'run through' your actions throughout the transition. Will you first remove your helmet and then change your shoes, or will you simply rack your bike, change your shoes and take your helmet off as you run? Practice and visualisation are key training for a good transition. Remember that it's all about time and these things need practice and training. Transition training can be a useful session on a recovery day. Simply spend a half-hour practising the change from one sport to the other, in each instance timing the process and working out how to save time.

Punctures fall into the same format. While a puncture can severely handicap a performance in an Olympic distance event, the impact on an Ironman event may be substantially less, providing you are adept at ripping out the tube and replacing it. This can only be learnt through practice.

RECOVERY OR TAPER PHASE

The stress of training increases gradually until you reach your period of peak training, after which you require a period of gradual recovery. Unfortunately, during this stage you may very well feel so strong that you want to test your strength, or indeed feel that you will benefit from 'just one last hard session'. Succumb to these temptations and you can wave goodbye to your long-term goal. The problem is it is so easy to do.

The importance of self-control and monitoring your body during the last weeks of preparation for an event cannot be overemphasised. Bruce Fordyce's suggestion that it is better to arrive at the start slightly undertrained must be remembered at this stage. It is during the final recovery or taper period that you gain the strength – physical and mental – which will allow you to dig deep in the final section of the event. This gives you the reserves that make the difference between finishing and succeeding.

Although triathlons remain a relatively new, complex and unresearched sport, the training procedures are similar to those of most other endurance sports. The difficulty is knowing where to begin and how to apportion our training. We seem to be running when our peers are cycling, or swimming when they are running. We continually question whether we are doing enough in any particular sport and even whether we are doing the right thing. It was confusing enough when we were only runners or canoeists or cyclists or swimmers, now the confusion is compounded.

The object of this chapter is to assist you with a more structured approach in establishing a suitable training programme, within your limits. Your training programme should make the most efficient use of your time within those limits. In doing this, combined with the basic training principles outlined here and elsewhere, you should have gained the confidence to know that without altering the priorities you initially set, you are on the right track to reach your long-term goal.

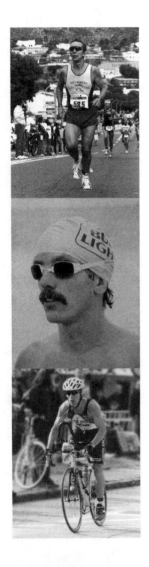

ABOVE *Triathlons comprise the disciplines of running, swimming or canoeing, and cycling*

PART 3:

MAKING THE MOS
OF YOUR TRAIN

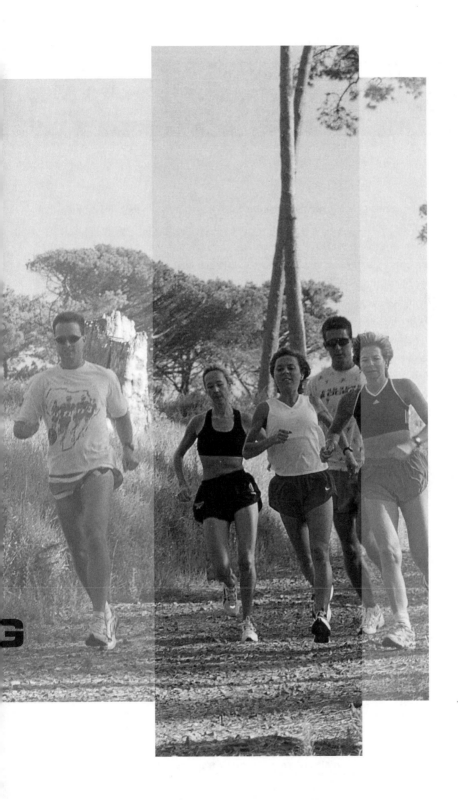

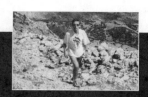

When runners really want to achieve their true potential, they programme their training and racing into segments, often called macro- and microtraining blocks, which means that they will peak for only a few races. With such limited opportunities to excel, it is important to take full advantage of your training during the build-up period. In the final weeks before a race, you need to give some serious thought as to how you will taper down for the race – your training is only as good as the rest and recovery that you allow your body.

Training is a form of 'breakdown'. When the muscles repair during rest and recovery, they grow stronger and it is this growth that improves your performance. Few runners dispute this fact nowadays, yet they still have insufficient 'courage' to rest properly. The question as to how to taper is still one of the great unknowns in sports science.

The taper is the period that allows you to recover from hard training. For a marathon this will probably be about 1–2 weeks, for 5 km or 10 km, this may only be 4–7 days. However, in the latter events, there is greater emphasis on speed and race tactics, therefore it is likely that your competitive period will comprise more than a single race.

Track runners, even for distance events such as 5 000 m and 10 000 m, use two or three build-up races in a one-month period, in order to 'peak' for the major race. They will establish a schedule during this period that is low on distance and high on technique sessions. The track sessions are short and are undertaken at a fairly high intensity with long recovery periods between the intervals. A marathon runner, on the other hand, is likely to reduce his distance in the final couple of weeks, and he will use fartlek and track sessions to put the bounce and spring back in his stride.

Under no circumstances must the taper period tax a runner; quite the opposite. The biggest problem runners are likely to experience at this stage is the temptation to 'test' themselves to see how they are doing, which inevitably leads to running too fast or too far. This effectively leaves their race out on the training roads. The taper should also be used as a period when a runner mentally prepares for, and concentrates on, the race, as well as the evolution of the game plan and tactics he intends using. It's an ideal period for mental strengthening.

While the effects of training sessions have often been researched, until recently the taper has always been left to the individual. Thankfully, recent research undertaken in the Netherlands has focused on this much-overlooked aspect.

THE TRIED AND TESTED TAPER

It is commonly held that the total quantity of your training should be reduced over the last week to ten days, that hard runs should be kept to a minimum, and that there is little chance of damaging your performance if you don't run at all over the last three days. Because the body takes 7-10 days to benefit from a training session, the purpose of the final taper relates more to 'active rest', circulation and psychological preparation, than physiological development. At this stage, the physiological improvement comes from the recovery, not from the training.

There was relatively little information on what speed you should run in the last week, or what percentage of your total previous weekly distance you should cover. Tapering was, and generally still is, a bit of a hit-and-miss situation with runners following a regimen that may have produced a good result in the past. They are unwilling to try much else in case it doesn't produce similar or better results. This is further complicated by the fact that it is virtually impossible to adjudicate the variations in taper, as the conditions of each race are different.

The long-term research conducted in the Netherlands has determined the type of training possible, without the risk of muscle damage. A group of 23 long-distance runners were monitored for an 18-20-month period, and their muscle damage assessed on a regular basis. In the first period, the runners trained lightly, averaging only 30 km per week, with a longest run of 12 km and racing a 15-km event after six months. The second period saw the training increased to 50 km with a maximum long run of 23 km and a 25-km road race. The final period of seven months averaged 79 km per week with a 32-km long run, and a marathon race at the end.

No runners sustained muscle damage after the first period of training, but 14% showed damage after the 15-km race. This is to be expected after a race. By the end of the second period, 33% of the runners had muscle damage both before and after the race, and by the end of the third period, this had increased to 57% with pre-race muscle damage and 62% post-race damage; 57% of the runners had damage BEFORE the marathon.

Remembering that many studies show that recovery from muscle damage takes between three and five weeks, it becomes obvious that there is a need to reduce severely the weekly mileage to 30–50 km per week over this final period if you are to line up with 'fresh' muscles.

This involves an overall drop in weekly distance and a reduction in the length of the 'long run'. From his experiments, Professor Tim Noakes has suggested that muscle damage increases exponentially when a long run exceeds 25 km. The last run longer than 25 km should, therefore, be about three weeks prior to the race. While this may seem ridiculously low, it must be appreciated that the South African running scene tends to be obsessed with distance. In most countries a runner will do one or perhaps two marathons a year, and the thought of anything longer remains that – a thought! In that context, 25 km is still a relatively long run.

The experience of the inaugural Durban City Marathon in 2002 reinforces such a recommendation. The marathon was organised for 29 September at six weeks notice and with only four weeks between the publicity launch and the race. As a result, few of the nearly 2 000 runners were able to put in the high-mileage training they would normally have done for such a marathon. Interestingly, many reported better than normal times or PBs, which suggests that it was because they arrived at the start with fresh, not overtrained legs.

One aspect that hasn't yet been discussed is the speed of this training, which is the secret to effective taper. You will remember that much has been proven about the worth of speed work. It is distance that causes muscle damage, not speed and it is important to maintain your average training speed. Within your reduced training schedule, maintain your 1 000–3000-m runs at 10-km race pace, and your intervals at 5-km race pace, and other such quality work. Your average training speed will probably increase, as it is the total amount of longer, slower runs that are 'sacrificed' in the weekly distance reduction.

Remember also that the fastest fall-off in fitness results from a reduction in blood volume and the resultant reduction in VO_2 Max. It has been found, however, that if one quality session of repeats of about 400 m at best 1 500-m pace is undertaken each week, the fall-off is counteracted.

From the above you will see that it is indeed possible to reduce your training safely over a 2-3-week period in this manner, before reaching the final week before the event. Further research assists us in the final week of preparation.

The same basic principles are supported by research that was conducted in North America, which suggested that a runner peaking for a 10-km or half-marathon should do only speed work during the last week. When first introduced, this was certainly a different viewpoint, and was summarily dismissed by some. However, my personal experience and that of numerous athletes I have coached at club and international level, is that this system works, not only for races up to half-marathon, but for all distances including ultramarathons. Consider the recommendations. The week starts with 6 x 500 m at best 1 500–3 000-m race pace with as much rest as you need between each. This is sandwiched between a warm-up and cool-down of about 1 km. Day two is 4 x 500 m in the same way, day three 3 x 500 m, etc. and reducing the total until only 1 x 500 m. The penultimate day is reserved for total rest.

Compare this to the 'traditional' recommendation of a longish run, seven days before a race, to help depletion of the carbohydrate stores, then three or four days light, easy running and two or three days of complete rest. In the speed taper, there will certainly be a considerable depletion effect in running 6 x 500 m, as the amount of glycogen burned up increases with speed and there is a greater depletion with short, fast intervals than with easier running.

Another benefit of this taper is that it prepares you for a race as it involves some anaerobic work. By comparison, light jogging is purely aerobic. Runners should have no doubts about their aerobic fitness by the final week of training for a distance event, or marathon. Running at the faster pace will make the race pace seem easy. The few kilometres put in during the final week of training will leave you feeling light on your feet – exactly as you do when you have completed a speed session. This will not only boost your confidence, but appears to give you a physical boost as well, which is exactly what is required before a race!

But what of the muscle breakdown associated with speed?

By putting in only 500 m and having long recoveries, there is little breakdown, as the muscles are not put under major stress. Furthermore, the total distance of the speed work in the week only adds up to about 17 x 500 m = 8.5 km. Add in the warm-ups and there is a weekly total of approximately 20 km. The only danger here is if you try to set PBs in each set, or allow yourself too little recovery between each 500 m. Limit your speed to your best 1 500–3 000-m race pace and allow a minimum of two minutes between each. It is recommended that the quantity of speed taper be only 9% of your weekly total, thus if you normally run 100 km per week, you should do 9 km of 400 m or 500 m over the full week. The speed taper is suitable for runners of all abilities as it is based on PB time, the only difference is the speed and number of the 400 m or 500 m intervals.

Again, compare this with the typical 'normal' and slower taper:

Day seven: 21–25 km, day six: 8–10 km, day five: 8–10 km with pick-ups, day four: 6–8 km, day three to race day: rest. This gives a total for the week of 43–50 km, most of which should be done at slower than race pace; not only is it a greater distance of work in the week, but also at a less 'uplifting' pace.

Compare this to running longer, slower easy runs during your final week. They make you feel sluggish, and create the temptation to 'test yourself' by running too hard. Have you noticed how your mind starts to play games, where doubt starts to creep in? Often during these runs you will doubt your ability by asking yourself, 'If this is what I feel like at this slow pace, how am I going to survive the race pace for longer?' Questioning your ability is the last thing you want on your mind in the final week. These are natural doubts, and probably unfounded, but if you do a quality taper, you will feel powerful, strong and psychologically upbeat. Isn't that how you'd prefer to go into a race?

The only drawback to the quality taper system is that runners should have gained some quality or speed work experience before undertaking this taper. However, a speed taper offers many advantages and has certainly delivered results for those who have used it.

You will have noted that the penultimate day is allocated as a rest day, and not the day immediately prior to the race. There is a good reason for this, relating back to the 'pendulum' or 'swing' theory (see chapter 21). The body has a propensity for 'overcompensation'. If the blood sugar level is raised, insulin brings the blood sugar level down – not immediately to normal, but first to a low blood sugar level and then gradually to normal. When you are dehydrated your body attempts to store fluid, in case there is another 'drought' (witness the swelling and fluid retention after air flights). I believe that the same applies to rest days. Often runners feel quite lethargic in the first run after a rest day, and only return to 'normal' running on the second training session. It is as if the rest day puts the body into hibernation, and a training session is required to awaken it.

It is, therefore, much better to have your rest day on the penultimate, or penultimate and third-last days before a race. The more intense (shorter distance) the race, the more intense the speed should be in the training session on the final day before the race. For very short events such as 5 km or short cross-country, not only should you complete a session of 2 x 500 m with warm-up and cool-down the day before, but also 15–20 minutes of easy warm-up and strides over 50 m on the morning of the event.

For longer events, another useful addition to the final training session on the final day, is to do about three or four repeats over 200 m at the same pace that you have calculated to be your average, predicted pace for the race. This allows you to mentally attune to the race pace in order to start the race at the correct pace.

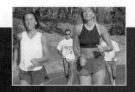

Some runners think that if they do the training, a result may be taken for granted. This is only true to a certain extent. The longer the race, the more planning it requires. Apart from anything else, the longer a race is, the more there is to go wrong. This would seem to be obvious, but an unusual set of circumstances in 1989 proved to me that many people have not come to terms with it.

In early 1989, I was preparing for a 1 800-km cross-Africa 'journey' run, which was to involve a number of large corporate companies, including Anglo-American, and was intended to be the launch of a new fundraising concept called ITHUBA. At that stage, it was planned to bring a number of top sportspeople, as well as politicians together, to commit to the future of South Africa, and in those dying days of Apartheid, it was one of the most exciting projects and concepts with which I was involved. I had structured my own programme so that my peak training was planned to build through Comrades and culminate in the journey race in August. As had been my routine for the past six years, I planned to train approximately 200 km in the week before Comrades. Typically, this meant a 20–25-km run three days ahead of the race, 1-km repeats two days prior, 10–12 km the day before (very easy), Comrades itself, followed by 10 km (very easy) the following day, and a rest the day thereafter. (My focus in the 1980s and 1990s was not Comrades. I used the latter purely as a training event in preparation for longer races.) As a result, I was satisfied with anything under seven hours and frequently ran with another runner most of the way.

In that particular year, however, I was told ten days ahead of the event, to hold back on the training as the journey run was to be delayed pending television negotiations. (It was apparently impossible to provide microwave links to large sections of the route through the western half of South Africa and the event was eventually changed to a relay from Pretoria to Johannesburg).

Because I was so unsure of the date of the run, I simply carried on with 100 km per week, and on Comrades day, I started out running with a group going for 6:30, passing the halfway mark at 3:12. At 10 km there must have been well over 1 000 runners ahead of me, therefore they obviously thought they were going to finish faster than 6:30.

By halfway, I was probably placed well around the 350th position, but was finding it uncomfortable to stay back with many of the runners. Without increasing my speed, I began to move forward through the pack. By Botha's Hill I still felt fresh and so increased the pace a bit and by the time I met my spectator friends at Kloof, I had moved up substantially, almost causing my triathlon teammate, Philip Kuhn, to drop his beer! At Cowies Hill I had left a radio with Mike Bell; I tuned in to hear the commentator saying that Frith van der Merwe (the leading lady who was to set a new course record) had passed Mark Page and was now in the top 20. I had passed Mark a few kilometres earlier and realised that I was quite high up, so decided to push a bit harder over the last 10 km. People who saw me at the finish commented on my fresh appearance, and indeed, I immediately ran to my car and went back up to Kloof to second a friend. My time was 6:07 in 27th position, and yet over 1 000 runners had been ahead of me through the bottom of Polly Shorts at the 10-km mark.

Equally surprising was the number of congratulations that were forthcoming in the following weeks – many from running administrators. Naturally, this was very welcome and gratifying, but it was for a Comrades time that, by comparison, was not as good as some of the 100-mile times that I had achieved in previous years. I had been tested by the University of Durban-Westville in March and was given a predicted time of a sub-six hours if I raced Comrades. As indicated above, however, Comrades was not my main focus at that stage in my career, as my preference was for longer ultra-events.

All of which highlights two main points: firstly, many runners had clearly not done their planning and preparation for the race day, as they never achieved the times their initial pace suggested; and secondly, a 100-mile race is twice the length of Comrades so there is twice as long for the weather to become adverse. It's estimated that any race run in an effective temperature of 25 °C will be 7% slower than the same race run in 20 °C or less. The 100-milers in South Africa that start during the day, frequently see temperatures of over 30 °C. Long races, in particular, must be carefully planned because the longer the race, the more there is to go wrong. Don't fall into the trap that double the distance means a straightforward proportion of time.

Race preparation may be classified into a number of subjects, the most obvious one being that of training (already covered in other chapters). Others are fluid and energy replacement (still to be discussed), as well as environmental conditions (see chapter 14) — all of particular importance in long races.

All of these factors must be taken into consideration in advance of the race, while on the day of the race, you need the planning, discipline and control to pace your way through it. For this to happen, you must set a realistic target time, after which you need to create an appropriate schedule, one that is flexible enough to allow for variations on the day.

The approach of lead runners will generally differ from that of back runners in as much as the top runners are aiming for a win, which makes racing that much more important than a finishing time. The object is to win! Of course the lead runner must still have some idea what he is capable of if he is not to fade. Armed with a realistic pacing schedule and a perception of his competitors' capability, a runner can decide whether to chase an early leader, or let him go, only to reel him in later in the race. The average or back runner may, however, concentrate on achieving a time goal, and will generally receive assistance from the runners around him.

Logistics planning is another area worthy of consideration. Most runners see this merely as turning up for the start of a race with sufficient time to enter and warm up. In general, the organisers cater for all refreshment tables, drinks, routes and other important requirements. If a runner is going for a win he may also organise someone to provide him with a split (the time taken to reach a particular intermediate point or the time difference between one runner and the next, ahead or behind) or other tactical information.

In longer events, however, there may be a need for seconds along the route; even a requirement for special drinks or food. Seconds also need food and drink if it is an all-day event. Vehicles may be required. In track ultras, you may well be required to provide two lap scorers for the entire length of the event. It is often difficult to find people to do this thankless task, especially since they will be asked to lap score for another runner they don't even know. Thorough logistical planning will give a runner confidence, as well as the ability to focus on the running, but peace of mind only comes with the knowledge that everything is in place.

Mental preparation is another important aspect, one that has never really been given its true place in coaching and training advice for runners. This will be covered in detail later.

To a large extent, if all these areas of preparation have been covered, a runner will have won half the battle in having a positive approach to the race. The knowledge that everything has been planned (and that all that's left to do is run the race), engenders much confidence in runners.

This is well illustrated in journey events where seconding is critical to a runner's performance, and must, therefore, be top class. I have been extremely lucky over the years to have Andy Booth as a second for many of my long runs. Andy was also my partner for three Duzi Canoe Marathons and was one of the first friends I made in South Africa. He knows me so well that he can actually predict what I will need. For instance, he frequently meets me with a cup of soup at a seconding point when I had been craving it for the previous 2 km. In journey runs, a competitor runs, sleeps and eats. EVERYTHING else is the job of the second. If my hat blows off, the second will retrieve it, otherwise I travel twice the distance before moving forward. Every metre counts. With that level of backup, who wouldn't be confident. Although much of this obviously relates to long events, the same principles and requirements should be applied to shorter, more common events from 5 km upwards.

SETTING A REALISTIC TARGET

Earlier on, we looked at the concept of maximum oxygen 'capacity' (VO_2 Max), which when combined with a measure of 'efficiency' through the threshold point, gives an indication of a runner's potential. As indicated, it is possible to train these factors to some extent, and there are tests that can measure such improvement.

When these parameters have been determined for an individual, it is possible to estimate his time for any distance of race using mathematical formulae. These times are particularly accurate between 5 km and 50 km, but are less accurate at either end, although corrective modification factors may be applied. I have written a computer program that allows runners first to determine their own 'profile' based on their previous race results, and then to predict their time for a distance. Thus without the services of a laboratory, which is the common way of determining VO$_2$ Max and threshold points, a runner will have an idea of his potential.

In many ways, this is more accurate than laboratory testing, although the figure for the VO$_2$ Max will only be indicative, and relative to others determined on the same program, because it makes full allowance for a runner's capabilities during races. Running on a treadmill in a laboratory requires a different skill and also involves heart monitors, breathing tubes and the very hot and humid climate of stationary indoor running, all of which can disrupt the runner's running style.

However, if I run three races 'all out' on flat courses, I am running with the same potential as when I run a race for which I want to predict my time. If a race is over a hilly course, I should use three race times over similar courses as the basis for my prediction. An additional benefit of the program is that once your profile is logged, you can use it to determine the time you need to run a distance at an 85% or 90 % effort, for instance. Alternatively, given a distance and a time, it will show at what percentage effort you ran, which may help you not to race during training.

Initially written in 1989, this program has been expanded to provide training, pacing, heart-rate and nutritional advice. Another runner, Anton Steenkamp, has developed other calculators and rewritten the program in a more computer-friendly format. I am sure that you will find it a useful training and racing tool – details may be found on my website (**www.coachnorrie.co.za**). For those who don't have access to a computer, **the table below shows some comparable times from 10–90 km.**

DISTANCE	10 km	21.1 km	42.2 km	56 km	90 km
10 km	1	2.187	4.65	6.445	11.36
21.2 km		1	2.133	2.95	5.195
42.2 km			1	1.42	2.42
56 km				1	1.763
90 km					1

There are other simpler calculations to assist runners in predicting race times. **They are less accurate but make good rule-of-thumb guides** (see following page):

EVERYONE'S GUIDE TO DISTANCE RUNNING

> ‣ half-marathon from 10-km time – double and add five minutes.
>
> ‣ marathon from half-marathon – double half-marathon time and add between five and ten minutes.
>
> ‣ 56-km time from marathon time – marathon time x 1.42.
>
> ‣ 90 km from 56-km time – 56-km time x 1.71.
>
> ‣ 90-km-time from marathon time – marathon time x 2.42.

In 1985 I recorded the times of gold medal Comrades runners and researched their best marathon times. By dividing their Comrades (90-km) time by their marathon time, I arrived at a ratio. Despite the fact that I made no allowance for either the direction or the ever-changing distance of Comrades, in statistical terms, the ratios were very close. I found the average of these ratios to be 2.42 and suggested that the best way of quickly predicting your Comrades time was to take your best recent marathon time and multiply it by 2.42. A similar method was used for the other factors identified above. I was flattered, when in an article in 2002 by a South African sports scientist, it stated that these were 'well-established figures'. I am not sure that the research background was as detailed as implied in the article, but they certainly work well, and that is the important part.

In early 1989 I was contacted by Jan Louw of Johannesburg, suggesting further modifications to this idea of predicting a Comrades time from that of a marathon. Jan had devised formulae that not only took into account a runner's ability in a marathon, but also the amount of training done by him between January and May. This made sense, as running a three-hour marathon in March and then becoming a 'couch potato' until race day (which in those days was 31 May), would certainly not give you a Comrades time appropriate to your potential.

In addition, Jan used a factor that made allowance for the number of years that a runner has been training, as well as factors allowing for a runner's sex, up- or down-run Comrades, etc. This table has been reproduced with Jan Louw's permission, as it is a very useful tool for the majority of Comrades runners.

One point I would draw your attention to is that a 3:00 marathon runner need only do a maximum of 90 km a week for a silver medal, and yet even if he trains at 120 km a week, he will only improve to around a 7:00 Comrades. The medal is

COMRADES TIME PREDICTION TABLE (DOWN RUN)

Current Performance / Race Distance (km)

Race Distance (km)	13.52	14.31	15.11	15.50	16.30	17.09	17.49	18.29	19.08	19.48	20.27	21.07	21.47	22.26	23.06	23.45	24.25	22.05	25.44	26.24	27.03	27.30
5	13.52	14.31	15.11	15.50	16.30	17.09	17.49	18.29	19.08	19.48	20.27	21.07	21.47	22.26	23.06	23.45	24.25	22.05	25.44	26.24	27.03	27.30
8	22.54	23.59	25.05	26.10	27.15	28.21	29.26	30.32	31.37	32.43	33.48	34.53	35.59	37.04	38.10	39.15	40.21	41.26	42.31	43.37	44.42	45.27
10	22.54	23.59	25.05	26.10	27.15	28.21	29.26	30.32	31.37	32.43	33.48	34.53	35.59	37.04	38.10	39.15	40.21	41.26	42.31	43.37	44.42	45.27
15	0.45	0.47	0.49	0.51	0.53	0.55	0.58	1.00	1.02	1.04	1.06	1.08	1.10	1.13	1.15	1.17	1.19	1.21	1.23	1.25	1.27	1.29
21	1.05	1.08	1.11	1.14	1.17	1.20	1.23	1.26	1.29	1.32	1.35	1.38	1.41	1.44	1.48	1.51	1.54	1.57	2.00	2.03	2.06	2.08
32	1.41	1.45	1.50	1.55	2.00	2.05	2.09	2.14	2.19	2.24	2.29	2.33	2.38	2.43	2.48	2.53	2.57	3.02	3.07	3.12	3.17	3.20
42	2.15	2.22	2.28	2.35	2.41	2.48	2.54	3.00	3.07	3.13	3.20	3.26	3.33	3.39	3.46	3.52	3.58	4.05	4.11	4.18	4.24	4.29
50	2.45	2.53	3.01	3.08	3.16	3.24	3.32	3.40	3.48	3.56	4.03	4.11	4.19	4.27	4.35	4.43	4.50	4.58	5.06	5.14	5.22	5.27
56	3.10	3.19	3.28	3.37	3.46	3.55	4.04	4.13	4.22	4.31	4.40	4.49	4.58	5.07	5.16	5.25	5.34	5.43	5.52	6.01	6.10	6.16

TRAINING GRID — KM PER WEEK

Jan & Feb	Mar & Apr	Total Jan–May	13.52	14.31	15.11	15.50	16.30	17.09	17.49	18.29	19.08	19.48	20.27	21.07	21.47	22.26	23.06	23.45	24.25	22.05	25.44	26.24	27.03	27.30
127	156	2600	5.15																					
121	149	2482	5.17	5.30																				
116	142	2374	5.20	5.32	5.45																			
111	136	2275	5.22	5.34	5.47	6.00																		
106	131	2184	5.25	5.37	5.49	6.02	6.15																	
102	126	2100	5.28	5.39	5.52	6.04	6.17	6.30																
99	121	2022	5.31	5.42	5.54	6.07	6.19	6.32	6.45															
95	117	1950	5.33	5.45	5.57	6.09	6.22	6.34	6.47	7.00														
92	113	1883	5.36	5.48	6.00	6.12	6.24	6.37	6.49	7.02	7.15													
89	109	1820	5.39	5.51	6.03	6.15	6.27	6.39	6.52	7.04	7.17	7.30												
86	106	1761	5.42	5.53	6.06	6.18	6.30	6.42	6.54	7.06	7.19	7.32	7.45											
83	102	1706	5.45	5.56	6.09	6.21	6.33	6.45	6.57	7.09	7.21	7.34	7.47	8.00										
81	99	1655	5.48	5.59	6.12	6.24	6.36	6.48	7.00	7.12	7.24	7.36	7.49	8.02	8.15									
78	96	1606	5.51	6.02	6.14	6.27	6.39	6.51	7.03	7.15	7.27	7.39	7.51	8.04	8.16	8.30								
76	94	1560	5.53	6.05	6.17	6.30	6.42	6.54	7.06	7.18	7.30	7.42	7.54	8.07	8.19	8.31	8.45							
74	91	1517	5.56	6.07	6.20	6.33	6.45	6.58	7.10	7.22	7.34	7.45	7.57	8.09	8.21	8.34	8.46	9.00						
72	89	1476	5.58	6.10	6.23	6.36	6.48	7.01	7.13	7.25	7.37	7.49	8.01	8.13	8.24	8.36	8.49	9.02	9.15					
70	86	1437	6.01	6.12	6.26	6.39	6.51	7.04	7.16	7.28	7.40	7.52	8.05	8.16	8.27	8.39	8.51	9.04	9.16	9.30				
68	84	1400	6.03	6.15	6.28	6.42	6.54	7.07	7.19	7.32	7.44	7.56	8.07	8.19	8.31	8.42	8.54	9.07	9.18	9.31	9.45			
67	82	1365	6.06	6.17	6.31	6.44	6.57	7.10	7.23	7.35	7.47	7.59	8.11	8.23	8.34	8.46	8.58	9.10	9.21	9.33	9.46	10.00		
65	80	1332	6.08	6.20	6.34	6.47	7.00	7.13	7.26	7.38	7.51	8.03	8.15	8.27	8.38	8.50	9.01	9.13	9.24	9.36	9.48	10.02	10.15	
63	78	1300	6.10	6.22	6.36	6.50	7.03	7.16	7.29	7.42	7.54	8.06	8.18	8.30	8.42	8.53	9.05	9.17	9.28	9.39	9.51	10.04	10.16	10.26
62	76	1270	6.12	6.24	6.39	6.52	7.06	7.19	7.32	7.45	7.57	8.10	8.22	8.34	8.46	8.57	9.09	9.21	9.31	9.43	9.54	10.07	10.19	10.27
59	72	1200	6.17	6.32	6.47	7.01	7.16	7.29	7.43	7.56	8.10	8.22	8.35	8.48	9.00	9.12	9.23	9.36	9.46	9.58	10.09	10.21	10.32	1039
54	66	1100	6.25	6.41	6.56	7.11	7.26	7.40	7.55	8.09	8.23	8.37	8.50	9.03	9.16	9.29	9.42	9.54	10.05	10.17	10.29	10.41	10.52	10.59
49	60	1000	6.33	6.49	7.05	7.21	7.37	7.52	8.08	8.23	8.37	8.52	9.06	9.20	9.34	9.48	10.01	10.15	10.27	10.40	10.53	11.06	11.18	11.26
44	54	900	6.41	6.58	7.15	7.32	7.49	8.05	8.21	8.37	8.53	9.08	9.23	9.39	9.53	10.08	10.23	10.37	10.51	11.05	11.19	11.33	11.46	11.55
39	48	800	9.50	7.08	7.26	7.43	8.01	8.18	8.35	8.52	9.08	9.25	9.41	9.58	10.13	10.29	10.44	11.00	11.14	11.29	11.43	11.58	12.11	12.20

the same and to a large extent, because Comrades distance varies, and the route and direction change, we must ask whether this runner is not better running his safe silver with as little training as possible and then saving his heavy training to improve his times at shorter distances. This will of course have the effect of improving his potential at the Comrades. It's all a matter of priorities. Likewise, anyone who can't manage around a 3:15 marathon, assuming it's been a flat-out effort, is not silver-medal material. Perhaps there is scope for adopting more of this approach to some of the events you want to run, but not race.

Stories abound of runners who contend that they were able to complete Comrades with less than the minimum 800-km training indicated in the table. This is by no means impossible. A look at the table will show that a runner with the potential to run a three-hour marathon can expect an 8:52 Comrades time with only 800 km of training, and would probably be capable of finishing in under 11 hours with only a little distance. The key, however, is still for him to set a realistic target in view of the training and to adopt a suitable pacing strategy.

Comrades is now in June not May

When Jan Louw compiled the chart, Comrades was on 31 May, and now it is 16 days later on 16 June. For this reason, the total distances for training should be increased by 90–180 km. These figures are based on two weeks' additional training in January, not at peak training. The reason for this is simple. The Comrades-specific training period should remain the same length as before, merely moved on by two weeks. The actual amount you can add will depend on your current standard as a runner. The easiest way is to take the recommended weekly training amounts for January for your current standard, and double it.

DECIDING ON RACE PACE

Even before you enter a race you should know how you intend running it. Perhaps you think that once you have a realistic target it will be easy to determine at what pace you should run. Divide the distance into your target time and you will know your pace – right? Wrong! You must also allow for the terrain over which the race is run, and what you should be aiming for is even effort, not even pace.

A classic example of this was Welcome Mteto who in 2000 was a member of the SA 100-km team to compete in Winschoten at the World 100-km championships. Welcome would admit that, in terms of actual performance, he was probably one of the last selection options for the team as he only had a 2:34 marathon PB. Other team members such as Donovan Wright, Andrew Kelehe, Russell Crawford and Colin Thomas boasted much better performances at that distance. Welcome and I knew that he could run just under seven hours for the ten-lap 100 km if weather conditions were good, and therefore set a schedule for this. The weather on the day suggested that the time should be a bit slower due to heat. We made the adjustment and Welcome kept to the game plan. I was able to second him every 10 km and he was last in the SA team, right through to 85 km.

By comparison, Donovan Wright led the race under the world best pace until 70 km, with Andrew Kelehe not far behind in about fifth place overall. At 85 km I told Welcome to run as he pleased to the finish, and he was able to carve his way through the field over the last 15 km, overtaking all the other South Africans except Donovan Wright. Welcome ran the last 4 km of the race with Andrew Kelehe helping him to keep going as he was struggling to match the pace. A last-minute sprint gave Andrew a two-second lead on Welcome at the tape, and the team took third place for the bronze medal, but Welcome had shown the value of even-effort running. I like to think that this was a lesson Welcome had passed on to Andrew. Perhaps it wasn't a coincidence that Andrew went on to win Comrades for the first time in 2001, and anyone studying his pacing on that particular occasion will see a much-improved distribution of effort compared to his earlier gold medal performances in Comrades.

This is certainly not a one-off example. Consider an athlete such as Marietjie Montgomery who used the same tactics in the 1999 (France) and 2000 (Netherlands) World 100-km Championships, becoming the second veteran in the world in 2000 and achieving eleventh place in Comrades in 2001. Another example is Carol Mercer who used the same advice to become the first South African woman home in the 2001 Comrades, and had enough energy left to sprint past Grace de Oliveira on the finish track at Kingsmead. At that time Carol had never matched Grace's times in either the marathon or half-marathon, but good pacing strategy took her to the 'goal', and in fact we had predicted a time of 6:40. She finished in 6:40:59, and so failed to meet the target because she had run through Hillcrest just over a minute too fast – and not because she was slow to that point. The point is, you can only do what you want to do at the end of the race if you reserve your energy during the first three-quarters.

Gather all the information possible about the course beforehand. You should be able to anticipate the hills, the corners, what effect changing weather conditions might have, etc. Try to live the race before you run it, and ensure that you have planned it. Apart from a good pace strategy, planning gives confidence, and confidence is something every winner needs. A sports psychologist has noted that winners are athletes who think that they can win before the race starts, and that is the truth of the matter.

In the shorter races and over flattish courses, it is fairly easy to keep a relatively constant pace, and this will deliver an optimum time because it uses up energy at a constant rate. As with cars, it is acceleration that consumes fuel, thus even pacing (or effort) is generally the most efficient approach to racing.

It is interesting to note that virtually all the track world records and world bests set on the road from 1 500 m upwards, are currently set by running the second half of the race at the same or slightly faster pace than the first half. This is known as a negative split, and proves that starting easy, saving energy and building up pace towards the end is the way to achieve optimum times. If that is true for the elite athletes, you may confidently assume that those are the same principles you need to adopt to ensure your best performance.

COLLAPSE POINT

'Collapse point' is approximately three times the daily average; maximum racing distance should be slightly below the collapse point. 20 km is slightly less than 13 miles, while the half-marathon slightly more; 30 km is a little below 19 miles; 31 miles is about 50 km. By implication, therefore, to race 100 miles: weekly distance = 234 miles = 375 km = 54 km per day. Even at 5 minutes per km = 270 minutes i.e. four-and-a-half hours.

(Extract from *Step Up to Racing*, World Publications, 1975)

COLLAPSE POINT TABLE – HOW FAR CAN YOU GO?

WEEKLY TOTAL	PER DAY	'COLLAPSE'	MAX. RACE
10 miles	1½ miles	5 miles	3 miles
15 miles	2¼ miles	7 miles	5 miles
20 miles	3 miles	9 miles	6 miles
25 miles	3½ miles	11 miles	8 miles
30 miles	4¼ miles	13 miles	10 miles
35 miles	5 miles	15 miles	13 miles
40 miles	5¾ miles	17 miles	15 miles
45 miles	6½ miles	20 miles	19 miles
50 miles	7 miles	21 miles	19 miles
55 miles	7¾ miles	23 miles	20 miles
60 miles	8½ miles	26 miles	20 miles
65 miles	9¼ miles	28 miles	marathon
70 miles	10 miles	30 miles	marathon
75 miles	10¾ miles	32 miles	50 km
80 miles	11½ miles	34½ miles	56 km
85 miles	12¼ miles	37 miles	
90 miles	12¾ miles	39 miles	64 km
95 miles	13½ miles	41 miles	
100 miles	14¼ miles	43 miles	
110 miles	15¾ miles	47 miles	comrades
130 miles	18½ miles	56 miles	

The distance you can race depends on the distance you have been training. The above table illustrates the American rule of thumb that relates average weekly

EVERYONE'S GUIDE TO DISTANCE RUNNING

training distance to a collapse point, and hence to the maximum distance you should race. To run Comrades according to this approach, you would have to train about 190 km a week at peak times. This is a realistic figure for dedicated gold medallists, but for most of us it is an impossible weekly distance. There simply isn't enough time to recover. If you intend tackling a race with a distance beyond your collapse point, I suggest that you try a run-and-walk schedule.

In 1989 I was asked to give a talk at a club in Durban, where my run-walk theory was fairly well known as a result of my newspaper articles. The speaker before me was one of KwaZulu-Natal's women runners, who had run Comrades around the 7:30 mark for a few years. I was horrified at her advice to aspiring Comrades runners, 'Start off running and keep running until you can run no more, then walk until you can walk no more, and then crawl if necessary.'

It is obvious that the majority of runners do not (and cannot) train sufficiently to enable them to run Comrades non-stop. If they try to do so, at some stage they will be forced to walk, knowing that they have used up their energy, and they are condemned to shuffling painfully to the finish. Such an approach is like tramping down on the car accelerator until the tank is on reserve and then hoping blindly that there will be enough petrol left to take you to the end of the journey. Or it's similar to lifting too much weight all at once and then being unable to lift even the slightest load, whereas lifting a lesser weight allows you to lift the same weight several times over.

It is the same with running. If your fastest 400-m run is 65 seconds, and after a flat-out 65-second effort you tried to run another fast 400 m, you would either start cramping or slow down to 80 or 90 seconds at best. However, if you ran ten runs of 400 m at 70 seconds, with a short break in between, it would be easy.

This is the principle behind the run-walk theory and it works. Club runners have used it to achieve their best marathon times, let alone Comrades times. Moreover, I convinced three back runners to use it during a hilly 5-km event, in which they improved their times by around 50 seconds, while another runner I coached had two walks in a 10-km event to record a PB of 33:50.

If you review the above accounts of Carol Mercer, Marietjie Montgomery and Welcome Mteto, you will see that the key to their success was consistent effort, and in each case we worked out a run-walk schedule to achieve their goals.

EXAMPLE OF A RUN-WALK SCHEDULE FOR COMRADES USING 8 KM RUN PLUS 3-MINUTE WALK SPLITS

DISTANCE	TIME	DISTANCE	TIME
8	45 mins	48.275	4:40:18
8.275	48 mins	56	5:23:45
16	1:31:28	56.275	5:26:45
16.275	1:34:28	64	6:10:13
24	2:17:55	64.275	6:13:13
24.275	2:20:55	72	6:56:40
32	3:04:23	72.275	6:59:40
32.275	3:07:23	80	7:43:07
40	3:50	80.275	7:46:07
40.275	3:50	88	8:28:00
48	4:37:18		

$$\frac{\text{MARATHON DISTANCE}}{\text{BEST MARATHON}} = \frac{4 \text{ hr } 05 \text{ min}}{3 \text{ hr } 30 \text{ min}} = 126 \%$$

= 26 % slower than best marathon

LOGISTICS

After the effort of training, it's important not to leave logistical details to chance. Make your travel arrangements well before a major race, particularly if the race is in another city and you need to book a hotel room. If you'll be sleeping in a strange bed, it's preferable to take your own pillow, as others are never as comfortable as your own. Use a 'blindfold' and earplugs (the sort they provide on international flights) when sleeping, to ensure that light and noise do not disturb you. It's worth sleeping with both of these ahead of a race so that you're used to them. What about eating arrangements? Will you be able to enjoy your favourite pre-race meal wherever you are staying? Should you take food with you? If you intend eating out, make a restaurant booking, so you don't have to wait or find that it's fully booked. In short, try to maintain your normal schedule wherever you go. It will pay off.

Even if the race is local, logistics are still important. Ensure that you arrive with enough time to enter, have one last visit to the loo, and warm up and change for the race. Have you put out all your kit the night before? Is the entry fee ready? Do as much as possible the night before.

Finally, on the subject of sleeping, don't worry too much about a restless night before the race; rather, ensure a good sleep two nights before. Few runners sleep well immediately before a race, but many of them lie in bed worrying about it. This additional worry makes sleep less easy, and the vicious circle continues. If you find yourself unable to sleep, lie back in the knowledge that it is the excitement of the race that is making it hard to sleep. Remind yourself how well you slept the previous night. Accept that you might not sleep much and tell yourself that you can simply lie there and relax. When you remove the pressure, you will be surprised how quickly you fall asleep.

RACE DAY

Have a plan for race day. Know the route to the start. If you use the lift in the hotel, remember that there will probably be many other runners doing the same thing and that will take time. What about your position at the starting line? Do you know where you want to stand? All these things need to be planned.

Helen Lucre tells a marvellous story of her 1985 Comrades. Although she lived in Westville, she thought it best to stay at the Royal Hotel, Durban, the night before. The starting line was right outside the hotel and she reasoned that staying there would be the easiest way of ensuring a good position, yet still allow time to lie in late. All went well until the morning of the race, when she opted to use the fire escape rather than wait for the lifts, which were full of other runners. Out on the fire escape, the door closed behind her. A few flights down she tried to open the door to go back inside and found that it would not open from the outside. Panic! Luckily she found an open door into the kitchen, which ensured her freedom, although it gave the chefs a start. She reached the starting line in time and went on to win that Comrades, but it could have been very different.

As you can see, planning is vital. You must know beforehand whether you will need to eat and make sure that you have a bottle of water to take with you to the start. Check that the fire escape doors open!

ALL WE NEED IS SOME INCENTIVE

The driving force of which we speak is linked to your 'need' to compete and frequently results from some success-linked incentive (see also the following chapter on mental preparation).

For an endurance athlete, there can be little doubt that South Africa is one of the finest countries in the world for training and racing. Apart from the fact that the climate is extremely conducive to encouraging runners out each day, I also firmly believe that the return to international racing will eventually prove that we have the world's best at every distance from 10 km upwards. Not all of these runners have come to the fore as yet, but with the sort of talent that put 11 South Africans in the top 15 fastest 15-km runners in 1990, and a world best from Elana Meyer in 1991, the signs are there. And there are many more examples to substantiate this train of thought.

Countering this, however, is the fact that past isolation, to some extent, robbed many of the top runners of the incentive to really produce their true potential. After all, racing at major events was always against the same competition, and most had predictable tactics.

For instance, Matthews Temane was known to wait before using his kick, a tactic that he in turn passed on to his protégé, Adam Motlagale; while the 1991 15-km champion, Xolile Yawa, used surges and the Tsebe brothers used 'team' tactics to destroy the opposition. There were few dark horses to really create challenges. Is it possible that the reason the 10-km and 21.1-km records fell in 1989 was because Colleen de Reuck was challenged for the first time in some while by Elana Meyer (then Van Zyl). Prior to that Colleen had dominated unchallenged, and as we all know, it's easier to cruise to the finish if there is no-one to challenge you. This is not to say that Colleen, or other athletes, had consciously put in anything but a 100% effort, but the extra 10% that sets records alight comes from the incentive of a challenger.

For this reason I didn't believe that we had seen the best of Colleen or many of the other top athletes, and this view seems to be vindicated by results since South Africa returned to international competition. De Reuck and Meyer have both competed in the Olympics and World Championships at 10 000 m and the marathon, Joshua Thugwane won the Olympic Marathon in 1996, and set a new South African record of 2:07 for the marathon in 1997. Ezekiel Sepeng not only broke the long-standing SA 800-m record, but also 'medalled' in a number of top international competitions. Why the sudden upsurge in South African performances? I believe it was the greater challenges and incentives of international competition, be it for money or medals.

How does this affect the majority of runners? Incentive and challenge are the essential driving forces required to attain top performances. Incentives can be anything... money, trophies, silver medals, even prizes not connected to the race, as offered by family or friends. If you are aiming for a best performance in an event, let your family and friends become part of the challenge. It will also force you to make an open commitment of your goals, which encourages pride (to do what you have said you will), and that, in itself, can be a great driving force. In addition, it involves these people in your sport and brings greater empathy from them regarding the time you spend in training. You find you are competing with them as your support team, and success or failure is something to be shared.

No matter how long the race, if you are running to your potential, you have to bite the bullet over the last quarter. In a 10-km race, this is only for 6–10 minutes, in a marathon it's up to six miles or about one hour, in 100 miles... it can seem forever! The support gained from friends, the need to run for them, desire for that incentive, the 'prize' – all of these keep you going.

Another way to improve your chances of realising your ambitions is to select other runners who you know will run around the time you are aiming for, and then set out to beat them. An evenly matched training partner is a good target, but it can also be a runner who is consistently just ahead of you over your target distance. It's probably safer to pick a few of these runners, in case they decide not to run your target race. Your 'incentive' could then be to beat one or more of these runners. When the 'going gets tough', you can draw on your competitive element to push you on – you have someone 'special' to pass. Planned carefully, this should also give you your personal best time.

Possibly the best-recorded use of this principle is Roger Bannister's attack on the four-minute mile. Training and racing in a highly competitive group assisted him through the historic barrier. Also of interest is the fact that, despite everyone saying it was impossible, once it had been achieved, the four-minute barrier was broken a number of times in the following few months. This reinforces the view that often, it is our belief in our ability to do something, or our perceptions of what is possible and impossible, that determine our ability on the day.

These strategies must be planned in the same way that you plan your training to peak at the race. Set your incentives, challenges and goals weeks in advance and then visualise and live your success during your training. Come the race, the stimulus, your correct training and the rewards of the 'win' will carry you through the 'darkness of the last quarter'. The motivation of large cash payouts, international competition, appearance money and recognition resulted in the highest number of runners breaking seven hours in a single 100-km race in Stellenbosch in 1989. It also resulted in a world best. Similar 'prizes' have resulted in many new South African records over the years, and have caused major upsets in many Olympics. The rewards may not be the same, but use of incentives and competition can take you to your goals. If you can dream your goal, you have every chance of living it.

Now you are ready to race. You have planned your training with a set goal, as well as intermediate goals along the way. You have trained – concentrating on your weaknesses – with an eye on the specific requirements of the challenge. You know the time for which you are aiming, you know the game plan you will use during the race, you know how you are travelling to the race, and you are mentally attuned and prepared for the challenge... it's in the bag! You are reliving it all. The race is the easy part — good luck!

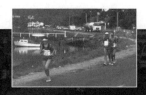

I am convinced that the difference between a win and second place, between achieving a goal and failing, is the mental attitude of the competitor. If you think something will go wrong, you can be sure it will. As a lecturer I believe that many students only reach the level their teachers expect them to reach, i.e. they sense the lecturer's assessment of their abilities and live up (or down) to them. If you know your coach does not think you are ready for a race, you are unlikely to do well.

YOU CAN DO IT – THE 'SECRET' IS HERE

Television is full of 'infomercials' that offer time- and mind-management packages that will 'change your life' – let you achieve your dreams, become prosperous and – that's not all – provide the 'heavenly' existence for which you long. Ironically, these are some of the few such commercials that really can and do work. Not because they offer anything revolutionary, but rather because they communicate the basic principles of a sound development strategy, with stepping stones to take you to your goal. With this you 'condition' your mind and attitude into a 'can – do' attitude, where you start to realise that your chosen goal is achievable.

I have seen it happen to athletes I have coached, irrespective of their standard. A woman who had battled with an 11-hour Comrades and was considered a poor runner by her local running group, approached me for advice. We decided on a totally different approach to the traditional training she had experienced with the group. We built a 'ladder' to her goals with small steps between each 'rung'. Less than a year later, she had achieved marathon times that surprised many of her previous running partners, completed a long-term goal of running a 100-miler, changed her body shape, and discovered a completely new confidence. Gone are the days when she timidly ran around the track, moving to the outer lanes when inconsiderate 'top' runners stood talking in the lane in which she was training. Now she considers herself worthy of equal rights and gives the track etiquette signal to move runners out the way. She hasn't reached the top of her ladder yet, but she has also realised that the ladder can take her to even greater heights than she imagined possible, simply with a realistic strategy and step-by-step approach – no hidden formulas, no secret approach, just logic and a building of self-belief.

Appropriate to my Scots 'heritage', I will save you the cost of those mind- and time-management packages. If you have followed the concepts and steps outlined in this book, you will already be building a realistic ladder to your running goal. This will give you confidence as you climb the ladder, and you will achieve your goal. What follows in this chapter will assist you to keep your goals in focus.

Here's the candid concept. There is no difference between the approach used to improving your athletic achievements and the approach you need to improve any other aspect of your life or business.

> ▸ Determine what you really want.
> ▸ Identify where you are now.
> ▸ Identify the small steps needed to achieve your goal.
> ▸ Focus on each step, one at a time.
> ▸ Eliminate things that distract you from achieving your goal.
> ▸ Keep reminding yourself of how good it will feel and why you want the end
>   goal, how it will improve your life and see yourself living that new life.

There are many ways of communicating these simple steps to people and that is what you pay for in those packages. We already know what we need to do. Usually, the biggest problem is that we want too much at once, and the clutter confounds a focused approach. In running terms, this is the confusion and temptation to which we subject ourselves each year by wanting to RACE Two Oceans, Comrades and a host of other events. Choose one at a time and you have a chance to achieve it.

I could name a number of athletes who never thought they stood a chance at provincial or national colours when they first commenced a structured programme. However, they had to sacrifice some events along the way, but now they are much happier with their achievements. Remember: winners make it happen, losers simply let it happen. Be a winner, you owe it to yourself to live your dreams.

POSITIVE ATTITUDE AND CONFIDENCE

Building a positive attitude towards your goal is an important objective throughout your training. This does not mean being unrealistic, but it does mean casting aside unfounded doubts and concentrating on your strengths. The concept I discussed earlier of building a ladder to success is the key to building a positive attitude. As each short-term goal is achieved, your confidence will increase.

The same applies during a race when you have worked out a realistic pacing strategy. As you pass each kilometre or landmark as planned, your confidence grows, and with each boost of confidence, the goal becomes ever more achievable, often leading to an even greater performance by the end of the race.

WHAT STOPS US?

As mentioned, clutter and a desire to achieve too many things at once can block your progress, but there is another complicating matter. We often have preconceived ideas of what we are able to achieve, based on our past experiences and sometimes even on the opinion of others. If we believe we are only capable of running 42 minutes for 10 km, it is highly unlikely that we will run under that time. We may even run the first 7 km at a pace that would result in a 41-minute 10 km, but if we look at our watch at 7 km and suddenly realise that we are on track for a personal best by one minute, it can result in a dramatic slowing down so that we finish in 42 minutes – AS WE KNEW WE WOULD. Sometimes it's worth running short events without a watch, or time and speed feedback, once a realistic pace is established.

Golfers often have the same experience when they play a great first nine holes, add up their cards and are surprised how well it has gone. Almost invariably, the second nine holes will take them back to their normal handicap. As discussed previously, the same mental 'block' prevented people from running sub-four-minute miles until Roger Bannister proved that it was possible.

At school I was always last in the 100-yard dash and last around the rugby field. Even my first 7:09 Comrades 'showed' me that I had endurance and not speed. After Richard Turnbull, a past coach of Willie Mtolo and Matthews Temane, suggested that I did have speed as well, I eventually started to believe it. Once I 'knew' that I had far more speed than I had previously thought, my times over the shorter distances went down. Even as I moved into the veterans' category (40 plus), I recorded times that were better than those I had managed when I was years younger. I believe that when I relinquish the longer distances to concentrate on the shorter distances, I will be even faster (age related) because I not only have speed, but also believe that I have it. It was my attitude that slowed me down in the past. I may not set any records, but I can still improve my relative times, and that will make running worthwhile.

Act your goal

People often comment that top sportspeople are arrogant, but it is difficult to draw a line between their self-belief and confidence, and the modesty the public expects. Because a sportsman needs to believe that he can win before he wins, it often comes across the 'wrong' way. If you ask runners in public how good they are, you will often receive a non-committal answer, as they try to dodge the question. Alternatively, they may downplay their ability, not wanting to appear 'cocksure', but are actually doing themselves a great disservice as they are preprogramming their own minds with a performance lower in standard than they wish to achieve.

If you want to be a silver medallist in Comrades, act and behave like a silver medallist. Walk, talk, eat and sleep like a silver medallist, not like someone who can't break 3:15 for the marathon, because if you do, that is all you will achieve.

Budding millionaires and successful business people exude that aura of what they want to be, before they actually achieve their goals. You can tell when someone is going to be successful in their business venture; they have passion, excitement and confidence as they discuss their plans and progress. Feel the same about your athletic goals. Use your training stepping stones to build your confidence, recognise your own progress and act the part.

Reset the thermostat

This refers to the 'thermostat' at the back of your mind that tells you what it thinks you can and can't do. You must programme that thermostat to reflect what you want to achieve. It can easily be done in two ways: firstly by completing a series of training sessions that physiologically prove you are ready to close in on the desired goal, and secondly by visualising yourself achieving that goal. Obviously, in both cases the desired goal must be realistic.

Visualisation

The technique of visualisation is used by top sportspeople. A sports psychologist who interviewed a number of sporting greats found that virtually all had the ability to imagine themselves competing in events beforehand. They would see themselves sinking a putt, putting away a backhand smash or running a four-minute mile. It's worth trying.

In road running it is necessary to visualise exactly what you intend doing when you come to a hill, how to handle the race and, most importantly, how you feel as you see yourself crossing the line within your target time. Do this in two formats. Firstly, see yourself running the event from 'outside' as a spectator watching the race. How do you look? How smooth is your stride? How is your pace? Is your breathing controlled? Secondly, go through the whole race again, but this time look through your own eyes, as if you are actually running the race in your own body. See the road ahead, the runner ahead and alongside, 'feel' yourself reaching for the water sachet from the table, biting it and drinking.

Don't shy away from the vision of things going wrong – the shoelace that is coming undone, your temptation to speed up when you know you shouldn't, the onset of sore muscles. Take each one in turn, stop the 'film', consider the corrective options, then rerun the 'film' with your chosen solutions. Each time you consider a potential problem you are being realistic, and by providing a solution you are solving it for the race day. In fact, you are eliminating a number of unforeseen items with which you'll be faced. Eventually, the race simply becomes déjà vu.

Relaxation

The best time for mental preparation or training is when you are relaxed. Relaxation is a skill that we often need to be taught, and there are several 'standard' introductory methods.

One typical method involves using a quiet and dimly lit room: sit or lie down in a comfortable position without legs or arms crossed, and alternatively tense and release your muscles – starting from the feet and moving up the body until you focus on the muscles in your neck and face. The protocols also concentrate on the rate of breathing and heart rate; a heart-rate monitor or other means of monitoring the status of your body is useful. (Such machines are termed biofeedback machines and are available in a variety of forms.) Once in a relaxed state, commence your mental training. Different people will find different methods more amenable to their lifestyles and you should read up further on this subject. The principles here are exactly the same for developing other aspects of your life – once you have mastered the techniques of mental training, they will prove invaluable in everyday situations.

At the end of this chapter, there is an introduction to one of the more technical methods to induce relaxation, which, because of the relatively strong link between sport and sound, may appeal to sportspeople.

Desire

It is claimed that we use only a fraction of our mental ability and that it is our mental view of ourselves which restricts our physical ability. I firmly believe this, and need only relate the story of the mother who lifted a truck with one hand to free her trapped son to show what our bodies can do if the desire and drive are great enough.

No matter what the event, an element of self-doubt can creep in while you are 'racing'; desire is the attribute that will take you through that wall. The desire to achieve the goal is the difference between making it or not, in many circumstances. The reason for that desire actually isn't important, or necessarily logical, but it is the catalyst to the force that drives you to keep moving towards the goal.

When preparing for a race, you need to identify that desire clearly in your own mind so that you can focus on it and 'feed' from it when necessary. However, you have to be careful that what starts as a desire does not become an overburdening stress, adding pressure to your goal. There is a subtle difference between something you WANT to do and something that you feel you MUST do. Wanting is an internal, positive ambition, whereas something you must do, tends to be a negative, external pressure that you impose upon yourself because you feel, for some reason, that it is expected.

Often focusing on the end goal for too long can turn desire into negative pressure. It is important to realise that there is a limit to your concentration span; to focus on one goal for months on end can become detrimental, as it can result in unbearable anxiety by the time the event occurs. You need to balance desire and anxiety. Intermediate goals and stepping stones help to keep this in perspective.

Moving from being a good club runner, to a provincial runner, to a national runner is a progression that can promote confidence and foster desire. Ultimately, the end goal is international competition, but each stepping stone provides a reassuring boost that keeps the desire alive, yet provides sufficient distraction and reward to control your motivation.

If you have seen *Chariots of Fire*, you will remember the scene in the changing-room after Harold Abrahams won the 100-m gold medal. He had spent years building to that goal. One of his team-mates wanted to congratulate him and give him champagne but others stopped him, saying that Harold should be left alone because he had just won a gold medal.

This might have seemed odd to some, but I didn't find it strange at all. When you aim for something such as a major win, your whole life becomes directed towards it. When desire is at a positive peak, it seems that achieving your goal is the only way to ensure another sunrise, that there is nothing more important in the world at that stage. However, as soon as you achieve it, you experience a sense of anticlimax that can be very hard to bear. It brings the realisation that, in fact, the sun would still have risen the following day, that it wouldn't have been an earth-shattering loss had you failed. It returns your perspective to normal. At the critical time, though, it was that exclusive focus and mental determination that made the difference between a good effort and the special 110% race. That is the power of desire. Desire and incentive are inseparable – it is the reward of achievement, what you perceive the changes will be for you when you achieve the goal that fuels your desire. Defining your incentive is important in developing desire.

DESIRE AND CONFIDENCE VERSUS PAIN

Every runner who attempts to push the envelope of his ability, experiences the tussle of pain and success, or comfort and failure. In many respects, it is the desire to test ourselves against this mental battle that entices us to enter races. Although it is evident at all distances from track upwards, it is more pronounced in longer events, particularly ultraraces.

Every ambitious Comrades runner wanting to achieve his potential, experiences a point in the race where pain dogs every footfall. There is no injury, it is simply the muscle damage of the previous kilometres. It is unchanging in intensity, and to continue, the mind must accept this 'sentence' of pain until the finish line is crossed. Ultimately, your ability to meet this pain 'head to head' will determine your performance in the race. If you grab it by the scruff of the neck and toss it out of your mind with the contempt it deserves, you will achieve your goals and possibly even exceed our expectations. If it becomes the focus of your existence at that time, if you permit it to erode the importance of the task at hand, you will compromise your goal or finish time. Every Youth Day in June, the road between Pietermaritzburg and Durban is littered with runners who have trained to be capable of a sub-nine-hour Bill Rowan medal, but eventually walk away with a 'compromised' bronze. The same can be said of every time slot in the Comrades, although it is probably more prolific between the eight- and 11-hour potential finishers.

The ability to 'override' pain is often inconsistent. In the case of Andrew Kelehe, it was claimed that he was fitter in 2002 than he was in his victorious year of 2001. Why in 2002 (5:45), did he fail to achieve a time comparable to his 2001 finish of 5:25? Even allowing for an extra 6–10 minutes (some believe the down-run to be this much faster), Andrew did not match his statistical potential. Yet we know he has the capability to be a champion. He had previously beaten almost every 2002 finisher ahead of him, so he could not have been 'overshadowed' by the competition. However, in 2001 Andrew ran in memory of his daughter and that was his 'driving' force. Perhaps his drive in 2002 was not an emotional one.

The three-quarter distance mark in long races is what I call the 'what am I doing this for?' mark. It is where physical fatigue meets mental muscle in a duel for supremacy. Why is it possible for the same runner to conquer this section of the race on some occasions, yet submit to some degree on others, even though it is the same event with similar competition?

Although I have no medical background, I find these aspects intriguing and, after discussion with other athletes, personal experience and reading, I have evolved an explanation and a way to prepare athletes for this tussle. I feel there are two describable attributes, which, when combined, are instrumental in determining how a runner will handle the situation.

Because 'desire' is an emotional attribute, based on the 'state of mind' of an athlete, it seems to me to be a measure of how much he wants to achieve his goal. Levels of desire may be influenced by the pure emotion of wanting to prove a point, or by major prize money, which can change standards of living, wanting to beat a particular competitor, or survival. The mother pulling her child from beneath a vehicle is an extreme example, in which survival was the driving force. In such cases, performances can far exceed the bounds of normal physical expectation. Her normal physical parameters were overridden by her 'desire' for the child to survive. Desire tends to be from the 'heart' and can reflect the emotion of the event for the runner. While it is possible to cultivate a level of desire, it is a volatile attribute that may be triggered by momentary changes in circumstance.

The second attribute is confidence. On entering a race you have a perception of your potential finishing time. In many cases, it can be fairly accurately predicted from previous statistics and your performances at other distances. In this respect confidence is more of a physical aspect that can be built up or eroded through analysis and comparison. Confidence is generally less volatile, and realistic levels are normally achieved through the analytical processes. Although a minimal amount of overconfidence can lead to exceptional performance, extreme overconfidence often leads to a below-par performance as you cease to have the physical attributes to support the expectations. For instance, it is not unreasonable for a 3:45 marathoner to expect a Bill Rowan (sub-nine-hour) in Comrades, but you would be exceptionally overconfident to think yourself capable of a silver medal (sub-7:30). In fact, if you run in search of silver, your end performance is likely to be far below both the silver and the Bill Rowan performances.

The four-quadrant graph on the following page illustrates the proposed relationship between desire and confidence for runners in distance events. It plots the likelihood that a runner who lines up in the correct physical condition to achieve a particular goal will survive the 'pain period' to achieve that goal. The darker the area, the more likely the runner is to reach the goal. It assumes that the pain experienced is fatigue-related and, as such, remains relatively constant.

Even if these assessments are correct, what impact do they have? Understanding these parameters is important for the coach and athlete, as techniques such as relaxation and visualisation may be used to improve confidence and desire. But there is also a message for race organisers: if they want to attract large fields of runners in long events, several levels of 'incentive' are needed, otherwise too many of the runners find themselves in 'no-man's land' without a realistic opportunity of

DESIRE AND CONFIDENCE – THE ABILITY TO ACHIEVE

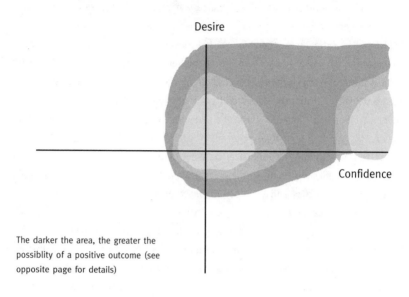

Desire

Confidence

The darker the area, the greater the possiblity of a positive outcome (see opposite page for details)

achieving the next level. For instance, a 4:10 marathoner is effectively stuck in an abyss between the 3:42 marathon required for the Bill Rowan Comrades medal and the 4:30 marathon that signifies a battle with the gun. If, however, a medal or incentive was introduced into Comrades for a ten-hour finish, these runners would find new zest to ensure they dropped under 9:59! In late 2002, Comrades Marathon organisers took the decision to reintroduce a 12-hour cut off for the Comrades Marathon, to open the challenge up to a bigger field. After the massive field of 24 000 runners that entered the 2000 'Millennium' Comrades (extended as a 'one-off' to 12 hours), entry numbers dropped to 12 000–15 000, which many put done to the fact that few people are confident of achieving an 11-hour finish. As a result, a new medal was introduced for 11–12 hour finishers and the qualifying time extended to five hours for the marathon. This will undoubtedly see not only a growth in Comrades, but also marathons and the sport as a whole. Similar splits can be identified for the marathon and 56-km races. Ultimately, a runner wanting to achieve a personal best must have either the confidence to achieve it or the desire. If you have both, you can move the world!

Where confidence is negative and desire is low or negative:

Here the runner simply goes through the physical motions and the chances of reaching true potential is minimal, as there is no real desire to reach it, and no belief that the goal is achievable.

Where desire is low or negative but confidence in ability is positive:

Low or negative levels of desire indicate that the runner is doing the event for some ulterior reason, perhaps having been committed by a club, coach, parent or school, or forced into a qualifier, or for social aspects after the event. As long as the runner's confidence level relates to a realistic performance, and levels of desire are virtually non-committal, there is some chance of relative success. However, at all other lower levels of desire, success is unlikely.

Where desire is positive or high but confidence is lacking or negative:

A slight lack of confidence may be an asset in some long events as it can result in a more conservative start and hence better pacing. For this reason, when combined with good desire, it can provide the required result. However, the basic principle that if you don't believe you can achieve something, you will have a problem reaching the necessary performance level, remains true.

When there is both positive desire and confidence:

This is the most exciting area and, as these attributes increase in strength, the potential performance level also increases, but guard against over-confidence as it can also cause a drop in performance. High levels of desire can result in exceptional performances.

ANXIETY

The subtle change from wanting to do something, to being forced to do it, takes positive energy and turns it into sour, negative energy. Our perceptions of what others expect us to achieve puts unnecessary pressure on us. If you look back at

Bruce Fordyce's reign as Comrades champion, each year the media would list him as the favourite, months before the race. Imagine the potential pressure of that. I recall listening to several interviews with Bruce over the years, and how each year he would identify his potential challengers. This not only acknowledged the talents of other runners, which promoted Bruce's public image as 'Mr. Nice Guy', but also deflected some of the pressure away from himself. But make no mistake, Bruce entered those races, not only with the desire to win, but also with the sacrifices and the planning that would give him the optimum chance of achieving his goal.

In comparison, in the 1980s, the very talented Danny Biggs commenced most years by stating that he wanted to win Comrades. In many ways Danny possibly had more physiological 'talent' than Bruce, but I think his main failing was the pressure he put on himself with his statements. Danny was not an arrogant man, but he believed he needed to state his intention to win. Perhaps in doing so, he crossed the bridge between doing for his desire and carrying his perception of what others expected of him. Thus, it isn't always what others expect of you, but rather what you think they expect of you.

Tackle goals because it's what you desire, not what others desire. When I first consider taking on new athletes, I ask them what their goals are. I am often asked what I think they can do and after discussion, I give them some alternatives. Some will ask what I think they should do, and I refuse to tell them. Quite simply, no-one can, or has the right, to give another sportsperson a goal. All you can do is show them the opportunities and listen to what they, in their hearts, want to do. Sometimes they opt for the 'wrong' decision, but they will achieve more by going with the wrong option than they ever would following someone else's 'right' option.

The balance between desire and anxiety is often described as an inverted U graph. If you are too far to the left, you have too little desire or arousal. If you are too far to the right you have too much arousal or pressure. The ideal is to be in the crown of the curve where the arousal is maximised in a positive way. Become aware of your feelings before events, and how much arousal is comfortable.

The optimum level of arousal will differ with race distance and individual. Normally, you should be more excited before a short event than a long event. As coach Sam said in *Chariots of Fire*, a sprint is run on nerves. Distance and ultra-distance is run calmly, with the head.

EVERYONE'S GUIDE TO DISTANCE RUNNING

THE PERFECT PERFORMANCE

Just as we have perceptions of what other people expect of us, we also have perceptions of what other athletes will do when they line up against us. This is one of the major pressures that athletes inflict on themselves. Instead of concentrating on our own race, we concern ourselves with other athletes in the event.

In the 2001 Spar Ladies Race in Cape Town, Elana Meyer only entered the day before the event. There is a group of 'elite' runners who always travels to the Spar series events, and a number of these women were annoyed because Elana had entered late. Clearly, it was going to upset the 'elite' athletes' mindset of who would win, come second and so on. There was nothing illegal about Elana's entry, the race is open to all, so why did these runners put such unnecessary pressure on themselves?

Carl Lewis gave me one of the most impressive and worthwhile concepts for racing attitude. He said he and his coach always pursued the perfect performance. They analysed the requirements of an event, what the perfect race should be from start to finish, and went in search of that. He relates the time he won his first Olympic medal. His coach shouted, 'You never left the blocks properly.' No congratulations, but a critical comment on his performance. He wasn't being derogatory, quite the opposite, he was saying 'there's more to come, you can do even better'. If you focus on your own perfect performance you will beat the people you want to beat and achieve what you can. Don't worry about who is in the race, simply race to your perfect performance. Too many runners try to outsmart the opposition with second-guessing tactics. Rather focus on how you can achieve your fastest time and the rest will take care of itself. Tactics only come into play in the final section, but you have to reach it with energy to spare to play that game.

Following on the comparison between Bruce Fordyce and Danny Biggs in Comrades, a look at past footage will show you that Danny frequently ran in the same bus as Bruce during Comrades. Presumably, he felt that this tactic would take him close to the finish with Bruce and then all he had to do was outsprint him. That was impossible in a long event, unless Danny was running so far below his potential to be jogging. Instead, it played right into Bruce's hand. When Bruce went through a bad patch all he had to do was slow the pace and the pack of runners with him would also slow the pace, thinking it was the right thing to do. On the other hand, in the last third of the race, if any of the followers showed signs of weakness or a bad patch, Bruce could simply ease the pace up and the stragglers would fall off the back. Who knows what might have happened if some of these talented runners had simply run their own perfect races.

LIGHT AND SOUND MACHINES

The use of light and sound as a means of mental stimulation has been around for a long time. Many moviemakers use it to take the spectator into the atmosphere and feeling of a plot. *Chariots of Fire* used music to stimulate the power of the runner and the patriotism of the challenge. This has become a traditional anthem of Comrades, even although it is over 20 years since the film was launched. Alfred Hitchcock used sound and light to good effect in his great thrillers. The combination of sound and strobe lights in discos and concerts were used to create different levels of arousal or calm in the 'psychedelic' 1960s and '70s. The rhythm of music and the pulsation or flicker of light can revitalise or calm the rhythm of the mind.

It has taken a while for psychological training in sport to be accepted, although most people (including scientists) agree that it is probably the area in sport with the greatest potential for progress. We already know that often it is our 'internal' doubt or disbelief in our abilities that restricts us to a lower level of achievement.

One of the greatest difficulties in advancing psychological training, is that many people are unwilling to admit or promote the subject, for fear of being branded mentally unstable. Sports psychology has gained ground, but only on a superficial level as far as the 'weekend warrior' or club competitor is concerned. Some competitors are aware of the benefits of relaxation, and perhaps even visualisation, prior to a match, and most know that it is beneficial to maintain a positive attitude. But the techniques to facilitate these states are almost a mystery. To most, relaxation means lying down at peace, or listening to some music on a Walkman.

Although available for some time, light and sound machines (mind machines) were expensive and cumbersome. Recently, smaller, more affordable machines came onto the market. Typically, they have a number of preprogrammed sessions so that a novice user can understand the principles from the outset. Programmes such as Athletic Warm-up, Visualisation, Maintaining Peak Competitive Posture and Body Mind Awareness are all directly relevant to sportspeople.

A machine normally comprises the central unit, a set of headphones, a set of glasses (not dissimilar to the running frames used by Nike) with four LED lights on each lens, and a cord for connection into your CD or hi-fi system. There may also be specific CDs or tapes varying from relaxation to learning languages. In normal mode, a user wears both the glasses and the headphones and is presented with synchronised pulsating light and sound. The frequency and brightness of these can be varied by controls on the machine.

In an experiment carried out by a Dr Thomas of Alberta in the USA, a control group was asked to relax and visualise a tranquil scene for 15 minutes. Simultaneously, another group was subjected to sound and light from a mind machine set to a frequency of 10 Hz for the same time. Comparisons were made in skin temperature, muscle tension and EMG readings. The control group said that they felt relaxed, but their muscle tension actually increased. By comparison, the 'sound and light' group not only reduced muscle tension, but continued to feel the effects for significant periods afterwards.

Most runners know that if they run in a group, all will tend towards the same cadence of foot strike. This is similar to the approach adopted for mental training using sound and light machines. When the frequency is set below the 'normal active' range, the tendency is for the brain's activity level to reduce to a matching frequency. Similarly, set the light and sound frequency to a higher level and the brain frequency also appears to escalate, to 'get in step'. This is referred to as brain entrainment. Not all areas of the brain operate at the same frequency simultaneously. Using the principles of brain entrainment, it is claimed to be possible to even out the frequency and make the brain more susceptible to creative and intuitive processes.

This is clearly an agility skill of the brain and, like other skills, becomes easier to do the more often you practise. As such, there are people who find it easy to achieve without a machine, presumably because they know how to recreate a 'feeling'. The novice, however, has no idea of the feeling he needs to duplicate, so the machine assists in accessing those frequency levels.

Different frequencies are associated with different activities and benefits. Our normal waking frequency is 13 Hz and above, called Beta. Between 12 and 8 Hz is the pleasant relaxed state of Alpha. At this level, we are calm but fully alert. Theta is from 7 Hz to 5 Hz and is the dreaminess we all experience before falling asleep. It is thought to be the zone in which, theoretically, we are most susceptible to behavioural change and learning. Delta is the level from 4 Hz and below during which time you are asleep. As you move up the frequency levels from 13 Hz, there is an alignment with traditional Indian chakras or energy centres: 16.5Hz – base chakra, 18.5 Hz – genital chakras, 19.2 Hz – solar plexus chakras, 22.0 Hz – heart chakras, and so on. It must be noted, however, that the frequencies above 17 Hz have been associated with seizures in photosensitive epileptics and should be terminated if there is any feeling of nausea.

How can this help the athlete?

The state of mind prior to competition (and training) can affect the level of performance. Ideally you should be at a level of 'arousal' and self-belief that gives confidence and control. Too low an arousal results in a 'lack of interest' when things are tough, too high results in tension that prevents the fluid movement of an optimum performance. What is too low or too high is an individual characteristic, of which you need to become aware (see desire and anxiety above).

One of the easiest ways to control the arousal level is by relaxation and focus. Using a light and sound machine such as an Orion will assist you in discovering your optimum level of relaxation and enable you to lock into that level of arousal.

Experience with some athletes has shown the following procedure to be useful – the initial setting is around 14 Hz (normal daily frequencies). Once your brain has 'engaged' to the machine for approximately five minutes, reduce the frequency gradually to 8–10 Hz. After a period of restful quiet, you may gradually increase it to a level of arousal appropriate to the type of competition.

We have identified that the first stage of visualisation is to reach a restful state of mind that will allow you to visualise. To achieve this, you will probably need to reduce the frequency of the sound-light machine down gradually to the 5–7-Hz level. Another area in which I have seen the Orion successfully applied, is in assisting an anxious athlete to sleep – the frequency level is gradually reduced towards the 4-Hz rate. This may include short periods in the other 'zones'.

These are by no means the only benefits of mind machines. There is significant scientific evidence to show that they can improve learning levels. Not only does it help repetition (rote) learning, but also increases the ability to apply learning to new problems and situations, and most impressively, the ability to take these concepts and extrapolate them into new and creative solutions. Experimentation suggests that the Alpha (8–12 Hz zone) is best for learning new facts or data that is required in the waking consciousness, whereas Theta (4–6 Hz zone) is more suitable for behavioural changes or those that you want to activate subconsciously.

In exercise, the physiological responses are said to continue hours after exercise has ceased. Similarly with mind machines, the effects continue; reading, studying and music can be most rewarding in the period after a session. Coaches may want to experiment with their athletes, trying a brief sortie into the Alpha or Theta zone prior to a session that introduces highly technical skills or new drills.

Whether to learn before or after a session will depend on the type of learning that you want to achieve. Simple rote learning where information is required for quick or short-term recall can be studied before a session. More complex concepts and learning are best achieved in the relaxed, synchronised, after-burn, using post-session learning.

It's only a starting point

This is by no means a complete summary of the opportunities and benefits that can accrue from mind training. It is purely an introduction to some practical experiences. Using such machines has reinforced my belief that our greatest improvements in sports performance are likely to come from improved manipulation and training of the mind. It is up to you to explore these opportunities and experiment with them.

FINALLY

Hopefully, all of the above has given you a taste of some of the mental preparation skills available. There are many techniques for accomplishing the correct balance of confidence, belief, arousal and focus – what is presented here is merely a glimpse and a starting point. However, no matter what you do, the key is to base it on something that is within realistic expectations. If you have followed the complete procedure of goal setting, phased training, basic training concepts, planning, nutrition, logistic preparation, pacing strategy, and covered all the bases, you are already 99% of the way to your goal. Race day becomes only the last small hurdle.

PART 4:

NUTRITION FOR HEALTH AND SP

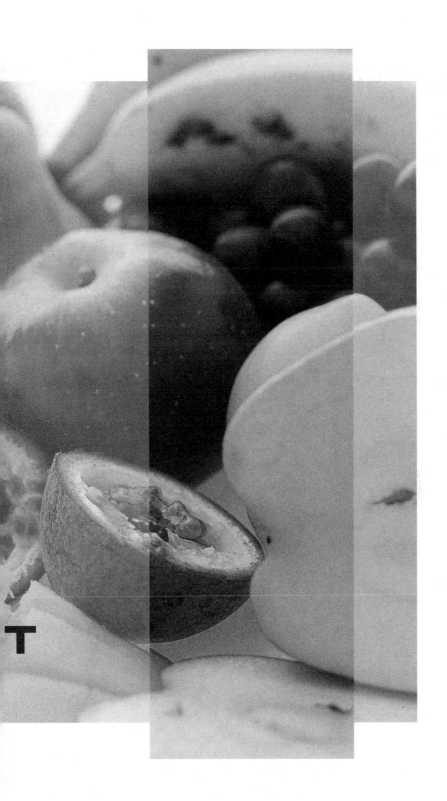

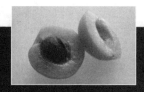

All too often we become aware of nutrition when something goes wrong. Only when we feel tired, ill or decide that we are too thin or too fat does 'eating' transform itself into the more scientific sounding term 'nutrition'.

Part of the reason for this is the marketing and promotion that goes into many of the food and sweet products on the market. Most food marketing is about taste, and revolves around the lifestyle associated with eating a product, rather than the actual content or benefits of the product.

We're all aware that we need energy to make it through the day, and you have no doubt discovered that certain foods give you a lift, so you reinforce this belief by eating or drinking them daily. Some of these energy 'lifts' are real, some short-lived, some can even be psychological, but you repeat the ones that taste good or make you feel good.

There is a reasonable probability that males are worse than females in this random selection of edible products, which relates to a general cultural trend for women to prepare the main meals of the day for her family. The modern lifestyle, which often sees both partners following a career, together with technological advances in foods and 'in-your face' advertising of fast/convenience foods, mitigates against the selection of a well-balanced eating plan. That doesn't mean that wives or mothers care any less care about what is prepared, but rather that they are presented (deliberately?) with a more confusing marketplace, less time, and even pressure from the children or adults to adopt trends that the marketing and promotional people have cleverly established as 'healthy norms'. The traditional 'meat and two veg' as the mainstay of three well-balanced daily meals is probably something few families can maintain throughout a normal week.

In many cases the description 'healthy eater' is used in relation to the quantity eaten rather than the quality, and may even refer to the size of a person, not the food selection. For many people, lunch is nothing more than a compromise as the days of staff canteens, luncheon vouchers, and even taking a lunch break, have diminished in the rush and bustle of commercial life. Such 'luxuries' have tended to become the reserve of civil services and major corporates. Other workers often have no choice other than fast-food outlets, or the nearby corner grocery store, or a 'snack' between meetings. Too few office workers take a mental and physical break from their desks, as the pressures of unrelenting e-mail, fast-track projects, deadlines and even ambition, have extended office hours beyond the standard 8:30 to 4:30 with an hour for lunch and two 15 minute breaks. Forget what the rulebook says, making progress means completing the job, NOW. It's even worse for the small businessperson, who can gain or lose a business opportunity in the time it takes to have a cup of tea and a sandwich.

Although we eat for energy and, socially, for enjoyment, most people's consideration of the overall nutritional balance is not as detailed as it was in years past. An interesting aspect to 'normal' eating trends is the fairly restricted nature and regularity of the range of foods that any one person eats. If you make a list of the foods that you consume in any given week, and list all the foods from another week, a month later, you will find that the overall intake is very similar and represents a relatively small selection. This, of course, excludes people who are involved in extensive entertaining or socialising. Even when offered a wide-ranging menu, most people will revert to their 'favourite' meals rather than try something new or varied.

A further change that has affected eating habits is the quality of our food. We are constantly bombarded by media coverage of another new technology that allows a larger crop to be produced from the same soil, or a new spray or dip that enlarges a fruit, or a new system for batch-rearing chickens or pigs. The problems of population increase, drought, famine and even the simple commercial interest of increased profit, force the focus on quantity of production.

Given these changes in lifestyle and production, the nutritional value of the average person's 'eating' has been compromised. These are not major changes, but subtle ones. It is easy to obtain sufficient 'energy' (kilojoules/kilocalories) from eating and relatively easy to take in a 'suitable' amount of protein and carbohydrate for a normal lifestyle, but it becomes harder to find the correct balance of micronutrients needed to match the extended lifespan that medicine and technology offer us.

These small daily or weekly depletions, combined with the loading of 'pollutants' and ingestion of artificial components such as preservatives, colourings, pesticides and hormone 'debris' from sprays and dips, can all affect us over a long period. A gradual reduction of a vitamin or mineral may lead to its depletion over a period of a month, a year or several years. Such depletion will result in one or more of several possible symptoms that can only be reversed by bringing the body's level of the vitamin or mineral back to 'normal' (whatever that is deemed to be).

It is this hypothesis that has spawned the mammoth industry centred on vitamin and mineral supplementation. The producers create lists of 'generalised' symptoms that result from low levels of each vitamin or mineral and 'brainwash' the public into believing that taking these will remove the symptom. The danger of this strategy is that any one symptom is rarely directly attributable to one specific vitamin deficiency, so the 'patient' is left totally in the dark as to which of a spectrum of vitamins and minerals to use. Vitamins and minerals do not act independently, but synergistically with each other, and selecting one single vitamin is unlikely to solve any problem unless that deficiency has been medically diagnosed. In fact, the exact opposite can be true, where taking a single mineral without the synergistic micronutrients, can cause further imbalance in the system and additional problems. These tend to be of a minor nature, and usually only result from relatively high dosages, which is why this sector of the supplement industry is allowed to sell these products over the counter in an unrestricted fashion. (Very often, the body excretes excess micronutrients.)

We are all conditioned to feel 'fatigued' or 'depleted' by marketing and promotional companies, each of which has a 'tonic, food, drink, vitamin or mineral' supplement to pick us up and revitalise us, and put cash into their company. The whole issue of 'eating' has become a complex fabric of reality, half-truths, and marketing 'hype' that makes it virtually impossible for anyone to fathom where one stops and the other starts.

Who is to say that the whole debate on decreasing soil quality was not started by the vitamin and mineral industry, which would clearly benefit from such a belief, or a food manufacturer who can show that his product is high in magnesium or calcium? The mere suggestion that calcium levels are linked to osteoporosis would bring a glint to the eye of any mineral marketing director.

In truth, the complexities of it all are impossible to explore here, and not that interesting to most people, therefore satisfying the 'pangs' of hunger in the most enjoyable and delicious way possible, is justification enough of the need to 'eat' – that is, until something goes 'wrong'.

Typically, people consider something to have gone 'wrong' with their eating when they fall into one of the following categories:

▸ too thin or have an eating disorder.
▸ too fat or obese.
▸ illness.
▸ nutritionally deficient.
▸ continually fatigued and unable to perform properly, either in normal life or in sport.

Another motivation for an interest in nutrition stems from the ambition to improve in sport. People become more aware of the role of nutrition from books, advertised products and their associated 'programmes', nutritionists, seminars and other educational vehicles. The volume of material and size of the industry that has grown around 'weight loss' is indicative of the level of poor 'eating habits' and lack of nutritional knowledge that exists, although it too has benefited from marketers who give credence to the lie that everyone should have a slender young figure, irrespective of their body type, size and age. Ironically, it is those who try to restrict their energy intake (either by weight loss or eating disorders) that have the biggest problem in maintaining a sufficiently balanced diet.

Because the interest in sports nutrition tends to be motivated by ambition, the levels of conformity to new knowledge are good because of the direct impact they have on performance.

In all cases, however, changes in nutritional habits take time to show results and require a heartfelt desire to be achieved. Motivational reinforcement of the goal can often be as important as the discipline to make these changes.

00:00:20
THE ROLE OF
SPORTS NUTRITION

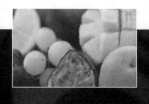

It has taken many years for the true potential of sports nutrition to be recognised, even by major sports; indeed, today many so-called minor sports are far ahead of the players in major TV sports. Average club athletes and triathletes often have greater knowledge of nutrition than many of the top-ranked team-sport players. I suggest that this is a result of the individual accepting full responsibility for the outcome of their performances, while teams often rely on the guidance of coaches and managers.

Good sports nutrition has both short- and long-term impact on performance, but more importantly, the adoption of healthy nutritional habits can impact on many other sports-related aspects, as outlined below:

Energy levels determine your ability to complete a training session

The human body is basically a machine – in many cases not a very efficient one – but a machine nonetheless, and in terms of energy, it follows the basic scientific rule of 'energy in should equal energy out'. If you attempt to train after failing to eat during the day, you will find that the quality of that session, and possibly the ones immediately following, are not up to standard. Without energy, your muscles cannot operate.

We will return to this principle in the section on weight control, as this is also the basis used to burn off weight, or to add weight in the case of those wanting to bulk up. The key to effective training, however, is to ensure you have the necessary energy before you start.

We need adequate fluid during training and racing to perform optimally

Our bodies comprise a very high percentage (80%) of water, and when these levels slip significantly out of the normal range, performance is impaired. This applies not only when there is a level of dehydration, but also when there is too high a level of hydration – hyperhydration. The reason for this is that water is the 'carrier' for many electrolytes and blood concentration; changes in the amount of fluid changes these concentrations.

Research shows that a 2% reduction in normal hydration levels can result in as much as a 20% reduction in performance. This clearly impacts significantly on the performance time or ability. However, for reasons that will be discussed later, endurance athletes will normally finish marginally dehydrated.

Although most people focus on the detrimental effects of dehydration, the more dangerous concern is hyperhydration, which can result in an athlete going into a coma. It is, however, more prevalent amongst runners/cyclists towards the back of a long endurance event.

Energy replacement is required in training and racing to maintain form

As indicated above, having enough energy is important for effective training and racing, throughout the event. If an event is long – over an hour – or perhaps has several heats or periods of play, replacing energy used during the event or training is also important. Failure to do so can not only cause impaired physical form, but also an impaired sense of judgment, both of which decrease the level of performance and increase the risk of injury.

Replacing energy after training is the first step in recovery

Shoe manufacturer Nike has a slogan that states, 'There is no finish line.' This is true. When you complete a training session or cross the line in an event, it represents the start of the build-up to the next training session or event. Replacing the energy used in a completed session is the first step you can take to impact on the effectiveness of the next session. It is one of the most powerful aspects of sports nutrition and one of the easiest to do, but you only have a limited period of time in which to maximise its benefit.

Optimal recovery requires the correct mix of time and nutrients

Most sportspeople focus on training instead of focusing on recovery. We train to improve so that we can perform better in competition, but both training and competition 'break down' our systems. It is only with adequate recovery that we benefit from the training or are able to 'bounce' back from the all-out effort of competition. Recovery is not simply having time off, but also providing the building block to 'repair' the damage done.

Nutritional supplements can boost performance

Supplementation can improve performance. By following procedures such as carbohydrate loading or using creatine, you can boost your performance in different types of events.

Nutritional supplements can boost the immune system and function as a prophylactic

Because the activities of training and racing break the body down, and can lower the body's immune system, it often means that a sportsperson in heavy training hovers on a knife edge between supreme fitness and becoming ill. Supplementation with certain nutrients can boost the immune system and also reduce the risk of illness or injury.

Nutrition can assist in injury treatment

In the same way that nutrition plays a role in repairing muscle damage after training or competition, it can also assist in speeding up recovery from injury.

Listed above, are just eight ways in which adopting good nutritional habits can have an impact on your sporting performance. Some are more evident in their action than others, which subtly provide the reserves and foundation on which a holistic and effective programme can be built. In sport, however, wins, losses and personal best performances are determined in split seconds, millimetres, and judgement and reaction time. It is the search for and the attention to the smallest detail that can make a difference between success and failure.

South Africans should be proud of the work done by Professor Tim Noakes *et al* who, in the early 1980s, researched the optimum type, quality and quantity of carbohydrates to be taken before and during endurance events. However, the commercial marketers have 'hijacked' this as a means of selling anything with the hint of sugar or starch in it.

Energy bars, heavily sugared drinks, sweets, pasta and pizza have all benefited despite many having significant drawbacks to their use in aspects of exercise. For instance, it is a myth to suggest that pizza is high in carbohydrate. The base may well be carbohydrate, but the layer of cheese and additional 'extras' such as salami and ham hardly contribute to the carbohydrates and change the overall combination of kilocalories to a minimum contribution from carbohydrate. Pasta is another problem. Yes, pure pasta is a good source of carbohydrate, but it is bulky and delivers very few grams of carbohydrate in a plateful. Not to mention that it is rarely eaten by itself, but normally with a cream or meat sauce, which again changes the carbohydrate contribution to overall kilocalories.

This induced 'obsession' with carbohydrates has led runners and other endurance athletes to overlook the vital role of protein and fat. To understand why these are important, it is necessary to go back to training basics.

WHY DO WE TRAIN?

We train to adapt our bodies gradually to the stress of the race for which we are training. A prime desire of training is to strengthen the muscles used in running, cycling or the chosen sport – runners train by running, cyclists train by cycling. In each case, as a rule, we need only concentrate on the muscles used in our sport, and minimise the weight in the parts of the body that are not used (and only 'taken along for the ride'). This is known as the rule of **'specific training'**.

How do you strengthen a muscle? In layman's terms, you need to damage the muscle (by overloading/working it), allowing it to repair and become stronger. The body works much like a pendulum or a playground swing. If a muscle is damaged, it rebuilds and recovers to be stronger than before, if it is to withstand that load again. In the analogy, the pendulum doesn't return to centre but overcompensates i.e. it swings up the other side. If training is seen as damaging the muscle on one side of the arc, then the rebuilding and muscle growth may be seen as overcompensation, taking the swing to a new height on the other side of the arc.

The swing (or pendulum) can only climb up the arc on the other side if it is left alone and there is no interruption to its passage, which means that it is allowed enough time to reach its maximum height on the muscle growth side before it commences back on a downward swing. This upward swing may be compared to the training recovery period. If you do not add any further stimulus as it passes through into the training side of the swing, it soon returns to a mid-point and the height gained (muscle strength), is lost.

To summarise, training damages the muscle but it recovers on the other side of the arc. If no other force is added, it returns to its original condition. This is the rule of 'use it or lose it'. If you don't continue to subject the muscle to a similar (or higher) level of stress, it will lose the strength gained from the initial training.

TRAINING DAMAGES YOUR BODY

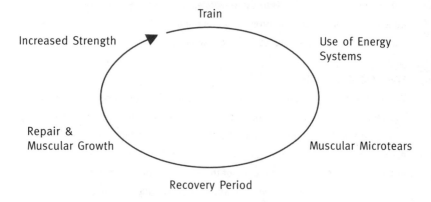

Train

Increased Strength

Use of Energy
Systems

Repair &
Muscular Growth

Muscular Microtears

Recovery Period

To continue developing the muscle it must be subjected to progressively greater stresses and loads, or there will be no further progression. Clearly, to progress, you must continue to train, allowing the muscle to grow and gain in strength.

By comparison, consider what happens to a swing when someone interrupts the motion by continually pushing it back up before it passes the mid-point. It is akin to putting in additional training sessions before your muscles have achieved their full growth and are still partly damaged. The additional 'impulses' push the swing ever higher on one side, effectively inflicting more damage on already damaged muscles. If more and more 'pushes' are used before the swing achieves full recovery, it will hit the limit of its range of movement and go no further. This results in over-training (or injury) as all the movement is on the side of damaged muscles.

Alternatively, if these impulses (training sessions) are injected into the swing at the correct time when the swing comes down from the recovery phase, the swing (muscle strength) can climb to a maximum on the side of growth. As any parent knows, the key is in the timing of when you apply the push to the swing. Likewise with training: applying training too soon after one session will result in additional damage and eventually in injury. If training is applied to allow sufficient recovery before another training load, the muscle will gradually gain in strength.

Another key requirement affecting the efficiency of the swing is a well-lubricated pivot point or bearing, which may be likened to the correct nutrition. If the pivot is rusted, the swing will never reach its full potential height. The correct nutrition must be present to rebuild the muscle. Carbohydrate is the 'oil in the bearing' keeping it loose and flowing, while protein plays the role of the bearings and housing that provide the structure. The reality is that carbohydrate does NOT build muscle.

Carbohydrate does provide energy to rebuild energy stores, but the 23 amino acids in protein are the building blocks for rebuilding and expanding the soft tissue. It is important to achieve the correct balance of carbohydrates, protein and fat to keep the swing in smooth efficient operation.

The simile may be taken further by considering the structure holding the swing. The main swing structure needs only four legs, forming two A-frames to hold the pivot-point in a 'pelvic-like' cradle at the top. If everything operates smoothly, in a line, this is all that is required, as everything is well balanced. The same applies to a runner who has good posture, without mechanical imbalances in running style.

However, it is normal to use two cross-supports, one for each pair of legs, to provide added stability to the structure. The reality is that the swing rarely operates in an 'ideal' situation and these cross-braces remove accidental side forces and wind, or other disturbing factors. These are like supplementary training, such as gym and plyometrics, which you use to complement your training. They aren't essential, but without them any weakness in your structure will quickly result in extensive damage.

As with a runner's body, the whole structure should be protected and maintained in good condition. With timber or steel, paint is used as protection against rust or rot. This is the role played by vitamins, minerals and micronutrients in ensuring a sound immune system with the ability to fight off illness.

However, even if a structure is solid, the swing will collapse unless the poles are well located into foundations. This is comparable to your running shoes and feet. If there is unnecessary movement in the foundation, as the swing moves back and forward, the entire structure will start rocking, joints will loosen, the structure will be damaged and the swing will not reach its maximum height. In the worst scenario, it might fall over and collapse – requiring a complete rebuild. Runners wearing the incorrect shoes, which will cause incorrect mechanical movement of the structure (at the feet), are no different: on landing, the small movements result in much larger movements at the knee and back. This shifts the load from one muscle onto another muscle, increasing the load. As training progresses, the muscle becomes overloaded and when it 'collapses' under the fatigue of the additional load, it shifts even more force onto other muscles. Like a house of cards, the walls collapse and the ceiling falls in – soon there is nothing left standing.

The swing simile works well: start everything swinging in a well-oiled, well-timed and balanced environment and you will achieve great heights, but let rust into the bearing or the structure, allow movement at the foundation, or simply mistime your pushes (training), and you won't allow the swing to reach its maximum height. If you don't address the problem, the result could be even worse – the swing can collapse and take a long time to rebuild.

Although this has been related directly to running, these principles hold true for any sport and for most other aspects of life.

00:00:22
ENERGY PRODUCTION
DURING EXERCISE

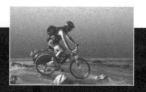

A key aspect to understanding the need for, and use of, sports energy drinks and nutrition lies in understanding the energy systems used during exercise. Briefly, it can be described in layman's language as follows:

Adenosine triphosphate (ATP) and creatine phosphate energy

Very short intense exercise, of a few seconds' duration (e.g. sprint starts), is fuelled by ATP, a chemical in the muscles, which allows them to contract. Such exercise does not require oxygen. From 2–45 seconds, the fuel required is a combination of ATP and creatine phosphate, which exists in the body. In sprinting terms, this will take an elite athlete around a 400-m track. (You may have recognised the term 'creatine', a popular sport supplement. Use of this is covered later.) Again, no oxygen is required and the body can produce ATP from other components, but at a slower rate than is used up in such high-intensity exercise as that discussed above. Exercise at such high-intensity levels results in high levels of lactic acid production.

Lactic acid is NOT the 'baddie' that some people would have you believe (see further in the chapter). Your body only has the capacity to process (metabolise) lactic acid at a particular rate and when it is produced faster than it can be metabolised, your muscles are unable to function properly as they become too acidic. This explains why a 400-m track runner is seen to 'tie-up' as he comes down the home straight towards the finish line. An example of a runner is used because the effects are more visible, but the same process happens in cycling, swimming or other continuous sports.

A key point to note is that this will occur after the same length of TIME, not the same distance i.e. after 40–45 seconds of FLAT-OUT effort in the sport concerned. Your capacity to cope with high levels of lactic acid can be increased to some degree, by training. A fuller explanation of the role of lactic acid is given later in this section.

Predominately carbohydrate energy

The next energy process relates to periods of flat-out exercise lasting 45 seconds to about three minutes. The amount of oxygen required increases as the length of exercise increases. It is used in the conversion of glycogen into ATP and hence energy, as before. An efficient method of fuelling exercise, this may be compared to 'high-octane' petrol. Energy can be derived from processes with (aerobic) or without oxygen (anaerobic). As the time increases, the proportion of anaerobic exercise decreases and aerobic exercise increases. For example, a 1 000-m race is about 50% anaerobic, 50% aerobic. By 5 000 m (typically 14 minutes flat-out exercise for an elite athlete), this is approximately 10% anaerobic, 90% aerobic, while a 10-km race (30 minutes), is 5% anaerobic, 95% aerobic. The higher the percentage of anaerobic work, the greater the build-up of lactic acid. Again it is important to recognise that it is the length of time, not the distance that is important in these percentages.

As the race distance increases towards the half-marathon distance, the rate of lactic acid production reduces towards a level that matches the rate at which the body can metabolise it and there is no build-up. The levels of lactic acid are measured in the blood as lactate and this 'balanced' level is often called the lactate turnpoint, and for a runner this occurs around the flat-out racing pace that can be sustained for one hour. For this reason, running as far as you can for one hour is a useful way to determine your lactate turnpoint pace. The 'lactate turnpoint' is one of the key training paces for most endurance sports. Many different terms have been used to indicate the point where lactate starts to exceed the point where it can be metabolised. Terms such as 'lactic threshold' and 'onset of blood lactate accumulation', are all used. These terms have evolved as the understanding of the highly complex chemical processes have become clearer, but for current purposes, it can be considered as the exercise intensity at which the amount of lactate production exceeds the rate at which the body is able to metabolise it. A key point is that this complex chemical process also provides ATP, which we have seen to be the key energy source. It is incorrect to think of lactic acid as 'bad', and this metabolisation can be considered as one of the body's 'recycling' processes.

Lactate is the outcome of a chemical combination with lactic acid and it is normal for the degree of lactic acid production to be measured by the analysis of lactate circulating in the blood.

Carbohydrate is stored as glycogen, in both the muscles and the liver. Muscle glycogen is used for exercise, while liver glycogen is primarily used to maintain normal blood sugar levels. Blood sugar is a vital fuel 'powering' the brain. Liver stores deplete constantly, even when sleeping. The maximum liver stores are around 150 g, which deplete at a rate of about 9 g per hour when resting. People who exercise or work in the morning without eating may only have 50% or less of their liver stores remaining after a night's sleep and before they take their first step. This can severely limit their resources unless they have breakfast before commencing an endurance event.

Muscle glycogen stores are sufficient for approximately 90 minutes of continuous exercise, after which the blood sugar is faced with the dilemma of trying to assist the energy requirements of muscle and brain activity. Difficulty in concentrating or doing simple mental calculations is a typical sign of the conflict caused by low blood sugar levels. It is referred to as the 'bear', 'bonking' or the 'wall' (different sports use different terms).

Exercise that lasts beyond this time, or is of a lower intensity, makes use of a combination of glycogen and blood fatty acids. The less intense the exercise, the higher the percentage of the energy that comes from the blood fatty acids.

Remembering that it is time and NOT DISTANCE that determines the sources of energy required in exercise, it is clear that high-intensity exercise, which can only be sustained for relatively short periods, will make a greater demand on muscle glycogen, hence those muscle stores are the first to be depleted. On the other hand, low-intensity exercise that can be sustained for considerable times will utilise higher percentages of blood fatty acids and make lower muscle glycogen demands, but in this case the critical energy source is liver glycogen.

Free fatty acid and carbohydrate as energy

Blood fatty acids are a very 'low-octane' fuel because they must first be converted to glycogen and only then into ATP and energy. Deriving energy from fatty acids uses an additional 10% of oxygen. This two-stage process means that energy cannot be produced fast enough to keep up with the demands of high-intensity exercise and therefore limits the speed of exercise. Fatty acids become an important energy source to those who race in excess of two hours.

It is possible to improve the efficiency of blood fatty acid conversion into energy through training, which is the purpose of a long run, cycle or back-to-back sessions. However, the major benefits of this are probably achieved in runs of 2–3 hours (3–4-hour cycles), and the length of long training (and the resultant muscle damage) needs to be balanced with longer recovery before training continues.

Lactic acid is produced during these low-intensity exercise sessions, yet the rate of production is low enough for it to be reconverted into useful energy. If your body is already depleted of glycogen, blood fatty acids will become your prime source of fuel. In theory, most people have an extensive supply of blood fatty acids and will never have insufficient stores of it for most events – you probably have enough to power you halfway round the equator. By comparison, you only have a limited amount of muscle glycogen stores and once exhausted, they must be replaced, which is difficult to achieve during exercise. The ability to replace energy also depends on the variety and content of the food or drink taken. Moreover, from the previous discussion on liver glycogen, it should be clear how important it is to keep blood sugar levels up to maintain normal brain function. Whereas muscle glycogen is difficult to replace during energy, taking carbohydrate drinks during exercise will assist in keeping blood sugar at a good level.

Lactic acid

Lactic acid is blamed for all manner of ills during exercise. In fact, we continually produce lactic acid in normal activity and it is simply converted into energy. A good way to understand the role of lactic acid is to consider a bucket under a tap, with a hole in the side, level with the bottom of the bucket.

At very low levels of activity, the lactic acid drips into the bucket from the tap and simply runs from the hole in the bottom. This indicates the metabolisation of the lactic acid back into energy. As the exercise intensity increases, lactic acid production is increased (the tap is opened) and the flow into the bucket increases. Again, the incoming flow goes straight through the hole in the side of the bucket. Eventually, the total incoming flow equals the amount of lactic acid that is able to exit through the side hole in the bucket – not less and not more – and the condition is balanced, which relates to the 'threshold' or lactate turnpoint. This is clearly a function of the size of the hole in the side. The bigger the hole, the more lactic acid that can be 'processed' to maintain the balanced condition. Trying to increase this capacity is the reason for the lactate turnpoint being a key pace for training. Because it is difficult to identify a person's lactate turnpoint intensity accurately in a practical situation, and because the time of training at this pace is limited, it is common for training sessions to be designed to 'cross' this intensity by running (or cycling, swimming, etc) at intensities known to be slightly higher or lower than the 'balance' exercise intensity.

If the tap is opened further (i.e. the intensity of the exercise is increased), the flow of lactic acid becomes greater than the flow out of the hole in the bucket. The result is that lactic acid 'backs up' in the bucket and the level rises. The length of time it takes for this level to reach the top and overflow the bucket, depends on the intensity of exercise (the higher the intensity, the sooner the overflow) and the height of the bucket.

When the level reaches the top and overflows, it is a sign that the muscles have become swamped with lactic acid and are no longer able to function properly. At this point, a runner will be forced to stop or drastically reduce his pace so that sufficient lactic acid is metabolised (flows through the hole) to drop the level in the bucket again. Clearly, if he could develop a 'deeper' bucket, he would be able to run with higher levels of lactic acid before tying up. This can be achieved with training that establishes high levels of lactic acid in the muscles, allowing them to adapt to operating in these conditions.

It's thought that the average runner has a capacity of about 21 litres of lactic acid before tying up. In an 'ideal' competitive situation, you would want to exercise at a high intensity that resulted in your lactic capacity only being reached one metre before the finish line, and your momentum would carry you over the line without any loss of speed.

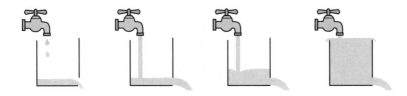

Training and energy systems

By now it should be obvious that the focus of your training must be on those energy systems you will require in the distance of the event for which you are training. A 3 000-m runner, or 1 000-m sprint cyclist, needs to be able to compete with large amounts of lactic acid in his muscle, and will focus on sessions that increase the depth of the bucket and the size of the hole in the side (increased ability to withstand high levels of lactic acid and higher lactate turnpoint). By comparison, an ultramarathoner will hope to improve his conversion of blood fatty acids into energy, increase their glycogen stores, and heighten his lactic threshold. The latter will require interval or track work. By increasing his lactate turnpoint, he can run at a faster pace before lactic acid builds up, which means that his training and racing pace during long runs can be higher, allowing him to undertake more training over any period of time and hence become stronger.

During training we deplete different energy stores, and before we can train again at that intensity we need to replace these energy stores. This link between energy (and nutrition), training and recovery is vital and probably the MOST IMPORTANT CONCEPT OF TRAINING to understand (and obey). Few people appreciate this link, and even if they do, it remains a major challenge to calm ambitious desires to allow sufficient recovery and adequate nutritional support.

Protein and amino acids

It should be clear from the previous analysis of basic training that although carbohydrates are required to replace energy burnt in exercise, protein is necessary to repair the damaged muscle and to increase the strength for which you undertook the training. Without the correct proportions of either, the process is less effective or impossible.

Yet the role of protein goes further. In very long endurance events, when alternative sources of energy are depleted, there is a tendency towards greater use of proteins, known as a catabolic action (as opposed to muscle building – anabolic). Amino acids and protein play a major role in exercise supplementation, because they are the building blocks to repair muscle damage and provide the growth we aim to achieve through training. Good supplies of protein are required to minimise the catabolic action.

WHAT WE HAVE LEARNT FROM RESEARCH

The aforementioned only relates to the energy expenditure in popular distance events, i.e. those that are commonly run. Most research and studies on exercise and sport are undertaken either on 'novice' exercisers or elite athletes over short distances, or 'mass' runners over distances generally up to 10 km, and less occasionally up to the marathon. The further the distance, the less invasive the study as the researchers try not to influence an individual's results. As it is impossible to run your best marathon every month, participants are less willing to sacrifice their performances to research, however a 5-km or 10-km flat-out effort may be undertaken at relatively close intervals.

The opportunity for in-depth investigations of ultrarunners is severely limited. While Comrades has the number of runners appropriate to a question-and-answer-type survey, few would be willing to undergo the invasive techniques of muscle biopsy or drawing blood during the event to determine exactly what is happening. Even if some volunteered, they would most likely be middle or back finishers, as elite runners can hardly be expected to sacrifice a top position (or prize money) for this. Therefore the research would be a test of what occurs in 9–11 hours of exercise, not at gold medallist level, or what happens after 14 hours in a 100-mile race (160.9 km). Most research for ultras is based on logical extrapolation from research at shorter distances. Those who can relate what actually happens, are generally those who have 'done the time'. It is surely no coincidence that Arthur Newton was heralded as the father of distance running and that many of his rules hold as good today as they did in the 1920s. Similarly, Wally Hayward, Don Ritchie and Yiannis Kouros all learnt the 'tricks of the trade' from 'being there' and their advice is often more practical than the speculated research. Of course, they may not understand the finer medical details of why their advice works, but experience has taught them how to overcome the hurdles of ultra-distance racing.

Naturally, it is important to keep abreast of the latest research, but also to bear in mind from where the research is derived. When it concerns short-distance events, the main focus only needs to be on the standard of the runner used in the research, and there is every probability that it has covered all levels of abilities. But as the distance increases, the impact of the research will diminish and more cognisance must be given to what the successful 'exponents' of that distance have to say. Once again, we should consider ourselves lucky in South Africa that scientists of the calibre of Professor Tim Noakes have gone out of their way to investigate and undertake research focused on the longer events and we have probably gained a better insight than many other countries.

Also remember that in runs over 12 hours the natural effects of 'fatigue' come into play and it affects people differently. For instance, Yiannis Kouros can run for six days, initially taking only 30 minute or an hour's sleep at a time. This would be a task in itself for a person who requires 10 hours sleep in a normal day. (Different people require different levels of sleep. Yiannos can manage with a few hours' sleep and will therefore not face the same challenge as someone who requires more. He can use more energy for a run and requires a different approach to a six-day race.)

It will be appreciated that the energy requirements for athletes racing longer than the 5–6 hours of a Comrades or 100-km gold medal, will differ dramatically from others in the same race. We have seen how a five-hour Comrades runner will focus on glycogen (mainly for powering the brain) and a mix of blood fatty acids and glycogen for low-intensity muscular movements. From what science has taught us, we can do this with the fat stores we already have, but it in no way accounts for the cravings for something more substantial that we experience when running for 7–12 hours. Yet back in 1924, Arthur Newton wrote that if he raced over 50 miles (80.45 km), which was six hours for him, he required something to eat at 40 miles (64 km). His choice included carbohydrate, but was also high in fat and protein.

My own experience in running multiday events has taught me the importance of protein and fat. I had started running as a front-row rugby player with good muscle definition, but an inability to supply sufficient kilocalories and protein during multiday and 100-mile runs, meant that I lost my muscle mass as the protein was 'eaten' up as I became catabolic in those events. The same thing happens to many distance runners who do not recognise the role of protein and fat, in the recovery process.

As discussed previously, we also need to consider recovery and repair to the muscle damage incurred during training or racing. Marketing people have overstressed the importance of carbohydrates to all endurance sports, and more attention must be paid to the role of protein and fat. The only reason for training is to inflict damage on the muscles that need to be strengthened, and when you understand this you will have a completely different view on how and when to train.

It should also be noted that much of the research is undertaken using undergraduate students, who either for educational or financial purposes, are often keen candidates in studies. In some cases, this might raise questions as to whether the extrapolations will apply directly to people in older age groups.

It is also important in the assessment of research studies to investigate who, and where the research was undertaken, and the funding mechanism of the research, as it is not uncommon for studies to be undertaken by 'in-house' research centres, or funded by companies manufacturing the product under discussion. In such cases a negative result may have significant commercial implication.

FUEL	TIME OF INTENSE EXERCISE (i.e. flat out for the time under consideration)
ATP	0–3 seconds
ATP and creatine phosphate	3–45 seconds
Glycogen	45 seconds to 3 minutes
Glycogen and blood blood fatty acids	+60 minutes to approximate threshold +90 minutes to depletion of glycogen stores

SUMMARY

In a simplified form energy production can be classified as follows:

It can be seen that carbohydrate plays an important role in all exercise and is essential if blood sugar level is to be maintained. Although these fuel systems tend to interrelate, the primary source of energy will be determined by the level of intensity of exercise and the length of time of the exercise (NOT the distance). Thus a two-hour marathon (42.195 km) runner uses the same energy systems (e.g. 80% glycogen, 20% blood fatty acids) as a two-hour half-marathon, (21.1-km) runner. The latter runner would take about four hours and 15 minutes if he attempted a marathon and would use approximately 60% glycogen and 40% blood fatty acids. For the same distances, the fuel requirements of these two runners are different, but for the same time of continuous flat-out exercise, their fuel requirements tend to be the same.

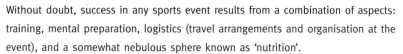

Without doubt, success in any sports event results from a combination of aspects: training, mental preparation, logistics (travel arrangements and organisation at the event), and a somewhat nebulous sphere known as 'nutrition'.

This is a book for winners – not necessarily event or competition winners, but rather runners who wish to maximise their performances, whatever their standard.

Energy replacement affects all sporting performance to some extent and if you can use and are willing to adopt and tailor the nutritional advice and suggestions in this section to your individual needs, you will have eliminated one possible source of misfortune from your competition. Correct energy and water replacement will lead to better recovery after training, leading to more effective training, better training results and improved competition results. Correct energy replacement in competition means better results. You can improve in two areas simultaneously.

It's not about eating X or omitting Y from your diet to become a champion. The objective is to give you a 'hands on' experience of how, when, what and how much use to make of the sports drink products that are available.

Most importantly, you need to know how to recognise your needs in your everyday diet. I believe that there is a need for most of us to modify our eating habits to return our energy intake back to the equivalent nutritional value of the 'three balanced meals per day'. But, even the concept of 'three meals' needs modification. Practical guidance is given later, on these basic requirements.

TAKING A LONG-TERM APPROACH

Lifestyles have become considerably more rushed than they were even ten years ago. There are so many more opportunities; technology has us answering the equivalent of bags full of mail in a day by e-mail, cellphones mean that we can be contacted at all hours, travel has become extremely accessible and normal office hours have ceased to exist for many people. A side effect of this is that our eating habits have changed dramatically. It is worthwhile consulting a good sports nutritionist for an analysis of your eating habits, at least once every 12–18 months. Lifestyle changes can make quite dramatic changes in your eating, and without the correct nutrition, you are wasting much of your training.

A nutritionist will ask for a list of everything you have eaten and had to drink over a three-day (or longer) period and this needs to be logged carefully with as good a measure of each item as possible. Compare this to your energy expenditure, not only in training, but also in everyday activity. From the combination of information and measurements of your body fat, height and weight, the nutritionist can determine what nutrients you require, how you are benefiting from the food you eat and what your deficiencies are. It is also possible to identify the proportions of energy you are receiving from carbohydrates, protein and fat, whereafter it will be possible to recommend changes in your diet.

While I respect the knowledge of nutritionists, I find that few really put it into a practical context. Many will provide a detailed diet made up of about 4–6 snacks and meals for each day, stipulating exact quantities and foods to be eaten (e.g. a green salad with half a cup of cottage cheese). This is where I have a problem. Unless you are willing to buy all these items and pack a suitcase of food to go to work each day and carry to and from meetings, it is an impractical solution. I rarely find myself somewhere after a morning meeting where I have the time to go in search of a green salad or skinned boiled chicken. This approach guarantees that I will fail to keep to the programme.

Instead, I try to work with basic guidelines that allow me greater flexibility. I know that I need 10–12 servings of carbohydrate and 4–5 servings of protein a day, and believe me, the fat will always take care of itself, although I try to opt for the essential fats as opposed to the saturated ones.

What follows is a description of a few quick calculations and rules to determine what you require. Once you have completed this and spent a couple of weeks familiarising yourself with the routine, ask a nutritionist for a more accurate assessment, but ask him to consolidate his recommendations into a similar set of rules. It will allow you the flexibility to build in that unexpected meal, or handle an extra slice of the cake on someone's birthday. The flexibility is the attraction.

HOW MUCH ENERGY DO YOU NEED?

Your body is a machine and to maintain your weight you need to take in (eat) the same amount of energy that you use each day. If you want to gain weight, simply eat more than you expend, and to lose weight, eat less than you expend. Weight loss can be achieved either by eating less or by exercising more so that you expend more energy. The best option would be a combination of both of these extremes.

As a quick estimate, you need around 40 kilocalories (kcal) per kg of body weight to maintain the energy balance. Using this, a 70-kg adult requires 2 800 kcal simply to maintain weight when not training. Remember, this is an estimate, as different jobs demand different energy expenditure. Sitting at a desk all day is much less physically active than being a bricklayer or delivery person.

You must add in the amount of energy used in training, which can be calculated exactly by adding up all the different exercise undertaken in a day. There are tables that detail energy expenditure at various intensities for various different sports or tasks, and one option is to detail out each 30 minutes of your day and work out an accurate energy expenditure.

However, a more simplistic method is to use your total weekly training distance and time to calculate an average daily training distance. Although the energy expenditure varies for different running speeds, use a mid-level value 1.028 kcal per kilogram per kilometre. (This value applies to speed from 4 mins per kilometre to 5.5 mins per kilometre – but remember, this is average training pace.)

It is worth noting that each runner will have a zone of speeds where he runs most efficiently, running either faster or slower than that which will cause greater energy expenditure. Let us assume our 70-kg runner covers 60 km per week in normal training: his average daily training distance is 8.57 km and his expenditure will be 6 16.8 kcal (8.57 x 1.028 x 70 kg). If, during peak training, this goes up to 120 km per week (17.14 km average per day), the energy expenditure also rises to 1 233.6 kcal (17.14 x 1.208 x 70). By adding this to the daily minimum, the total daily requirement for this runner in peak training is 4 033.6 kcal if he simply wants to maintain his body weight.

It is obvious why merely increasing training can cause runners to lose weight. However, be aware that long, slow distance running is not the best way of losing weight for the average person, as we will see later.

Having worked out that our runner needs about 4 050 kcal per day, we need to consider the split of nutrients that make up the total. It is generally recognised that an endurance diet needs to be high in carbohydrates and therefore a split of 60–70% carbohydrate, 15–20% protein and 15–20% fat is recommended.

These splits are given with a variation of percentages in order that they may be matched to the period and emphasis of training. When you are doing more speed and strength work, your protein intake will increase towards the 20% with the carbohydrates dropping towards the 60% mark. Conversely, when you are doing the maximum endurance work, the carbohydrate intake moves closer to 70% and the protein requirement drops towards 15%. The reason for this (covered in the previous chapter) basically relates to the amount of muscle damage incurred as a result of the strength work being more than that inflicted during endurance work.

At peak distance training, a 70-kg runner requires 2 835 kcal in carbohydrate form (4 050 x 70%). In more recognisable terms, convert it to grams or carbohydrate by dividing the number of kilocalories by 3.81 (the kilocalories generated from 1 g of carbohydrate). This gives a daily requirement of 744 g, which can be 'translated' into popular food items. For fruit (apples, oranges or bananas), you would need 44 pieces per day. In a less nutritious food such as marshmallows, it would take 148 marshmallows to satisfy these needs or about 40 baked potatoes per day. This is clearly unachievable, which is why sports supplementation and liquid are key.

Protein requirements

A runner in peak endurance training requires approximately 607 kcal (4 050 x 15%) from protein sources. This can be converted to grams by dividing by 3.76, which means that the runner requires 161 g of protein.

However, there is a second rule of thumb to check the relative accuracy of an estimate. A sedentary person requires about 0.75 g of protein per kilogram of bodyweight to maintain muscle mass. A runner in training requires between 1.2 g and 1.6 g per kilogram. As a guide to where you are on that scale, consider that a cyclist in the Tour de France needs 1.8 g per kilogram, so the 1.6-g region only applies during your heaviest training period. If we apply this to a 70-kg runner, we find he needs 112 g of protein. In food terms, this equates to approximately 12 eggs or 700 g of cottage cheese or a 400-g (cooked weight) steak or 450 g of chicken.

This is certainly more achievable, and applied kineticist Ron Holder uses the fist or open palm of the hand as a guide to the amount of protein-rich food, which roughly equals 25 g of protein. This makes it easy to gauge and our runner needs about 4–5 'fists' or palms of protein per day. Excuse the pun, but that is a very handy way to monitor how much protein you are absorbing.

Protein quality

Having determined the amount of protein, the next consideration is the quality. Initially, eggs were seen as the most complete protein and everything else was related to eggs as a percentage. Eggs led the field at 100%. However, recent developments and improved understanding now see some proteins ranking higher than eggs. There has been a move to 'regrade' proteins, but the egg is still the point of reference with a 'biological value' (BV) of 100.

The higher the value, the better the protein, and currently, top protein supplements such as whey and ionic whey are graded as having a BV of 159 – a staggering 60% improvement on the egg. Ionic whey is refined by a process that involves bombarding the protein with ions and selecting specific sections of the whey. Whey has a high percentage of three amino acids, known as branched chain amino acids (BCAA). Although there are 23 amino acids and the body's muscles contain around 70% of these three BCAAs, it is important to have a high percentage of BCAAs in the protein you select. Because whey proteins are products of processed milk and cheeses they contain small amounts of fats, and carbohydrates that assist in absorption.

When to take protein

Because we need carbohydrate for energy, your carbohydrate intake for the day should be weighted more towards meals and snacks taken at the beginning of the day. By comparison, protein should be spread so that most of the day's requirement is in the meals and snacks eaten after training and towards evening. However, all meals should have some protein, carbohydrate and fat.

If you are using a protein supplement, it can be split with half in the hour after strength or intense training and the other half as a pre-bedtime drink. Evening is an ideal time to take some protein, because that is when hormone activity is at its peak. The prime time for rebuilding and repair of muscle is while we sleep, so it makes sense that we should ensure that all the necessary building blocks are present for this to take place.

Fat requirements

We need about 20% of our kilocalories in fat, i.e. in this instance 810 kcal. However, the energy value for fat is significantly greater, so conversion to grams is calculated by dividing by 9, to give a daily requirement of 90 g. Considering the amount of food that needs to be consumed to meet carbohydrate and protein requirements, taking in sufficient fat is rarely a problem. One reason for this is that fat often gives food its taste, so the problem is not taking in enough fat, but rather trying to ensure that it's the right type of fat. Steer away from saturated fats such as butter, meat fat, and move towards the 'essential fats', also known as omega 3 and omega 6 fats. Fish oils such as salmon oil, flaxseed oils and evening primrose oils are excellent examples.

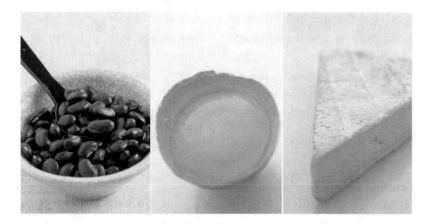

ABOVE *Not always what they seem – for instance, beans are not only a source of carbohydrate but also protein; eggs are one of the best sources of protein but are relatively high in fat; cheese is high in fat but is also a protein – the key to a healthy diet is to achieve the correct balance*

TO CALCULATE YOUR ENERGY REQUIREMENTS

1. **Multiply your body weight** by 40 to obtain the total resting energy requirement.
2. Calculate your **average daily training distance** – work on a 7-day week.
3. Your **energy requirement for training** is: your weight x your average training distance x 1.028. The answer is in kilocalories.
4. Add **1.** and **3.** together for the **total daily requirement.**
5. The **carbohydrate requirement** is: total daily requirement x 60%.
6. To turn the **carbohydrate requirement into grams** of carbohydrate divide **5.** by 3.81.
7. Keep a **daily track of your eating** by considering each piece of fruit or potato equal to just less than 20 g of carbohydrate, and a marshmallow equal to 5 g.
8. The **total protein** is: total daily requirement x (15 to 20%).
9. To **turn the total protein amount into grams,** divide by 3.76.
10. To **double-check your total protein requirement:** take your overall body weight x 1.2–1.6 (depending on the training intensity).
11. Take the lesser of **9.** and **10.** as your **daily protein requirement**.
12. **Divide the protein requirement by 25;** this gives the number of open palm, or fistfuls of cooked protein food you require per day.
13. The **fat requirement** is: total daily kilocalorie requirement x 20%.
14. **Convert the fat requirement to grams** by dividing by 9.
15. Aim to **reduce saturated** fats and **increase the essential fats**.

THREE WELL-BALANCED MEALS

Many people (even medical personnel) refer to 'three well-balanced meals', and many of us remember our mothers chiding us not to snack between meals as it would spoil dinner. Our bodies are clever and our natural desire to 'graze' throughout the day is exactly what we should do. Instead of three main meals we should be spreading our kilocalorie intake throughout the waking day in a wedge-like fashion.

The most important meal is breakfast, which should have a high percentage of carbohydrates for energy with small amounts of protein and fat. A mid-morning snack will take you through to lunch, which is probably the most balanced meal between protein and carbohydrate, while a mid-afternoon snack will keep your energy level up for early evening training, prior to the main evening meal. Your evening meal should have the highest percentage of protein of the day (but still be less in amount than carbohydrate), as it provides the building blocks for recovery overnight. As a point of interest, this process should be reversed for nightshift workers (or night races).

Following this routine means there is never more than about two hours between meals and snacks, which means that the blood sugar level is kept fairly constant. Moreover, the total kilocalories can be spread over more intakes, each of which is easier to digest. It will also be discussed later how the type of food you eat has an impact on your blood sugar levels.

Swings in blood sugar levels are a serious problem with the 'three meals' approach, where large kilocalorie intakes are taken at 4–5-hour intervals. Each meal sees a rise in blood sugar, causing the body to produce insulin to reduce the blood sugar level. However, it operates like a pendulum, so it is not brought down to 'normal' but to low blood sugar levels, which initiates a craving for more sugar. The natural reaction is to indulge in a sugar snack, which 'pushes' the blood sugar level back up and before you know it, the entire day has become a 'swing' between high and low blood sugar levels – and also high and low levels of production in whatever you are doing.

Try to develop the habit of 'grazing' throughout the day – small amounts more often, rather than the 'dump truck' approach of eating everything at breakfast and supper, which has become the trend with many busy sportspeople juggling work, family and training.

THE ROLE OF SPORTS SUPPLEMENTS

The above calculations show why sports supplements should be an important part of the endurance athlete's armoury in day-to-day eating. Some people consider these supplements as a 'magic formula' that you take only in the final days before a major event. This is totally wrong; they must be used on a daily basis.

Consider only the requirements for carbohydrates in the above example, and as opposed to peak training, look at the same runner in normal training at 60 km per week. His carbohydrate drops to 2 050 kcal, which converts to 540 g or 27 baked potatoes or pieces of fruit per day! Even at this level it is unlikely that he will take this in via normal food, which results in a number of problems. Firstly, the amount of energy consumed is less than he expends, causing a weight loss. While that might be considered a good thing, if the proportions of fat, carbohydrate and protein are incorrect he may break down protein from his muscles rather than surplus fat. Secondly, he will not have enough carbohydrate energy to perform the following training sessions properly and will not derive the best benefits from his training. Indeed, he may inflict more damage because of poor form. If there is insufficient energy and/or protein, the recovery of his muscles will be delayed and the next training will be on damaged muscles – a sure recipe for injury. This problem becomes greater as each day of insufficient intake passes.

A sure test of this is simply to take a day off and see if your energy levels, and hence your standard of training, returns. If so, the chances are your daily energy intake is insufficient.

Sport supplements are called 'supplements' because they supplement your daily food intake, i.e. when you have analysed your requirements and compared them with what you are eating, you will find that you are short of certain components, such as carbohydrate, protein, or possibly vitamins and minerals. You should then use the supplements to correct these deficits.

This is where your nutritionist can help; he can accurately calculate and analyse what you are eating, then identify the shortfalls. However, start with this rough analysis for a couple of weeks, so that you go there with a basic understanding of where you currently stand.

Inadequate eating negates your training, can lead to illness and injury, as well as long-term problems.

GLYCAEMIC INDEX

The speed at which a carbohydrate is absorbed in your system and the effect it has on your blood sugar level relates to something called the Glycaemic Index of the food. Each food is ranked in relation to glucose or white bread, which has a value of 100 as the high end of the scale. Because you should have a consistent blood sugar level, your preference for normal eating should be towards low glycaemic foods. Some examples of this include apples, oranges, porridge oats and flavoured yoghurts. However, even making a list of items is not that simple, as one brand of oats may have a high index while others are low, and even the heat of some foods changes the index rating. Unfortunately, there are no rules to guide us on what foods have a high, low or medium glycaemic index. The best is to buy a book that lists the foods you commonly eat and to become more aware of when and what to eat. The website www.gifoundation.com is an excellent source of information on glycaemic index.

There is one occasion when the production of insulin is quite desirable – immediately after training. Insulin is part of the process used to assist absorption of nutrients into the muscles to promote recovery. The faster we can deliver the nutrients to the damaged or depleted muscle, the faster it will recover. It is in our interest to create insulin after training, and one way of doing that is to induce a high blood sugar level, therefore it is useful to take high glycaemic foods such as corn flakes, crisped rice, instant mashed potato and jellybeans, immediately after training, to commence the energy and nutrient replacement.

Muscles are particularly receptive to this replacement in the first 15 minutes after training, which is why a quality carbohydrate drink immediately you stop training is recommended. This not only begins the replacement of energy, but also induces the insulin reaction. Thereafter, it is useful to have food or a sports supplement with high-quality protein to provide the building blocks for muscle repair. (However, read the following section on weight control if trying to lose weight.)

RESULTS TAKE TIME

Anything to do with nutrition takes around 3–4 weeks to show benefits, so don't expect overnight results. For instance, if you are diagnosed as iron deficient, the doctor prescribes iron pills. When you take one, it's not like an aspirin; the problem doesn't disappear immediately. Instead, it takes 2–3 weeks before your iron reaches new levels. The same applies with vitamin, mineral, protein and essential fat deficiencies. Ensure that you keep to nutritional changes for a significant period of time before you judge their benefits.

LOW FAT, NOT NO FAT

Fat has been given a bad bill of health, and once again, marketing has convinced people to cut out fat altogether. In our favour as runners is that we need to eat so much that we tend not to eliminate fat from our diet. However, many people, believing that all fat is bad, go to extremes to cut out fat. This is not the case – a group of fats called essential fats are required for hormonal balance. Although this has mainly been given exposure for women, particularly those suffering from premenstrual syndrome, it is important to all. The essential fats are key to the cascade involved in the production of hormones and testosterone, which is vital in muscle repair.

As noted above, you need approximately 20% fat, but it should be the right type of fat, and that is the challenge. Primrose oil, the fat in salmon and flaxseed oil are typical of the directions in which you should be moving, but try to reduce the amount of saturated oils by trimming meats and selecting lean cuts.

WEIGHT CONTROL – NOT LOSS

Every runner quickly recognises that being lighter seems to make them faster, and as a general rule that is true. However, there are a few things to take into account on this subject.

From the section on daily eating, it seems that all we have to do to lose weight is to run more. Furthermore, the section on energy systems showed that during long, slow, easy running we burn high percentages of blood fatty acids. For these reasons, many people (even personal trainers) and magazines promote slow, easy running as a good means of losing weight. At best this is poor advice. Although it is true that you will burn fat while running slowly, the distance required to make a useful loss in weight is too great to be the only action to follow in a weight-loss programme.

Let us assume that our 70-kg runner runs a 56-km race in five hours; 72% of his energy would come from fatty acids. The total energy expended in the race would be 4 030 kcal, of which 2 900 would come from fatty acids, i.e. 317 g. Thus running Two Oceans will result in less than 0.5 kg loss of fat weight. Compare this with the personal trainers who put their 'protégés' on a stationary cycle or a treadmill in order to lose weight.

In both of the above cases we will assume that it was an easy pace for the runner, so his heart rate would not have been pushed above about 75% of maximum, which means that it would quickly return to normal.

Now consider someone who trains in the quality sessions, such as those recommended in the programmes in this book. For instance, a runner does a session of 10 x 1 000 m at his 10-km pace of 3:45 per kilometre. He also does about 6 km in warm-up and cool-down at five minutes per kilometre. The total expenditure of this will be around 1 153 kcal with about 20 g deriving from fat. The total session will take only around 90 minutes, of which only 70 will be spent on actual running, the remaining 20 will be in the recovery periods between the efforts, and during this time additional energy will be burnt. Furthermore in this session the runner's heart rate will have been taken up into the regions of 90% of maximum. When he stops it takes a long time to return to 'normal' so there is an after 'burn' as his metabolic rate gradually reduces. If no carbohydrate is ingested during this time, then additional energy will be supplied by fatty acids, depleting his stores even further. Thus there may be up to another 90 minutes to two hours of time where the metabolic rate is increased to levels that will continue to burn fat. This may double the total fat burnt.

Compare it another way: assuming that the runner takes a long, slow run of 90 minutes, also at five minutes per kilometre, he would only burn about 1 220 kcal of which 30 g is fat. Such examples show that it is better to do high-intensity exercise to achieve weight loss. Of course, the runner must have trained sufficiently to be able to handle the more intense work (see graph of exercise heart rate versus time on the following page).

Finally, you don't have to achieve these speeds to make these losses; you can do exactly the same by using speeds relative to your own standard of running – the above is purely an example to show the principles. Conversely, it shows why runners (who do not need to lose weight) should take energy on board as soon as they finish their training, to start the process of replacing lost energy.

When such an intense training approach is combined with a restricted diet, weight loss can be quite dramatic and initially it will produce faster times as the strength of the leg muscles propel the body through the air more easily, because there is less weight to move. However, a restricted diet, if not properly

EXERCISE HEART RATE v TIME

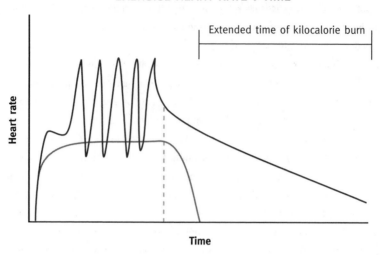

proportioned, or is eaten in such a fashion that recovery is not completed between training sessions, is just as likely to be short of key ingredients and possibly even protein. The result will be diminishing muscle strength, which will compound into further destruction. This is evident with many female athletes in particular, where their initial rocket to faster times, only encourages them to reduce weight even further. The social pressures of looking thin add further stimulus to lose weight, all of which can lead to even more hazardous eating disorders – something to be guarded against, particularly in young female runners.

A final point on weight loss: DO NOT mix diet pills with athletic training; it is a recipe for disaster and death. The combination will increase your metabolic rate and can take it to the point where your body can simply not handle the pressure. Read the section on diet pills and caffeine in chapter 25 on what to take before the event.

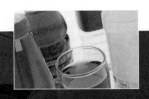

00:00:24
THE MINEFIELD OF
SPORTS SUPPLEMENTS

There is overwhelming scientific evidence to support the use of sports drinks and energy products. As a result of various marketing claims, the market has become a minefield of information and misinformation. This chapter aims to guide you in recognising the types of products and ingredients to look for and their purpose in your nutritional armoury.

The need to keep blood sugar levels up during endurance events has been witnessed by millions who have seen disorientated marathoners and ultrarunners stagger in, in total oblivion of the crowds, determined only to make the tape. The previous chapters have explained why it is impossible to obtain all the carbohydrate energy required each day from solid food, which is where sports energy and replacement drinks play an important role.

Although many of the current sports drinks were developed through the sport of running, and latterly triathlons, most sports participants will benefit substantially from the correct use of such products, before, during and after an event.

To understand their benefits, a basic knowledge of carbohydrates is necessary. A layman's approach to energy systems is covered in chapter 23, but if you require a more detailed description, read Professor Tim Noakes' book, *Lore of Running* (OUP). Basically, your body has two carbohydrate fuel tanks: the liver and the muscles.

LIVER STORES

The liver uses glycogen (stored carbohydrate) to keep blood sugar levels up. This primarily fuels the nervous system and brain. Only a small amount of this fuel is used for muscle energy and thus, once the muscle stores have 'run dry', the muscles must find an alternative source of energy to keep them working.

The liver is constantly depleting because it is always working, and even while asleep you burn about 9 g of glycogen per hour. Typically, your liver has a capacity of 150 g and if not refuelled – even if you only slept for 16 hours – would be drained. This happens even faster during exercise or in the case of anxiety. Hence any sport that requires large amounts of nervous energy, or work by the brain, will benefit from the use of energy drinks.

This also highlights the importance of ensuring a good carbohydrate store in the liver before examinations and the importance of eating a good breakfast. Many sportspeople find breakfast before events impossible and again, this is where sports drinks fill a need as they provide a much better rate of absorption, as well as energy while leaving a relatively empty stomach.

MUSCLE STORES

The use of muscle stores of glycogen are basically restricted to the use of the muscles in which they are stored, i.e. glycogen stored in upper limbs cannot be used to fuel the legs, but the driving of your arms will, to some extent, help you to keep your legs moving. Thus there is some benefit in ensuring that all muscles are loaded to their maximum.

In general terms, muscle glycogen cannot be used to fuel the nervous system and the liver glycogen cannot be used to fuel the muscles.

Assuming a normal diet of about '40%' carbohydrate, which accounts for most of the western world, and assuming that a participant has rested for at least a day before an event, normal muscle glycogen stores will last 60–90 minutes. The rate of glycogen use will vary with the intensity of the exercise (speed).

An athlete completing several series of sprints will burn glycogen faster than one using a more uniform and lower rate of exercise. This is one reason why it is better to taper with quality running rather than long, slow running (see chapter 16 on taper). Glycogen depletion of the muscle stores is likely in events lasting longer than 75–90 minutes at a more uniform effort, or in competitions that require a high number of high intensity efforts.

Although the liver stores or blood sugar may be supplemented during the course of an event to maintain normal levels, muscle stores do not accept significant supplementation during exercise. This implies that during events in which muscle store depletion is likely, a participant should use carbohydrate-loading (popularly referred to as 'carbo-loading') techniques to maximise muscle stores. These stores can be increased 2–3-fold above normal when carried out correctly. In events in which your liver glycogen could be depleted before your muscle glycogen, you will benefit from a combination of carbohydrate loading and energy supplementation during the event.

USING SPORT SUPPLEMENTS – MORE CAN BE TOO MUCH

Even though there is substantial scientific material to support the use of sports energy products by athletes, why do we hear of people for whom experiments in this area have proved disastrous?

If we examine a field of runners at any road race, and in particular those runners who are trying the carbo-loading and energy-replacement techniques for the first time, there will be several different outcomes from these 'experiments'. That is not to say that the runners should be trying these solutions in races for the first time. Indeed, everything should first be tried in training, before being used in an important race. However, people often approach races differently to training, which results in a different reaction. Race anxiety also has an influence.

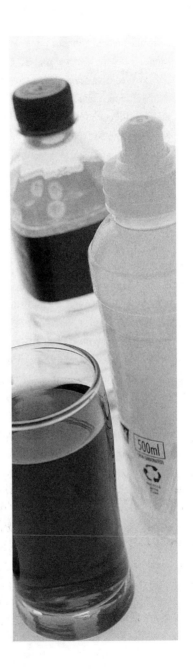

RIGHT *A wide range of sports supplements are available – some good, some bad*

In our field of runners there will be a few who have an allergic reaction to the products in the energy drinks. This should be determined during training. The complex carbohydrate polymers used in many sports drinks derive from maize starches, which can cause an allergic action in a small number of people. Similarly, many products contain small levels of fructose (should not be more than 2–3%), which can also cause gastric problems for some runners, particularly if the percentages are high.

Others in the field will experience no benefit from the energy-replacement techniques. They may have been too cautious, opting to use a much lower carbohydrate-loading scheme, and may have reduced the carbohydrate content of their drinks during the events. Although they will still have benefited to some extent, they will not notice it as they will still 'hit the wall' at some stage. These runners will dismiss the techniques and products as useless.

Finally, there are those who believe that 'if one dosage makes you fast, double or triple will make you a world champion'. This is DEFINITELY NOT THE CASE. While overdosing on these drinks is not physically dangerous, it is very likely to ruin your sporting performance, in dramatic fashion.

Sports products should be approached in the same manner that cyclists set their saddle height. There is a rule of thumb that determines the saddle height from the centre of the crank, and initially you use this to set the saddle height. After hours of riding, a cyclist makes a few millimetres change to the height. Some hours later, another slight adjustment is made and so it continues until a specific saddle height is established. This process takes much time and distance, and in the end is only fractionally different from the 'ballpark' rule of thumb used originally.

Approach sports supplements in the same manner. Commence with the 'ballpark' advice, then tailor the recommendations to your specific needs. Runners who work in this way will benefit significantly. Those who use the 'overloading' technique will probably be left behind in the bushes. Overuse is abuse and will result in negative consequences.

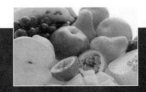

It is said that prevention is better than cure. From chapter 24, you have seen that, when muscle glycogen stores are depleted during an event, there is no cure. Hence, the best and only solution is to prevent it from happening by using a technique known as carbohydrate loading. An average runner, competing in an event greater than 15 km, is likely to benefit from carbo loading.

However, it must be remembered that, even though you can improve these stores by two or three times their normal capacity, there will still be events where this will be insufficient to see you through to the end. The amount of glycogen you require will vary with the intensity and the length of the event.

For instance, compare the effect of intensity over the marathon distance in two runners. The runner who completes the 42.2 km in under four hours, will enhance his performance by carbo loading, due to the increased muscle glycogen stores. This runner's performance is limited by the amount of glycogen in his muscles. However, a runner slower than 4:30 faces a different problem: that of liver glycogen depletion, because he will burn a higher percentage of fat to fuel his muscles and thus has a lower carbohydrate requirement. The full carbo-loading diet is of little benefit, and a shorter version of carbo loading may be used to ensure liver loading prior to the event.

There are a few drawbacks to the carbo-loading diet, which suggests that the slower marathon runner *may* (personal preference is also involved) be better off with a 'normal' approach to his diet before a race.

Obviously, the same type of approach applies to ultra-distance events. Your main concern in such events should be to ensure a full liver store prior to the race, and with food and drink to maintain your blood sugar level during the event (this is covered in more detail later).

The following table gives an indication of **the speeds and distances where carbo-loading diets are beneficial:**

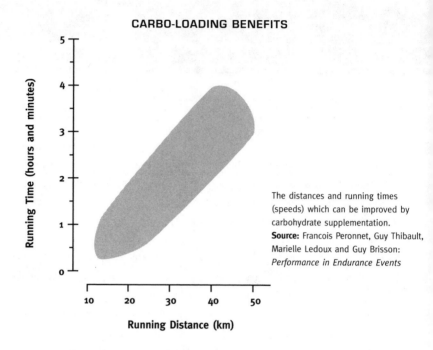

CARBO-LOADING BENEFITS

The distances and running times (speeds) which can be improved by carbohydrate supplementation.
Source: Francois Peronnet, Guy Thibault, Marielle Ledoux and Guy Brisson: *Performance in Endurance Events*

Top runners may find this less accurate at both ends as one of the natural attributes of top runners is their ability to absorb and store muscle glycogen.

MAXIMISING MUSCLE STORES – PRACTICAL CARBO LOADING

The original practice behind the carbo-loading diet was as follows: a runner depleted his existing muscle stores with a longish run of 90–120 minutes at a medium- to high-intensity (below competition) pace, seven days before an event. Having drained these stores, his body's system 'craved' carbohydrates. (It has been found that muscles synthesise the glycogen storage best during this craving period.) The craving was maximised by following a diet very low in carbohydrates for a further three days subsequent to the depletion run.

Yet another reason for the three-day low-carbohydrate period was to schedule the exertion of a long depletion run a full week before the race, allowing additional time for recovery.

As we have seen, it is possible that many heavy trainers may inadvertently be experiencing this 'depletion procedure' on a regular basis during their training routines, despite attempting to replace the carbohydrate straight away. This may result in an adaptation to carbohydrate loading and improved carbohydrate uptake.

The carbo-loading diet continued on the fourth day with a swap in diet emphasis, to a very high-carbohydrate diet of 70–80%, which resulted in the satisfaction of the 'craving' and supercompensation of the muscle stores, so that 2–3 times the normal quantities were stored in the muscles over a period of three days. Achieving these high percentages of carbohydrate in the diet is a major problem, as, by nature, most truly high-carbohydrate foods are bulky, particularly the unrefined ones. The problem is that we feel full long before we have taken in enough to satisfy our loading requirements.

It was never intended for the diet to be 100% carbohydrate, as there is still a requirement for fats and protein during this phase. However, the human tendency to believe that more is better, has led competitors to concentrate solely on carbohydrates. The massive 'swing' to an almost exclusively carbohydrate diet, without sufficient protein and fat, can result in gastric problems and an uncomfortable feeling from the loading phase. Such dramatic changes in diet immediately before a competition should be avoided.

The high-carbohydrate sports drinks that contain long chain carbohydrate polymers are ideal for this situation. Typically, 1 litre of these products, when mixed at 10–20% solution, (i.e. 100–200 g powder to 1 litre liquid) delivers just less than 200 g of carbohydrate.

As indicated, there is still a need to maintain a level of protein and fat in every diet. For this reason, I use a daily serving of a quality sports meal replacement drink, which provides not only an extra dose of carbohydrate (about 60 g), but also some high-quality protein (30 g) and some quality fats. This allows a runner to obtain the remaining carbohydrates from a diet that still resembles normal eating habits. Thus a daily regimen of two carbohydrate drinks and one meal replacement, added to your normal diet, can provide the basis for carbo loading during the three days prior to an event.

Although glucose polymers are at the leading edge of the products currently available in South Africa, recent research from Leeds University in the UK, and on

Scandinavian skiers, suggests that galactose polymers included in sports drinks may be of even greater benefit. However, these products have only been marketed in the USA and may take some time before they are commercially viable for the South African market. Galactose is a sugar found in nuts, fruit and other foods, but is thought to have a greater rate of absorption and lower insulin reaction. The existing product range comprises four categories: a hydration and pre-event drink, a drink for exercise lasting 1–2 hours, a drink for more extreme events, and a recovery drink. Studies have compared these drinks with some of the best quality drinks currently available and it seems that statistically significant increases in performance are noted with the use of the galactose-based products.

CARBOHYDRATE LOADING – HOW MUCH CARBOHYDRATE?

Runner's weight = 65 kg

Body fat $\longrightarrow$ Muscle = 26 kg

Max glycogen/kg = 36 g

Total loaded muscle = 26 x 36 = 936 g

Liver depletion (3 days) = 3 x 24 x 9 g/hr = 648 g

Exercise allowance (60 min) = 60 x 3 = 180 g

Hence total = 936 + 648 + 180 = 1764 g

$\longrightarrow$ **600 g per day**

100 g baked potatoes = 19 g carbohydrate $\longrightarrow$ 30 per day

Banana = 19 g $\longrightarrow$ 30 per day

Pasta 100 g $\longrightarrow$ 23 g $\longrightarrow$ 2.8 kg per day $\longrightarrow$ 5 packets

ALTERNATIVELY

2 drinks of quality carbohydrate (1 litre) = 150 g

1 drink quality meal replacement = 40 g

Normal diet with emphasis on quality carbohydrates

Note: You still need protein and fats – meal replacement ensures a balance.

A major practical problem is determining just how much carbohydrate you need during the loading period. Use the calculation on the previous page as an example for a runner. From this calculation, it is obvious that unless a runner uses a combination of sports supplements and food, it is highly unlikely that he will achieve the carbo-loading targets. Attempts to do it with food only are likely to cause gastric disturbance due to insufficient protein and fat intake over the three days. This is probably the likeliest reason for the 'failure' of carbo-loading diets.

REFINED OR UNREFINED CARBOHYDRATES?

Recent years have seen much debate on whether refined carbohydrates such as jams, syrup and white flour, or unrefined carbohydrates such as beans, apples and potatoes are better from a loading and energy perspective. The debate continues in light of inconclusive evidence.

Over the years, my practical experience suggests that the best solution is a combination, commencing with a predominance of refined carbohydrates and completing the loading with more unrefined carbohydrates. However, unrefined carbohydrates have high fibre levels that not only fill you up, but also promote a full bowel, which is uncomfortable during a race. Initially, this was further complicated by the glycaemic index (GI), but in fact the concept of GI may actually explain the apparent conflict of research as to whether refined or unrefined is better.

As noted earlier, GI is an expression of the rise in blood sugar level after the consumption of a particular food. High blood sugar levels trigger a rise in insulin and are also thought to promote the storage of energy as fat.

Dr Michael Colgan, author of *Optimum Sports Nutrition*, recommends that preference be given to foods with a lower GI. For example, use rolled oats, apples, oranges, lentils and whole-wheat bread in preference to bananas, raisins, honey, white potatoes, white bread and white rice. By looking at this list you will see that both refined and unrefined foods are on both the high and low GI lists. Obviously, if the initial research simply classified foods as being either refined or unrefined, the results would be confusing as they could both contain a mix of high, medium and low GI foods.

Unrefined foods such as rolled oats release their 'energy' over a longer period, whereas refined foods tend to cause major surges in the system. After exercise you

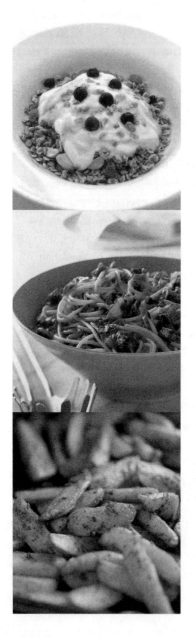

should aim for high GI foods, as they will promote faster uptake of the nutrients, but on the day of an event, keep to low GI foods to maintain as stable a blood sugar level as possible.

In summary, current thinking suggests the use of high GI foods after any training session or effort during the carbo-loading period and low GI foods throughout the rest of the day. Within each of these categories, use a balance of refined to unrefined to ensure that you ingest enough kilocalories and carbohydrate without the bulk or being restricted to fibre-packed, unrefined foods. The move towards carbohydrate selection based on GI is further supported by the latest galactose research, as it also has a lower GI.

WHEN TO START LOADING

Because the body absorbs carbohydrate best when the demand is greatest, the best time to start loading is immediately after exercise. The typical protocol is to start loading in the morning after a shortish, medium-intensity training session. My personal preference is to

LEFT *Cereal, pasta, potatoes – always remember to check the glycaemic index of your carbohydrates, relevant to your specific needs*

extend the loading phase by one evening and to commence the loading with a carbo-loading drink immediately after finishing a short track session. The benefits of this are that the evening session can be more intense, hence I will burn more glycogen, as my body has loosened during the day. Moreover, in the final days before a race, I can extend my rest by lying in bed a bit longer, which works well with the recommendations on tapering.

Research has shown that synthesis is greatest in the first 15 minutes after training has ceased. Many people find it impossible to eat so soon after training and this is where the commercial sports drinks with long chain carbohydrates come into their own. It is easy enough to swallow 500 ml of fluid, which delivers just under 100 g of carbohydrates. An hour or so later, you may continue loading with solid food. For effective carbohydrate loading, you will need between two and four drinks of a 10–20% carbo-booster solution each day for the three days. Each drink should be just over 500 ml.

THE FINAL DAY

We have already determined the amount needed to carbo load, the type of carbohydrates to take, when to start, and that loading should continue for three days before an event. What follows for the final day will depend on the starting time of your competition.

Often, this will be in the morning and for many that means that the last meal will be the night before as anxiety, pre-race nerves and the desire to feel 'light and mean' renders solid food on race morning impossible. The problem is that your liver doesn't know that it has to store glycogen for the competition, so even as you rest (if you can rest the night before a major event), you are burning up at least 9 g of your 150-g liver store every hour.

A quick calculation will show that if your event starts at 09:00 and your last meal was 21:00 the night before, you will start the race with only 42 g of glycogen in your liver, i.e. it is three-quarters empty and needs to be topped up. Often the temptation is to take a carbohydrate drink such as Coke or Lucosade, or a glucose tablet immediately before the event. After all, sugar gives us go… isn't that the message? This may be true, but it is not a wise move immediately before a race because these are all high-glycaemic drinks. Ingesting high-glycaemic drinks or foods will result in the insulin reaction explained earlier, and by the time the race begins, you will have a low blood sugar level that will result in the same feelings you experience after competing for over 90 minutes.

If this is the practice you have been used to, try the following approach, which will probably bring an instantaneous improvement in performance. There are two alternatives for events lasting up to four hours.

Firstly, you can rise early enough to have a meal, which should be light but high in carbohydrates e.g. cereal, whole-wheat toast with jam or honey, followed by fruit juice or water. This meal would be timed such that, despite your anxiety, you are able to digest the meal and allow sufficient time for your blood sugar level to return to normal before the event – probably 3–4 hours before the start.

The second alternative is to rise later and then to recoup your overnight carbo depletion with a large glass or two, of carbohydrate glucose polymer. Being both fluid and a glucose polymer, it is easily absorbed and will not cause an insulin reaction. Ideally, this should be about 90-60 minutes before the event starts. We calculated that your liver will have depleted about 110 g overnight, therefore 700 ml to 1 litre of the drink prior to the event will satisfy your requirements and ensure that you are topped up for the start. Even if you have taken an early meal with a 500-ml drink as a carbo boost, one hour before the start, it will be good insurance.

EVENTS LONGER THAN FOUR HOURS

Most runners running 56 km, 60 km or longer, will be out on the road for over five hours, and this needs greater consideration. The importance for them is not with carbohydrate loading for maximising their muscle stores, but ensuring that they have sufficient stores in the liver. The length of the event also affects the amount of time between meals and the composition of solid food.

Consider a typical day: you start with breakfast, go on to mid-morning tea, lunch, afternoon tea, supper, and often round the day off with a snack. Yet many runners think that on the day of an ultra-competition all they need is fluid and some sort of sugar intake in drinks. While this may be sufficient for shorter events, even up to the marathon in four or five hours, most runners will benefit from some additional nourishment in longer events. Beginning with a more substantial pre-event meal would be the first step.

Furthermore, because longer events have a lower intensity (e.g. Comrades pace is about 20% lower intensity than 10-km race pace), the need to be fully carbo loaded is less critical as much of the energy source will come from blood fatty acids. It stands to reason, then, that a more substantial meal will be required prior to the longer events. Wally Hayward, the famous South African runner who set world bests at 100 miles, 24 hours, London to Brighton, and who won five Comrades races, used to eat a steak three hours before a race.

Given that most race organisers do not provide savoury food, or protein and fat snacks during a race, it makes sense to commence these events with a well-balanced meal, as the only other intake for the following 5–7 hours will be carbohydrate.

During long events you will find a craving for 'substantial' food – normally of a savoury variety. Your body has an ingenious ability to let you know what you need, and my own experience suggests that the use of similar food for the final pre-race meal works well before these longer events. The slower pace of such races allows digestion of the meal. (See also chapters 22 and 27.)

REMEMBER THE NOVICES' RULE

There is a simple rule that all runners pass on to novice runners – 'don't change anything for racing', but it is a rule many runners break when it comes to nutrition.

Often, they alter their diet from balanced meals with carbohydrate, protein and fat, to one comprising only carbohydrate for three days. Or they change their normal eating habits of snacking every 2–3 hours by going for seven or more hours with nothing but coke and water. It is just as important to keep to normal eating habits, as it is to other normal aspects of running. Once you have planned your pre-race meals and drinks (and your energy intake during the event), review the plan to see if there is any other practical way in which it can closer reflect your eating habits in a typical day. The less you change, the more successful you will be.

CARBO LOADING, WATER AND WEIGHT

Carbo loading results in an increase in weight prior to a race – often perceived as a drawback. The major portion of the weight increase results not from the carbohydrate, but from the 3 g of water required to store each gram of carbohydrate, thus each gram results in a total of 4 g of weight increase.

An immediate benefit of this is that it allows you to monitor your carbo loading to ensure that you are achieving your target. For example, a 65-kg runner who needs 600 g of carbohydrate per day for three days, will increase his weight by around 2.3 kg over the three-day loading period, which relates to the amount of additional storage in his lower muscles. Although the extra weight may appear to be a disadvantage, the additional water supply at the start will be useful in extending your ability to cool and remain hydrated. Remember that your performance drops off substantially when you lose over 2% of your normal body weight in sweat. Greater loss can see you suffer heat stroke and exhaustion.

Considering the problems with 'energy surges' associated with the consumption of high-glycaemic food or drink before the start of an event, it is clear that the safest drink in the last hour is water. The best absorption rate of this has been found to be water at a temperature of around 10 °C – you may have to add a few ice cubes to your water bottle.

CARBO LOADING CAN BE DEHYDRATING

In 2000 I had the honour of being the senior manager for the SA 100-km team to the World 100-km Championships in Winschoten. As part of the pre-event logistics, I arranged for the team's hydration levels to be tested using a sophisticated body fat analysis machine from Graeme Homman of Nutrition Matters. A number of the team members were below normal and we pushed their fluid levels up to normal before flying out the following day. After the flight and train journey to the race venue in Europe, we tested them again and this time they were all dehydrated to some extent. Again, over two days they returned to full hydration, after which they started to carbo load. Many started showing signs of dehydration again, this time because they were not drinking enough water with the additional carbohydrates; 3 ml per gram of carbohydrate means adding around 2 litres per day to your normal fluid intake. In the Netherlands we normalised everyone's hydration levels and that year we brought home the men's team bronze, a top ten finish, second women's Veteran, and a top five place for the women. Once again, attention to preparation and planning paid off. From this, I hope you can see that even if you carbo load, you can still compromise your performance by applying only the principle of the system, but not the detail.

EVERYONE'S GUIDE TO DISTANCE RUNNING

FAT LOADING AND FAT BURNING

Sports science is in continuous evolution, operating as a kind of 'vicious circle', i.e. sports scientists research subjects to assist athletes. However, by the time athletes gradually accept this advice, technology and understanding have moved on, scientists have modified their thinking and athletes are required to change their understanding further.

Another way of looking at it is that athletes spend lifetimes in search of methods that work for them. Scientists then take on the challenge of proving why they work and extrapolate new methods from the same principles. Such a situation occurred with the subject of fat burning in long distance events, i.e. any distance that requires a runner to be out at racing pace for longer than four hours, and applies equally to a 4:30 marathoner, and an elite athlete racing 60 km or further. In 1985, on the eve of the Durban launch of Tim Noakes' first edition of *Lore of Running* (OUP), he and I spent the night in a local gym doing tests as I ran over 160 km on a treadmill. The object was to determine what fuel I was burning on long runs.

Tim noted Arthur Newton's 1924 observation that he needed a meal when he raced over 40 miles and highlighted the carbohydrate content of the meal. My experience of such distances told me that I needed something more substantial, but I could not put my finger exactly on what it was. What I did know, however, was a continual stream of sweet food was particularly unappealing to me.

The treadmill test confirmed in my mind the need for more fatty and protein foods during these longer runs, and indeed, closer inspection of Newton's 1924 recommendations confirmed that his meal was significantly high in fat.

Incidentally, when I visited the *Guinness Book of Records*' office in London in 2002, I realised that my treadmill run was a world record. Although Tim and I only continued for 18 hours, eight minutes and 25 seconds, the record is based on 24 hours, which was only surpassed in October 2001 when New Zealander Gavin Smith took 24 hours to cover 170.29 km. Some would argue that there are not many mad enough to attempt this!

More recently, scientists have suggested the use of a 'fat-loading' diet for two weeks in the final preparation for races of 80 km or longer. These recommendations are targeted, I believe, at the more elite runner. I am sure that this advice will be proved to be more dependent on length of time spent running, rather than distance, and will, therefore, benefit any runner requiring over four hours to complete the chosen race distance. This means that a slow marathoner, Two Oceans runner and Comrades runner faces the same problems as an elite runner in Comrades or 100-km events.

The purpose of the high-fat diet is to train a runner's energy system to 'mobilise fat' into energy and appears to fly in to the face of all previous advice. However, it should be remembered that whenever you run in excess of four minutes at race pace, your energy comes from a combination of glycogen and fat. The longer you exercise, the greater the percentage of fat. As this percentage increases, you are forced to slow down because the conversion of fat to energy is a two-stage affair: first to glycogen then to energy, and is less efficient than using glycogen. Obviously, the more efficient you can make this energy system, the less effect the slowdown will have and is the purpose of a two-week high-fat diet; it forces the body to adapt to training without the readily available carbohydrates.

This research is still in its infancy and many alternatives have yet to be tested. I consider it only one method of improving the fat-burning systems, although I can see there may be some benefits from this concept.

It has already been shown that heavy training on consecutive days can cause a significant reduction in glycogen levels, and indeed, the failure to ingest carbohydrate within 45 minutes of completion of exercise will further delay this. If you study my recommendations for training for longer races, you will find that there are two recognisable features.

Firstly, established runners follow a 'quality first – endurance second' format in their build-up to a race, which means that during the final six weeks, the training emphasis is on relatively low-intensity training and higher weekly distance. Secondly, during this period, weekends alternate between long runs, and back-to-back runs of around 25–35 km. Because of the limited recovery between these back-to-back runs, and the increased total weekly distance, I think that runners will find they are partially carbo depleted for much of each week. Recovery of the carbohydrate stores is only really achieved during the rest day. It is during this 'depleted' stage that a similar adaptation to the high-fat diet has been achieved.

An aspect that concerns me about the 'fat-loading diet', is that such sudden changes to the composition of daily diets may cause gastric reactions.

Remember that one of the key reasons for long runs is to improve fat-burning efficiency. However, a drawback of long runs is the damage done to muscles, which becomes substantial the further past 25 km. It would be a big advantage if the fat-burning system could be improved without having to do a long run too close to an event, as it would assist a runner to arrive at the race with fresh legs. A 'high-fat diet' may well provide the solution.

An interesting facet of this research is that the high-fat two weeks is thought to be necessary only about 2–4 weeks before an event, after which a 'normal' diet may be resumed. If this is the case, is it not possible that a runner who specialises in multiday ultraraces will be able to forgo such dietary manipulation as his systems will be almost permanently adapted to such efficient fat burning? Such runners would be undertaking the same type of 'depletion' training in the multiday journey events in which they compete. The answer to this will no doubt take another few years to determine. In the meanwhile, we must continue to 'play' with this idea. There is no doubt that in longer runs there is a need for substantial food intake and that some of this must come from fats as well as carbohydrates.

A last point on a 'high-fat' diet: there are over double the number of kilocalories in a gram of fat compared to a gram of carbohydrate, so if you try a high-fat diet, you must be careful not to increase your overall kilocalorie intake substantially or you will put on weight.

CAFFEINE

Coffee and alternative caffeine sources have been promoted for use before races, because caffeine is known to encourage the burning of fat in preference to carbohydrate and thus saves carbohydrate stores for later in the race. Although this is true, there are some negatives to the process, which you need to be aware of before deciding in which events you will benefit from taking a pre-race caffeine drink. There are also a number of 'natural' caffeine sources such as guarana, kola nut, and Ma Hung, but it is important to treat these in the same manner as coffee or caffeine pills.

Caffeine is a diuretic, i.e. it increases the production of urine and can further promote dehydration during a long race. Clearly, you must find a balance between the performance advantage that caffeine provides for some distances, with potential disadvantage of dehydration. Nor is it merely a matter of distance, as the heat and humidity will also alter this balance. As a rough guide, I imagine the balance point to be between 70 and 120 minutes. It is a case of determining what distance you can race in this time period. In longer events, the dehydration factor is likely to be of greater concern, but weather conditions must also be taken into account.

If you use caffeine, there are a couple of points to remember. Firstly, and most importantly, caffeine is a banned substance, but only over set levels. Drinking one cup of coffee before a race is unlikely to take you to those limits. If you discuss the quantity of caffeine required with various medical professionals, you will receive a wide variety of answers – from four cups to 22 cups or more. There is some truth in all of this. The amounts you require to exceed the limit will vary from day to day, depending on your hydration levels, what and how much you have eaten over the past 8–10 hours, how much sleep you have had, among others. Even the type of coffee used is relevant. A cup of filtered Java may represent 100 mg of caffeine, whereas a chicory-instant coffee blend may be well under 50 mg per cup. Know what you are drinking if you use this 'legal' method of performance enhancement.

Don't forget that many other products also contain caffeine, such as Coca-Cola and other soft drinks. As drugs tests are held at the end of races, I can only speculate what some runners' levels may be by the end of the race, when Coca-Cola is provided by all race organisers in South Africa. While short events may not present a problem, races such as Comrades could see substantial intakes, particularly by those running for more than ten hours.

If you are a big coffee drinker, the effect of one or two cups before a race will be negligible. One way to enhance the 'buzz', is to abstain from coffee and caffeine products for about a week before an event. You will have to be careful about everything you eat as even products such as chocolate contain caffeine.

Another benefit of the early morning cup of coffee is the promotion of a bowel movement – one cup equals one trip to 'the big white telephone'. You will find similar reactions with most early morning hot drinks; rooibos is a great alternative if you want to avoid caffeine prior to a race.

It's worth noting that a small amount of caffeine, supplied in its natural form such as kola nut or guarana, taken during an event is of benefit, but the emphasis is on 'small', typically in the region of 25 mg per hour. It is also found in a number of quality sports drinks. The levels, if used as directed, are generally lower than those in Coca-Cola. I think the use of green tea extract will grow over the next few years as it not only provides the natural caffeine effect, but is also a good anti-oxidant to combat the action of free radical damage.

DIET PILLS AND FORMULAS

I include this here, because some people have been known to use them for the 'buzz' often associated with such supplements, while others simply follow the instructions that typically suggest a number of capsules or tablets, about 30–60 minutes before training.

The use of diet pills is dangerous to the training runner. The majority of diet supplements consist of the 'ACE' formulation, often in natural products. ACE stands for aspirin, caffeine and ephedrine. The purpose of this formulation is to increase metabolic rate, thereby burning more kilocalories, even while sitting. It's often suggested that they be taken before exercise, as that will increase the metabolism even further. But this assumes that people wanting to lose weight will not participate in *vigorous or intense exercise*. If they do, these tablets are LETHAL! The tablets increase the metabolic rate, which is further pushed up by the exercise, creating a heat build-up, all compounded by the level of dehydration generated by the exercise and the diuretic effect of the constituents. This causes the heart rate to climb, often reaching a point where the body can no longer handle the pressure. Many deaths have occurred from the incorrect use or abuse of diet pills. Avoid these formulas. If you have followed the advice on day-to-day eating, and balance it with exercise, you will quickly reach your correct weight.

00:00:26
OPTIMUM FLUID LOADING

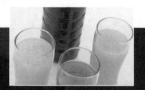

In their search for an 'edge' to performance, athletes typically overlook the most common component of the body – water. Water accounts for around 80% of total body weight, in a number of forms, including blood plasma. It performs a wide range of functions that are vital to an athlete's performance.

Ironically, as a solvent, water is key to the effectiveness of many other supplements that an athlete may take in the search for performance advantage. Most nutritional supplements require closely defined concentrations, often balanced with complementary vitamins and minerals for optimum performance. Relatively small changes in the body's water content can easily upset those balances and lead to a less than optimal performance.

SWEAT LOSS

One of the major roles of water during exercise is to aid cooling, thereby maintaining body temperature in a narrow band of efficient operating temperature. A key procedure in the cooling system is the evaporation of sweat from the skin. This water is lost to the system and there is a limited amount of water that can be released for this purpose before the efficiency of other operations is sacrificed.

The rate of perspiration depends on various factors including the environment, and intensity of exercise. Though warm temperatures can increase sweat rates, high humidity can reduce the rate of evaporation and hence restrict the cooling effect.

Winter training can result in similarly high water losses. Not only is water lost through breathing, but also in the micro-environments created by more protective clothing. Typically, outside training requires a windproof jacket or top. As exercise increases the body temperature, the air within the jacket increases both in temperature and humidity. This temperature increase intensifies the need to cool. An increase in humidity restricts evaporation, demanding a further need for cooling, and hence more sweating, all of which leads to greater water loss.

Another consideration is core body temperature; as the intensity of exercise increases, so too does the core temperature and the need to perspire, leading to dehydration, which in turn results in an increase in body temperature in an ever-increasing spiral.

LOSS OF PERFORMANCE

Aerobic endurance exercises, such as cycling and running, are typical of activities that promote extended periods of sweating. Although typical perspiration rates are in the region of 1 litre per hour, athletes have often lost as much as 2 litres of fluid per hour. Alberto Salazar has the highest recorded level of 7 litres. Normal rates equate to a 1 kg per hour 'weightloss', which can quickly add up.

Research has shown that performance can drop off by 20% when fluid loss reaches 2% of total body weight, which in practical terms means that a 65-kg runner need only lose 1.3 kg of sweat. In adverse conditions this can be reached in the first 90 minutes of exercise.

MAINTAINING FLUID LEVELS

There are basically two remedies to control loss of sweat:

> ▸ Adopt a rehydration programme that will keep your fluid levels topped up.
> ▸ Use a 'water-loading' technique to provide a larger starting base before commencing exercise.

In competitive situations it is highly unlikely that fluid levels can be maintained throughout a long event. Research has shown that, even with the recommended 250–300 ml per 30 minutes of exercise, it is unlikely that the fluid can be absorbed at a rate that equates with the rate of loss.

In practice, however, it has been found that the majority of runners imagine that they drink more than they actually do. The voluntary drinking rate is closer to 500–600 ml per hour, which compounds the risk of performance loss and dehydration. Therefore long, intense exercise will lead to a degree of dehydration for most people and partial dehydration automatically results in a reduction in exercise intensity.

The potential for dehydration is further compounded by the fact that water alone is not easily absorbed and, ideally, should contain some electrolyte to assist in absorption. This can be achieved by adding about 1 g of salt to a litre. This is not a new concept, but one that Arthur Newton noted as far back as 1924 with his special 'corpse-reviver' drink. He also added sugar and bicarbonate of soda, which were diluted into old-fashioned home-made lemonade. Interestingly, the constituents of his drink form the basis of most of the high-quality modern sports drinks, which also contain electrolytes and sugar. Only the more technically advanced drinks have made use of lactic buffers, which was the purpose of the bicarbonate of soda.

Even in 1924 Newton knew that water by itself is not absorbed. In the early 1980s, sports science condemned the use of salt tablets during races, mainly because runners had overdone it and were using abnormal amounts of the tablets during events. Furthermore, salt was generally denounced, even in normal eating, as a cause of high blood pressure, which caused runners to reject all forms of salt – a big mistake. The swing away from salt tablets was so significant that many of 'big name' brands were no longer stocked by pharmacies. The effect of electrolyte-less water provided in races can often be seen in longer events where runners become bilious, and vomit fairly large volumes of water.

Electrolytes are necessary for the absorption of water – in training and racing, so the idea of stopping at water taps every 4–5 km in a long training run is of little benefit unless steps are taken to take in salt at the same time.

Runners who competed in long ultra-events quickly learnt that the 'no-salt' advice was flawed, and recognised Newton's wisdom. Now there is a move back, but remember that more is not better. We require some salt, NOT large amounts.

Eighty years after Newton, a 'new' capsule has come onto the market, which not only offers the right quantities of salt, but also the acid 'buffering' effects that Newton identified in the 1920s. One capsule, with water, every hour to 90 minutes improves absorption and hydration levels. Many runners also report additional benefits of improved recovery (a logical effect from better hydration) and a general improvement in performance.

As a contrast to those runners with average and faster race times, it is worth noting that cyclists do not experience the same reduction in voluntary drinking rate, nor do those who exercise at low intensity.

There have been several cases of slower ultramarathon runners suffering from 'hyperhydration' in races of 50 km and longer (as well as marathoners finishing in over four hours in hot conditions). Hyperhydration occurs when very high levels of fluid are drunk along the route. It is speculated that these runners may also have trained inappropriately for the events, and were in a stage of extreme fatigue for the latter section of the races. Runners who have difficulty in passing urine during exercise may also be susceptible to hyperhydration.

Sometimes, as slower runners tire, they spend more time at refreshment tables and use the drinking of fluid as a 'reason' to delay their progress, leading to excessive fluid intake. (Ironically, the symptoms can often be mistaken for dehydration and there have been cases where medical staff applied drips at the end of the event.) Thankfully, this condition has received greater awareness due to research in South Africa, primarily by Professor Tim Noakes and the team at the University of Cape Town.

Studies conducted in the South African Ironman, and other long events, found that competitors with low sodium blood plasma levels performed poorly in comparison to those with normal sodium levels. It was also noted that the fastest runners were those who finished the event slightly dehydrated (which prompts higher sodium levels). The most important finding of these studies is that runners who drink too much water, lower their sodium levels dramatically, which can (and has!) become a life-threatening condition. Although dehydration will generally only result in a runner recording a less than optimum performance or grinding to a halt, runners who overhydrate, risk death.

The current recommendation is to drink as you please, and while this might work for short or medium events, most runners will be safer using a more specific guide in longer events. The old standard of 250–300 ml per 30 minutes is still a good starting point and well below the amounts that induce overhydration.

For the majority of runners in most races (i.e. all runners in short events and most runners in a marathon), the greatest threat to performance comes from dehydration. Although hot fluid is obviously not desirable, it has been shown that there is little difference in absorption rate between warm and cold fluid. The main benefit of cool drinks is taste, as well as the overall cooling effect. Studies indicate that 10 °C is the most attractive water temperature to runners, therefore

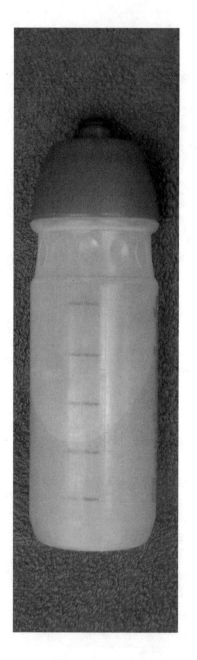

they voluntarily drink more. By comparison, if too cold, drinks can have side effects that include headaches and stomach cramps.

KEEPING TRACK OF HOW MUCH YOU DRINK

The best absorption rates are obtained by taking small, regular amounts of fluid, i.e. sipping 100 ml of fluid every ten minutes, rather than drinking 250 ml at the end of each half-hour. The importance of water with energy gels, and drinking, is emphasised throughout the nutrition section, but do you know how much you are drinking during a race?

Try the following: take two glasses, one full of water and the other empty. Swallow from the full one and hold the water in your mouth. Now spit it into the empty glass and measure it. You will find that your swallow is only about 20–25 ml. Even if you pick up a full bottle of water during the race, you probably only take three or four swallows, which amounts to a total of 60–75 ml. At the time it will seem as though you are drinking a lot, but in reality, it may be

LEFT *Indicating time and amount, this bottle developed by Norrie Williamson assists runners to pace their drinks*

substantially less than you need. The situation is aggravated if you use energy gels because they typically need 150–250 ml of fluid to be diluted correctly (see the following chapter), and explains why some people have problems with energy gels.

Counting mouthfuls is a simple and useful way of ensuring that you keep to a practical fluid intake. A simple calculation can guide you as to how many mouthfuls to take at each table. For instance, if you plan to run your race at five minutes per km, and the refreshment tables are set at 3-km intervals, there will be a water point every 15 minutes. Using the previous advice, it means you need 125–150 ml. Converted to mouthfuls it shows that you need about six mouthfuls at each table, which is all you need to remember to ensure a reasonable level of hydration.

PRE-EVENT FLUID LOADING

The problem remains, however, that competitive athletes find it extremely difficult to replace fluid at an adequate rate during intense exercise. This leads to a second option – preloading. Most authorities extol the virtues of drinking prior to exercise and steering clear of diuretic drinks such as coffee, tea and alcohol. But the body is a clever machine that, in normal conditions, maintains a natural balance; drinking extra water prior to exercise merely increases the rate of urine output.

However, a major benefit of pre-event hydration is that some fluid in the gastric system appears to facilitate absorption. The virtues of carbo loading as a means of boosting energy stores prior to an event have been fairly well documented. A similar, but less well-known technique is available for boosting hydration levels.

In the late 1980s, the University of New Mexico undertook a number of studies to show that it is possible to increase the body's ability to hold fluid with the ingestion of glycerol. The benefits of this are clear. By increasing the total body water prior to exercise, the effects of sweat loss during exercise are reduced. Hence, blood plasma levels are maintained and the core body temperature is stabilised for longer, as is the balance of electrolytes, allowing performance levels to be maintained for longer periods.

The New Mexico study revealed a reduced urine volume of approximately 50% in exercise lasting two-and-a-half to four-and-a-half hours, which are typical finishing times in a marathon. They also proved a 60% increase in water retention and lower core temperatures. The latter was associated with higher rates of sweat loss.

Although New Mexico led the research, similar results have been seen with cyclists in a variety of studies reported in *Medicine & Science in Sports & Exercise*, the official journal of the American College of Sports Medicine, and the John Stuart Research Laboratories in Illinois, USA. As a result of that research, there has been a move to put glycerol onto the market for sportspeople. Use a pharmaceutical-quality glycerol as it mixes easily with water or your favourite carbohydrate drink for easy absorption.

To some extent, the benefits of 'fluid loading' have been around since the adoption of carbo-loading protocols. When storing extra carbohydrate (stored as glycogen) in the muscles, it is necessary to increase the amount of water absorbed; each gram of glycogen requires 3 ml of fluid to be stored, which explains the increase in weight that athletes detect in the final days of carbo loading prior to an event. Thus a 65-kg runner, who takes about 600 g of carbohydrate per day to ensure a full energy store, will experience a weight increase of 1.5–2.3 kg over the three days, from water bound into the glycogen. The difference with glycerol is that fluid is 'pulled' into the spaces between the cells, packing even more fluid into the body. For this reason there is less of the 'bloating' associated with carbo loading but there will still be an increase in weight.

Although little has been published on the subject, there is reason to believe that a combination of carbohydrate and glycerol loading will provide the highest gains. Whereas carbohydrate loading commences between seven and three days prior to an event (see carbo-loading section), glycerol loading is undertaken in the hours before an event. Thus, when combined with a suitable carbohydrate drink, it offers an opportunity for a final 'top up' of energy stores.

The glycerol-loading protocol varies from athlete to athlete, but the instructions in the table on the following page provide a good starting point for evolving your own preference.

In all, a 60-kg athlete will have consumed 1.26 litres of fluid in the 90 minutes of loading. If mixed with a 10% carbohydrate solution, it will also have added another 100 g of glycogen to the energy stores.

While this is primarily a pre-event procedure, it is possible to use the glycerol in longer events. In such cases, try taking 1 ml of the 20% solution per kg of body weight, every 30 minutes. Using glycerol in this manner during an event has been

A SAMPLE GLYCEROL-LOADING PROTOCOL

1. Mix a 20% solution of **glycerol and water** (or carbohydrate drink such as Viper), i.e. 20 ml (4 tsp) of glycerol with 100 ml of fluid. In total you will need 500–800 ml of solution.

2. Two-and-a-half hours prior to the event, **drink 5 ml (1 tsp) of the solution** for every kilogram of body weight, therefore a 60-kg athlete requires 300 ml, a 70-kg runner needs 350 ml, etc.

3. Two hours ahead of the race, **drink 5 ml (1 tsp) of water** (or carbohydrate drink) per kilogram of body weight; which represents 300 ml of water for a 60-kg athlete.

4. After another 15 minutes, **repeat with another 5 ml (1 tsp) of water** per kilogram of body weight.

5. With 90 minutes to go, **return to the glycerol solution** and drink 1 ml per kilogram of body weight (i.e. another 60 ml of glycerol and water for the 60-kg athlete).

6. As the last hour approaches, **drink another 5 ml (1 tsp) of water** per kilogram of body weight (another 300 ml for the 60-kg athlete).

evolved by runners themselves, rather than by scientific research. You will more than likely need to adjust the amount or frequency to your personal requirements as you determine its efficacy. This intake is, of course, additional to your normal event drinking protocol.

If you want to maintain a high level of performance, you must maintain high energy and fluid levels for the length of a competition. Your ability to do this is a function of the amount of fluid and energy you consume during the race, and the amount of fluid and energy with which you start the competition. If you don't start with a 'full tank', don't expect to reach the end.

The fluid-loading protocol should not be attempted by back runners in races where there are adequate refreshment points, because that would increase the risk of hyperhydration.

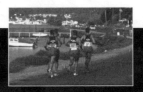

Remember that we have two types of carbohydrate stores: those in the liver, which primarily fuel the brain and nervous system, and those which fuel the muscles in which they are contained. There are effectively three types of events to consider: where muscle and liver stores are adequate for race duration; where muscle and liver stores become depleted; and where liver stores are likely to deplete first.

ADEQUATE MUSCLE AND LIVER STORES

Normal muscles stores are adequate for most events that a runner can complete in under 75–90 minutes, assuming he has followed a reasonable training diet and has had a few easy days prior to the race. This time can be extended for longer events where the normal muscles stores may run out before the finish time by carbo loading in the three days prior to the competition. According to one school of thought, there is very little advantage to be gained by ingesting carbohydrate during an event to increase muscle glycogen, as scientists have suggested that it cannot be absorbed through the 'muscles filter'. This is, however, a subject of some controversy, and more recent research suggests that there may be some absorption by the muscles, although this is limited.

Thus, in any event for which you have amassed sufficient muscle stores and will not run out of liver stores, there is no advantage in taking energy drinks during the competition. In which case, all efforts should be set on replacing water lost through sweat. (Note: this applies to all distances that a runner can complete in 2–2.5 hours. This is time-, not distance-orientated, so while a world-class athlete may almost reach 50 km, a good club runner may only complete a marathon, and an average runner may find that 32-km races are his limit on this protocol.)

Research indicates that most runners prefer a water temperature of about 10 °C, possibly because the water feels more refreshing, but in normal weather conditions, temperature is not too critical. In adverse heat, cool drinks are preferable.

As we have seen in the previous chapter, fluid is required at a rate of 250–300 ml per half-hour, and a low concentration of minerals added to this water will aid absorption. It is also worth considering the use of the new salt and buffering capsules discussed in the previous chapter, which cover all the aspects relating to fluid replacement before and during races.

MUSCLE AND LIVER DEPLETION

Events that require both muscle and liver stores to be greater than normal tend to last from two-and-a-half to five hours in duration, i.e. a Comrades winner at elite level, but a tail-end marathoner at the other end of the field. Once again, this highlights that not all Comrades runners will benefit from following the energy regimens or products used by leading runners – it's about time, NOT distance.

If you expect to deplete your normal muscle stores, carbo load in the days prior to the event; it will also ensure that your liver stores are at a maximum at the start.

There are two requirements to be met during a race. The first and most important is to ensure proper fluid replacement. No-one ever died of starvation in a race – you simply grind to very slow plod, walk or halt. However, a lack of water (dehydration) can result in heat exhaustion, or more dangerously, heat stroke. Put fluid replacement at the top of your list and energy replacement second.

In hot conditions, try wetting your vest before you start. It may not look too smart but wouldn't you rather perform better because you are cooled as the air evaporates the fluid?

There is also a need to supplement blood sugar levels, and to exploit any opportunity to supplement glycogen to the muscles. This is a fairly complicated subject physiologically, but what counts to the runner is the practical application. If you want to delve deeper into the science, consult Professor Tim Noakes' *Lore of Running* (OUP).

Water with small amounts of electrolyte is the best fluid absorbed from the stomach. When carbohydrate is added to the drink, the absorption rate will reduce, and if the dilution of the solution goes above 5%, there is a considerable drop-off in the rate of absorption. Therefore, you may not be replacing the amount of fluid, i.e. water, that you require and may very well experience excessive dehydration and a drop in performance.

However, in 1984 Professor Noakes was a world leader in the identification of long chain glucose polymers as suitable for use in higher concentrations, without adversely affecting the rate of absorption, which led to the development of glucose polymer sports drinks. When first launched in 1984, Leppin FRN Enduro-Booster was a world first and subsequently became the market leader. Most quality sports products now use similar glucose polymers as the base of their energy source.

The use of glucose polymers allows the concentrations to increase to around 10%, although individual preference will determine the maximum that can be handled. The intensity of an event also has an impact and the normal protocol is to suggest a 7–10% solution for normal races. If the event is long, the running intensity drops and the ability to absorb higher concentrations increases, although about 12% is probably the highest that should be considered without thorough testing over the full event distance. It is important that the drink should have sufficient electrolytes to aid absorption.

In powder form, 10% means using 100 g with 1 000 ml of water. If you choose to use another fluid as a base, e.g. fruit juice, reduce the amount of powder by the amount of carbohydrate already in the other fluid. If the base fluid is a simple sugar, it will slow down the absorption rate from your stomach if it provides over 5% of the carbohydrate in the solution. It isn't that complicated if you think it through.

As indicated in chapter 26, recent research suggests that galactose-based carbohydrate drinks may be even more efficient and you would be well advised to keep track on new developments in this field.

Mixing the powder is not difficult, but the inevitable lumps frustrate some people. The trick is to put the water into the bottle first and then add the powder slowly, allowing the powder to 'fold' into the water and mix easily. (Of course, using a blender is the best solution.)

In events where a runner may be seconded, it is simple enough to hand him a constant supply of water and energy at the designated areas.

Energy gels and goo's

However, seconding is generally banned in road running and it is impractical to carry bottles of energy with you or to leave energy drinks beside the road or along the route. For this reason sachets of concentrated syrup were developed and it is possible to carry several sachets. An athlete can dilute these during an event at the appropriate refreshment tables. It must be clear, however, that the development of the energy gel was a compromise to allow energy to be carried. The rules regarding energy replacement remain the same, and, for instance, you should dilute the gel to the same 10% level.

This provides another challenge as gels are typically packed in 25 g sachets, which means that you require about 250 ml of fluid for one sachet. That is quite a substantial amount of fluid to take at one time in a race as the sachet size is basically set on a 30-minute dose, which is why gels don't work for some runners – they don't take the time to ensure the correct dilution.

Recently, it was suggested that a solution as high as 20% of glucose polymer may be absorbed at relatively normal rates, provided some fluid remains constantly in the stomach. But this sort of concentration is better suited towards the end of longer events and may also be easier in sports where there is more body support such as cycling and kayaking. The implication of this is that an athlete should maintain a steady, constant fluid intake at short intervals throughout a race, drinking several small drinks at short intervals rather than bigger drinks at greater intervals. The side effect of this – not acceptable to all – is a sensation of swilling fluid discomfort during a race, which I call the 'pea soup syndrome'.

Another problem is that many gels are thick and viscous. Do the following experiment. Take a sample of the different types of syrup available and pour each into an empty glass. Add the stipulated amount of water, normally 250 ml, and see how well they mix. This is quite a good representation of the way in which many people take these syrups during competitions. They bite of the tops, swallow the syrup contents and then drink some water. Frequently they fail to take the minimum 250 ml of water, thereby decreasing the dilution ratio considerably. Some people suggest that the action of running will have a mixing effect, so take each glass and turn it upside down, with your hand sealing the top and see what happens. In most cases, there will still be a major 'blob' of syrup stuck to the bottom of the glass – not the desired effect, as ideally, you need a well-mixed solution.

Clearly, it makes sense to select free-flowing or 'runny' syrup that will mix well with the water you swallow after the syrup. The alternative is to take the syrup in small bits in your mouth, hold it there, take some water, and then mix it in your mouth before swallowing. This may be possible during less intense races, such as an ultra and possibly a marathon, but it will destroy the breathing rhythm in something more intense, such as a half-marathon.

If the syrup is not properly mixed, a blob such as the one in the glass will exist in your stomach and you would then have a highly concentrated solution in your stomach. This can be further exacerbated by insufficient water consumption. Your body senses that there is a 'meal' to digest and thus absorption drops dramatically, while blood is diverted to the stomach to aid digestion.

If the concentration is high enough, absorption of fluid may cease entirely. Either way, fluid will no longer enter your system at the correct rate, but initially, will still exit the system through sweating, creating the threat of dehydration. There is also the possibility of nausea and a series of 'pit stops' depending on your reaction to a very sweet solution.

At this stage it is unlikely that you will realise what is happening and you may be tempted to try some more solution, as you experience a 'tingling' sensation and a fall-off in performance, which you might attribute to low blood sugar. This will further compound the problem and a downward spiral commences.

The ideal way to take energy drinks is in a solution of about 10% (possibly 20% towards the end of an ultra), providing it is a glucose polymer. To do this with a gel would ideally mean using half a sachet every 15–20 minutes with 100–150 ml of water, which is a much more manageable amount to consume at any one time.

There are a number of commercial products on the market that claim to be energy drinks, which are suitable for events of up to four or five hours' duration. It is simple to identify those that are of use. Look at the table of ingredients: the carbohydrate content per 100 ml should be close to 10 g; and there should be zero, or negligible protein and fat, as well as a reasonable amount of electrolytes. Also look for a mix of short- and long-term energy. The short-term energy should only account for around 2–3% of the total carbohydrates, and the remainder should be long chain glucose polymers. Beware of high levels of fructose, as many people can not tolerate levels above 2%.

Some manufacturers also produce electrolyte drinks, which have very low carbohydrate contents. Do not mistake these for energy drinks; they are best suited as post-event drinks, or for use in longer events or hot and adverse conditions.

Carrying gel or goo energy in an event or training

In a long event, you may require a number of gels or goo sachets, which means you must find a convenient way to carry them. Although there have been belts on the market for a number of years, they have a tendency to chafe, move or bounce around as you run. This problem has been overcome with the development of energy shorts, which are designed to carry energy gels. They hold up to five hours' worth of energy gels, so in longer events it may be necessary to 'reload' along the way from a friend or one of the official tables.

Another popular way to carry your energy replacement, particularly in hot climates, is by means of the Tripper Fluid supply system. It is available in different sizes, with the runner/triathlete version having 500-ml flexible fluid bags positioned back and front. These bags are on a specially designed harness that ensures that the weight is transferred directly down through the vertical axis of the body. Because they are flexible, the bags mould themselves to the body and therefore there is no bounce.

The 'two pack' version is superior to the single fluid pack (which some cyclists use) from a running perspective, as a single pack alters running style and position. The fluid packs are also insulated and use separate supply pipes, permitting the use of hot and cold fluids or two different fluids at one time. In some countries the Tripper may be worn in place of a vest in triathlons.

Choline

For many years there has been a controversy over the requirements of minerals in replacement drinks. Calculations on the amount of potassium, salt and magnesium lost during an event show that, under normal conditions, it seems unlikely that any mineral supplementation is required other than electrolytes to assist with absorption. If your chosen event is a marathon or longer, some research suggests that ingesting 2 g of choline chloride prior to the race, and again

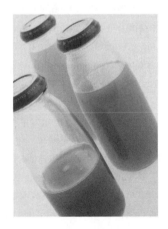

at the halfway mark, will assist muscle performance and reduce fatigue in the latter stages of the race. I have found this beneficial, but suggest that you experiment with it in training on a long run. A drink or a capsule with additional choline may be worth trying.

EVENTS WHERE LIVER GLYCOGEN IS CRITICAL

If the time taken by a runner to complete a distance increases, the intensity of his running drops, the percentage of energy from blood fatty acids increases and his glycogen muscle stores decrease. When that happens, it is the liver glycogen stores that are likely to run dry first. Thankfully, this can be 'refuelled' during the event with the use of carbohydrate drinks and gels as indicated above. However, in events that take longer than six hours to complete, the benefit of energy from more substantial meals is worth consideration.

Events, such a 100 km or 100 milers, have abnormal requirements in that they are far in excess of our normal training distances or times and, as such, they require us to think about how they alter our normal day. Consider, for example, an ultra of 100 km, which will take an average runner 9–11 hours. Using the previous recommendations, a runner will have only water and energy drinks for that length of time. In a normal day, however, he would probably have had three meals and two or three snacks in the same period.

There aren't any training protocols to adjust to such an 'abnormal' regime, yet for some unknown reason, competitors seems to think their bodies will be willing to accept this abuse without grumble on race day. It doesn't make sense. In my view, any event requiring constant effort over a period of time greater than six hours, requires a competitor to give significant thought to a more substantial form of food. The longer the event, the greater the reason for more substantial food.

I cannot claim the following idea, but I'm at a loss to explain why it needs 'reinventing', considering that the great Arthur Newton wrote about it in 1924, 'If I race over 50 miles I need something substantial to eat around 40 miles.' Why do we keep ignoring the lessons from others?

As you increase the length of events in which you participate, the number and type of 'walls' that you experience become greater. The 'wall' in the marathon is said to be at 32 km, which equates to approximately 2.25 hours in any endurance event.

There is another at 4–5 hours (the one that Arthur Newton referred to), and others as you move beyond 100 miles.

The need for more sustenance was regularly highlighted when the top South African Comrades runners first graduated through to 100-km races. Despite their exceptional talents over the gruelling 90-km Comrades course, which they typically completed in 5.25–5.5 hours, they often floundered over the final 45–60 minutes required in the 100-km race. In reality, they finished Comrades just after they reached the 65–81-km 'wall' that Arthur Newton had identified, but by this stage, the crowd, the excitement of the runners and the drive of being at the front enabled them to 'hang on' for the final 8 km or so. However, in a 100-km race they still had another two hours to go and could not continue at the same pace, because they had ignored the different energy requirements of the longer event. This became patently obvious in the World 100-km

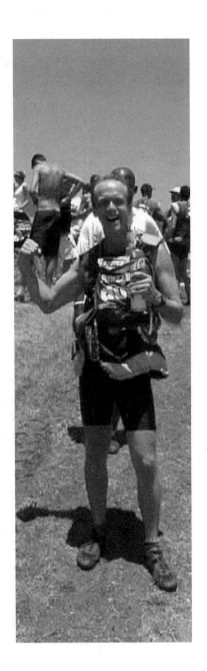

RIGHT *Bruce Fordyce, nine-times winner of the Comrades Marathon and three-times winner of the London to Brighton, pictured here at the end of the first day of the Duzi Canoe Marathon*

Championships of the early 1990s, when the South African team often dominated the race up to 80–88 km, only to grind to a halt. Other top runners, who had taken regular amounts of food throughout the event, had the sustenance to move through and take the lead.

One of the greatest short-distance ultrarunners of the 1980s and '90s was Bruce Fordyce, who won the Comrades Marathon nine times, London to Brighton three times, and set a world best for 50 miles and 100 km. Bruce suffered the same fate when he first moved up to 100 km in the Stellenbosch 100-km Challenge in 1989. Having run a tactical race early on, he moved into the lead just after 80 km and was over ten minutes ahead of the then world best road time, with only 15 km to go. This meant that he had run at an average pace of under three minutes, 45 seconds per kilometre to reach 85 km, but in the final kilometre he battled to stay under five minutes per kilometre, and eventually only shaved one minute from the previous world best.

By comparison, Scots and Greek ultrarunners Don Ritchie and Yiannis Kouros, commence eating right at the start of their ultras. Between them they hold or have held the world bests for every distance from 50 miles to 1 500 miles, so it's safe to assume that they know something about long events.

One of the attributes that made Bruce such a talented performer was his ability to listen to others' opinions, whether they were novices or experienced runners. He would evaluate each piece of information as it related to him, discard the rubbish and modify his approach to training and racing in the light of what remained. He was constantly able to learn and keep abreast of developments, and his preparation for an event was thorough – an approach that is worth emulating. In ultra-events, it's even more critical because the longer an event, the more there is to go wrong, and the greater the impact will be of elements such as weather, crowd support and seconding on in the outcome of a competition.

The fact that some runners are able to manage Comrades or a 100-km race without eating does not mean that they, or you, wouldn't perform better by including more substantial food. For a top runner, who will finish in less than eight hours, it may be sufficient to simply add a liquid food in the form of a quality sports meal replacement along the way. However, a 9- or 11-hour runner, may need a few sandwiches and soup, which was one of the meals that Arthur Newton used.

TIME	A – GOLD/SILVER MEDAL	B – BILL ROWAN MEDAL	C – BRONZE MEDAL
SPREAD OUT YOUR ENERGY THROUGHOUT THE RACE			
0:45	Gel or carbo drink	Gel or carbo drink	Gel or carbo drink
1:30	Gel or carbo drink	Gel or carbo drink	Gel or carbo drink
2:15	Gel or carbo drink	Gel or carbo drink	Gel or carbo drink
3:00	Meal replacement	Meal replacement	Meal replacement
3:45	Gel or carbo drink	Gel or carbo drink	Gel or carbo drink
4:30	Gel or carbo drink	Food/meal bar	Food/meal bar
5:15	Meal replacement	GU/cytomax	Gel or carbo drink
6:00	Gel or carbo drink	GU/cytomax	Meal replacement
6:45	Gel or carbo drink	Meal replacement	Gel or carbo drink
7:30	Finish	Gel or carbo drink	Gel or carbo drink
8:15		Gel or carbo drink	Food/meal bar
9:00		Finish	Gel or carbo drink
9:45			Gel or carbo drink
10:30			Meal replacement
11:15			Finish

Remember that in low-intensity events, after substantial lengths of time, you will experience a protein breakdown. Doesn't it make sense that some of this should be replaced in long events?

The table above provides some suggestions on how to spread out your energy requirements for Comrades. No doubt you will have your own preferences, but this is a good starting point, and you will generally find that the timing of the necessary drinks and food will fit in with the easy location of seconds or helpers along the way. The reference to carbohydrate drink and energy gels means using high-quality products; many of the commonly available 'energy drinks' are not suitable for such use.

Cycling, canoeing, adventure racing and triathlons require a similar approach. Take advantage of the opportunity to eat during longer events. In some sports eating is less of a problem than it is in running, because there is less bouncing and stomach discomfort. In a triathlon, for instance, it makes sense to eat early on the bike, as you have an ideal opportunity to digest the food before the rigours of the run leg. Of course, in all cases, food should be as easily digested as possible. The less energy wasted in digestion, the more there is available for competing. Select foods that won't upset your stomach.

It may be beneficial to start such events with an adequate breakfast. Over the years I have had the honour of coaching and assisting a number of elite runners both in the UK and South Africa for ultra-events. One of the first things that I teach them is how to run immediately after a good breakfast, usually comprising buttered bread, a boiled egg and a hot drink of their choice, plus a glass of Metabolol or some other quality meal replacement drink. After a few attempts they can usually run at 100-km or Comrades race pace within 30 minutes of eating this meal.

Between 1999 and 2001, Marietjie Montgomery, Welcome Mteto, and Carol Mercer all ate during the World 100-km events – to great benefit. Montgomery was the second-placed veteran woman in the World 100 km, while Mteto powered his way through the field and helped a struggling Comrades gold medallist, Andrew Kelehe, through to the finish, to secure the bronze medal for the South African team. Kelehe went on to win Comrades the following year and has stated that the fact the Mteto was able to pace himself and still have the energy to catch up to him in the last lap of the 100 km, convinced him that he needed to review his race eating and pacing strategy.

Carol Mercer, who was nineteenth in the World 100 km at her first outing, had the most consistent pacing of the whole field (men and women), and went on to become the first South African woman to finish Comrades in 2001. In each case, the runners achieved these honours by maintaining their energy levels, and hence their running pace, throughout the event. Each of them beat potentially more talented runners by understanding and adopting a better energy replacement protocol.

1 000-MILE RELAY

In August 2002 I was involved in the technical aspects of an attempt on the World 1 000-mile relay record. A talented ten-man team of South Africa's top distance runners ran in relay for 99:03:27, from Cape Town to Johannesburg. They averaged 3 minutes 40 seconds per km and typically were running between 2 km and 3 km at a stretch before handing over to the next runner. Once again, the secret of their success in maintaining energy levels was not in drinking energy drinks, but rather sports drinks that contained protein, and eating regular meals (at roughly three-hour intervals) that contained protein, fat and carbohydrate. Only with a mixed diet was it possible to replace the required kilocalories and reduce the effects of the regular bouts of high-intensity exercise. The key was not the carbohydrate, but the fat for kilocalories and the protein to prevent them becoming catabolic. The carbohydrate assisted with energy and keeping blood sugar levels up, and hence mental fatigue at bay.

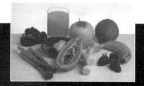

As competitors, we gear ourselves up for the big event, we compete to the best of our ability, and with an interest in detail and preparation that would put an army to shame, and when it's all over and done, we forget everything!

CARBOHYDRATES – THE FIRST CHOICE

If we build ourselves up to a peak with the 'right' foods, surely it stands to reason that competition will deplete these foods, and we should replace them afterwards. The type of food we require will depend on the type of event in which we competed, and strange as it may seem, our bodies tend to tell us if we are making the correct choices. Instinctively, your body will 'crave' for the carbohydrates, proteins or fats you need, and be repulsed by the things you don't need. That said, however, **an item that you will need after most events is carbohydrate, for the following reasons:**

> ▸ it is the first line of energy source.
> ▸ the depletion of carbohydrates in the liver has probably been substantial.
> ▸ the need to induce an insulin reaction in order to assist the transfer of protein and nutrients into the muscles, which will start the process of recovery and rebuilding.

Glycogen synthesis is most efficient when the demand for glycogen is greatest, and this generally occurs within 15 minutes after the end of an event. For this reason, keep an extra bottle of a carbo-boosting solution available to drink as soon as possible after a competition.

If you have been involved in an ultra-event, or possibly even a marathon, your desires may well stretch to a steak or high protein or fat meal. Even if this is not your usual desire, there is nothing wrong with it under these conditions. This is not only indicative of depletion in these areas, but also the need to commence muscle repair. Cravings are your body's way of obtaining the necessary fuels and nutrients to recover.

A point to consider is the type of drink that you have been using during your event. Many of the drinks we use are of a slightly acidic nature and by the end of the event we have an acid build-up. Try taking your first few drinks in a more alkali form, e.g. milk, or Rehydrat. Water is, of course, neutral. Most meal replacement drinks will have a neutralising effect, with the added advantage of offering quality carbohydrates, as well as proteins that will assist with recovery.

As a guide, to determine what you should be taking, remember that energy used should equal energy replaced.

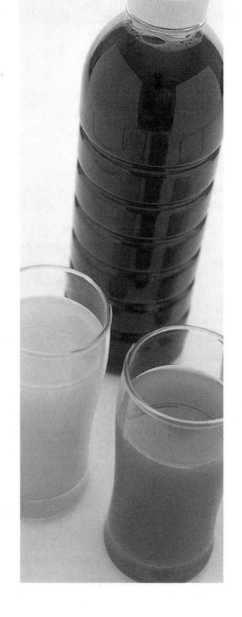

RIGHT *Try to avoid drinks with an acid profile immediately after a race*

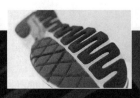

Your ability to recover from training sessions, and therefore your ability to perform the next session, is based on the recovery of your glycogen stores. A similar approach should be used after all training sessions. In the first 15 minutes after training, ensure that you have approximately 25 g of carbohydrate – most easily achieved by taking 250 ml of a quality carbohydrate sports mix. Failure to do this will result in a gradual depletion of stores over a number of days and your training will become increasingly less productive. There can be few things as frustrating as ineffective, non-productive training sessions.

For many years, Olympic coach Frank Horwill insisted that his athletes carry an apple with them to their training sessions so that they could commence 'loading' immediately afterwards. Although this is a good starting point, there are now even better options. Firstly, from the information on the Glycaemic Index, it is clear that an apple has a low index and that jellybeans would be a better option. Even better would be a carbohydrate drink, which does not require digestion time and replaces fluid. But why does an Olympic coach insist on this approach by his athletes?

During periods of heavy distance training, runners are presented with an ideal opportunity to experiment with various methods of maintaining their energy stores during a run, as well as carbohydrate-loading procedures prior to a race. The training sessions are, however, only stepping stones in reaching their goal, which is to recover from the stress of the training session as soon as possible. The depletion effect of training is so dramatic that the old 'Eastern bloc' countries deemed it necessary for athletes to take a day of complete rest after every third training day. Omitting this was found to leave an athlete incapable of training effectively on the fourth day.

In the quest for the best recovery methods, research has proven that if carbohydrate is not consumed immediately (during the first 45 minutes) after the completion of exercise, the replacement of normal glycogen stores is likely to take up to 48 hours. The rate of replenishment is also a function of the carbohydrate composition of food intake. Greater glycogen absorption will occur with a higher carbohydrate content.

The outcome of this is that international athletes now consume food such as apples or commercially available energy drinks almost immediately after completing their training, i.e. they are already concentrating on recovery and preparation for the following day's training; the better the recovery, the better the next intense training session. This concept of faster recovery allowing a faster return to training (or more intense training), is the reason some athletes have been tempted to use drugs. Ironically, many would achieve better performances legally if they paid more attention to their nutrition habits and post-training recovery.

ALWAYS KEEP THE FOLLOWING RULES OF THUMB IN MIND:

1. Consume some **high-content carbohydrate food** or **drink** within the first 15 minutes of stopping exercise (certainly no later than 45 minutes).
2. The **higher the carbohydrate content**, the faster you are likely to reach normal stores.
3. Drinks comprising **long chain carbohydrates** are most efficient in absorption, but **high Glycaemic Index (GI) drinks** after the event are more effective in raising insulin levels (see protein on the following page).
4. Particularly after quality sessions and long runs, follow up with a **quality meal replacement drink** within the first hour, to provide the necessary building blocks for the repair of damaged muscle.
5. If you feel particularly jaded during a training session, look back over your previous few days of training and eating to see whether you could be a victim of a progressive depletion of carbohydrate stores. **If so, take a day's rest and some carbohydrate drinks.**
6. Likewise, in the joyous aftermath of the next race, or after the next sweat-drenched training session, make a beeline for a **cup of the carbo-boosting solution** you used for loading before the race. In this way you will prepare yourself for the next day and the next challenge.

PROTEIN FOLLOWS THE CARBOHYDRATE

As discussed, racing and training induce microtears in the muscles and although carbohydrate will replace the energy used during an event, it does not repair or rebuild muscle damage. However the carbohydrate will raise the level of insulin and that, in turn, will assist the absorption of protein and other nutrients that are required to repair the damage.

Because high GI carbohydrates are highly effective in raising insulin levels, they are ideal for use immediately after training, and provide an excellent preparation for the next stage of post-event nutrition, which is to take in some protein. During the first hour, the most effective is to use a quality, broad-spectrum protein supplement. These two stages – carbohydrate then protein – may be combined if a quality meal replacement drink is used. Taking 30–40 g of protein in the first hour after the event is a good starting point and it should be remembered that the leading protein supplements provide a better quality of protein than food. However, the use of liquid meals must never be considered as a complete solution, as there is still a need for solid food. Liquid is simply easier in the first hours after a taxing session or race.

When checking the labels of quality supplements, also look for high quantities of glutamine, HMB (see page 308) and the branched chain amino acids, all of which have been shown to assist in post-event recovery.

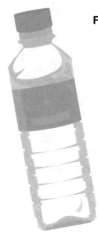

FINAL THOUGHTS ON EVENT NUTRITION

It is almost impossible to list the requirements for each event and specific details of the ideal drinks, amounts, consistency, and where and when to take them. As philosopher and runner Dr George Sheehan noted, everyone is an experiment of one – what works for you, or me, will not necessarily work for the next person. However, the 'rules' and advice in this book will provide a good, practical, starting point for all runners (and, in fact, all sportspeople). It's now up to you to plan your requirements for your chosen event.

One thing is certain: if you attend to your energy and water requirements in a more professional manner than you did before, your performance and recovery will improve, and that, in turn, means better training and better competition. I believe that is the goal towards which all sportspeople strive.

Several of the suggestions and information need to be modified for your individual needs. For example, the principle that glycogen synthesis is greatest when the demand is greatest, indicates that in events with multiple heats, or multiple efforts (such as track events, multiday stage races or parluaf cross-country), it is important to drink some carbo-boosting solution as soon as possible after each leg of the competition. This permits recovery in time for the next leg, even if it is on the same day.

Moreover, the advice given here must not be considered as the final word. There is so much more still to be learned and research is an ongoing process. 'There is no finish line!' Although the basics may not change, newly discovered subtleties may result in a slight improvement in performance, which can make the difference between winning and losing, whatever that means to you.

It is important to put winning into perspective. Winning is not necessarily about those who take home the trophy or cross the line first. A winner, by my definition, is someone who achieves his target and ambitions in sport by reaching his potential within his own limits. We can all strive to be 'the best we can be'. Remember, a runner who undertakes the detailed preparation will frequently beat more talented runners who simply rely on their inherited skills. Winners make it happen – losers let it happen!

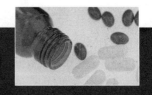

Whether we actually need vitamins is yet another contentious issue in the worlds of sport and nutrition. One argument says 'no, because the average person absorbs enough from three well-balanced meals per day'. It has been proved that if the average person has the nutritional equivalent of three well-balanced meals per day, supplementation is unnecessary.

The issues here though are whether the 'average' person trains for marathons or other endurance competitions, or trains in adverse weather conditions. We know that the training athlete burns more kilocalories than the average person, and we know that protein intake rises as training intensity increases. In fact, these requirements can be 2–3 times the amount deemed necessary for the average person. The counterargument is that the extra food intake should more than cover the vitamin and mineral requirements.

Because it is a major challenge for runners to consume the necessary quantities of carbohydrate in solid food, they make use of sports drinks, which typically do not contain vitamins and minerals. The prestigious British Milers Club warns its members and coaches that one aspect separating the average man from a runner is that a runner sweats 4–7 litres of fluid in a week's training, and that's for a middle-distance athlete in the relatively cool climate of the UK. However, anyone who eats the 'basic four' every day is at little risk of being low on vitamins or minerals.

The four basic components are:

> ▶ one meat meal or its protein equivalent e.g. milk, cheese, dried beans, nuts.
> ▶ 5 cups of fruit and vegetable.
> ▶ 1 litre of milk (including milk in tea, etc).
> ▶ 5 slices of bread, and a plate of WHOLE-GRAIN cereal.

The next question is, 'How many "athletes" are certain that they managed that in a day, let alone every day?' Forget three meals – with work and training, as well as other chores, many runners have little more than one and a half meals per day, and the need for supplementation becomes more serious, particularly in adverse climatic conditions.

Athletes are definitely not average. If you consider that Britain sends a team of athletes to the Olympics, which represents about 0.0003% of the population, it is hardly reasonable to equate them to the 'average' person in the country, whether in diet or anything else. Even if you add up all the participants in Comrades, Two Oceans, Duzi, Argus Cycle Race and Midmar Mile (i.e. the major participation events), it will be around 70 000 participants, and this still only represents 1% of the South African population. The training distance runner is NOT average.

Naturally the weather conditions and status of the food we eat varies from region to region in the country, and affect your requirements. For instance, the humidity and year-round heat of Durban, combined with the low levels of magnesium in the soil, present a different picture on how depleted runners will become in coastal KwaZulu-Natal compared to runners in coastal Cape Town where the weather is cooler for a significant part of the year.

HOT AND ADVERSE CONDITIONS

According to Dr Steve Browne, author of *Running in the Heat*, 'hot' is when the effective temperature is above 25 °C. However, a more expressive guide can be found in the 1990 New York Marathon entry form, which details time incentives for runners. Incentives are paid to runners breaking 2:12 for the marathon distance in normal conditions and 2:18 when the temperature is above 19.5 °C AND humidity above 65%. In addition to the $23 600 prize-money, the winner also receives a new Mercedes-Benz and, if he sets a new course record, he adds a further major bonus. If it's classified as 'hot', this incentive is increased by another $10 000. The influence of heat on your training and your body cannot be spelt out any clearer than that, and it is another reason to desist from long training in seasons of adverse conditions. Although a single long run in the heat and humidity is not that much of a problem, combining a number of these in continuously poor conditions will take its toll.

It is no longer unusual for major championships such as the Olympics and Commonwealth Games to be held in adverse climates, particularly for endurance runners. My experience as a coach of international athletes, and in team management, has taught me that a surprisingly large number of team managers have little 'hands-on' experience of the true effect these conditions can have on runners. Such teams are not prepared for the challenge they are scheduled to face. Perhaps the most amazing case concerned a team from Great Britain during my three-year stint in Scotland from 1995 to 1998. Surprisingly, the team manager was also a highly respected coach, but this was by no means an isolated incidence.

VITAMINS

What types of vitamins and other supplementation would I suggest? This needs to be answered on an individual basis, particularly because most people have strong likes and dislikes when it comes to food.

A good starting point for most sportspeople in heavy training is a multivitamin and mineral pack – ideally a slow-release formula, or split across the whole day. This can act as an

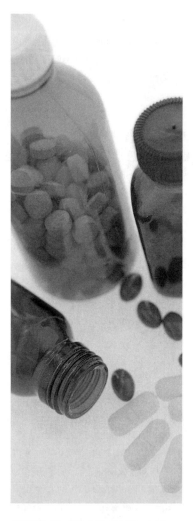

ABOVE *Vitamins and minerals work in synergy – it's no use simply taking a range of pills in the hope that you will achieve the correct balance*

insurance policy; it will cover most needs and the majority of excesses will be urinated away at the next opportune moment. However, if there is a need, it will be satisfied. Assuming that you follow the basic instructions on the pack, the only danger of intoxication is with the fat-soluble vitamins such as A and D, but very large amounts are needed to reach toxic levels – far more than that contained in a multivitamin pack, so generally, this can be discounted.

What may be even better is to use natural supplements such as the greens and spirulina, which contain a synergistic combination of vitamins, minerals and micronutrients. Although the quantities of nutrients are considerably smaller, the fact that they are integrated into one naturally occurring supplement in natural proportions possibly leads to more efficient absorption and more effective action than chemically manufactured single vitamins, or combinations.

At the time of writing, I have been using SA Natural Spirulina over a period of six months during which time I have not experienced any illness and have enjoyed a high level of immunity despite going through the rigours of Comrades training and running. I recommend following such a broad-spectrum 'insurance' approach for 8–12 weeks before a major event. For a normal club runner, this is only required during heavy periods of training.

Yet a further area to consider is that of your eating preferences. If, like me, you limit your intake of red meats and also have a strong liking for vegetables and cereals, you may easily find yourself deficient in some areas and even low on protein. However, this can be redressed by the additional intake of amino acids and vitamin B-complex.

ANTI-OXIDANTS

In recent years there has been significant research done in the area of anti-oxidants and their beneficial effect on free radicals. Air pollution and training are just two elements, which are known to increase the amount of free radicals in the body. It has been shown that these have a negative effect on cell repair and growth. However, studies have proven that increased levels of anti-oxidants can 'negate' the free radicals by soaking up the free oxygen molecules. Vitamins A, E and C, together with selenium, are a powerful combination and should be a feature of any selected vitamin supplementation.

INDIVIDUAL VITAMIN SUPPLEMENTATION

The synergy between the levels of vitamins is important, therefore I do not believe that is particularly useful to take one specific vitamin unless it has been medically proven that you have a deficiency. There are a number of water-soluble vitamins, including vitamin C, and studies have indicated that supplementation of this at levels of 1 g per day have improved endurance. Vitamin C is also thought to assist in the defence against colds, although recent research suggests that it is more effective in combination with zinc.

A disturbing side of supplementation and sport is the use of vitamin B12 injections, particularly by swimmers as young as 12 years of age. If they have been introduced to the concept of a needle improving performance at such an early age, what is the next progression? Even more worrying is that some coaches and parents endorse this practice.

MINERALS

On many a summer morning in Durban (South Africa), I have watched the thermometer slowly creep up, starting from sunrise just after 5.15 a.m. With it comes the escalation in humidity. In February, a notoriously hot month in Durban, those who are involved in endurance training such as running leave themselves open to the problems of dehydration and mineral depletion. The latter can be a slow, virtually unnoticed, problem.

Ironically, about the same time of year in the very cold climates of the northern hemisphere, runners can induce the same type of conditions while wearing rain jackets or similar protection on top of their running gear. Although this keeps out the wind and rain, it also creates a very humid microclimate inside the jacket and simultaneously reduces the amount of sweat that can be dissipated. The removal of sweat is a prime method of cooling. This causes a runner to sweat more than normal and hence greater quantities of fluid and minerals are lost than in spring, or even summer.

The following information should give you an idea of some of the more common minerals used in supplementation, particularly those that you need be concerned with, especially in the 'hot' months of training, or in conditions that promote a high rate of perspiration:

Calcium

Calcium is indicated when suffering from allergies, joint pains, lead poisoning (have you run in traffic recently?), and lack of Vitamin D, among others. Calcium absorption, even if you achieve the recommended levels, is greatly hampered by phosphorous, which is found in all soft drinks. For example, 12 sufferers of chronic shin soreness were all found to be calcium deficient even though their intake was adequate. All drank an average of three litres of soft drinks per week. Many runners will drink that in a single race, particularly in events where Coke is provided as a sugar drink on refreshment tables.

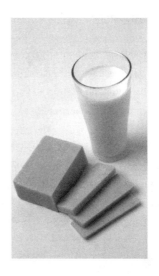

Magnesium

Like calcium, the absorption of magnesium is hampered by a high-bran diet, particularly in conjunction with highly processed and refined foods. Magnesium acts as a pump within cells and distributes calcium, potassium and sodium in the body. This highlights the fact that a deficiency in one mineral (or vitamin) can have a carryover effect to other minerals (or vitamins). In many areas, low magnesium content of soil exacerbates magnesium deficiency, which results in foods that are normally prime sources of magnesium, being low in this mineral. Such a situation occurs in Durban, where bananas have a lower than expected magnesium content.

Magnesium is also involved in glycogen metabolism in the muscles and is thus of immense importance to those needing to carbo load, or compete in endurance events. Its deficiency has also been associated with cramping. Only five members of a 14-strong French football squad were found to have 'normal' magnesium levels. After supplementation, not only were their stores replaced, but their recovery times and match results also mproved. Studies with the French footballers were also used to substantiate the use of uvi-mag supplementation, which combines vitamin B6 and magnesium. The results were quite remarkable. Runners using uvi-mag in the build up to the 2001 Comrades claimed similar results.

Potassium

When Steve Ovett collapsed in the 1984 Olympics, his heart beat raced and he was heading for a cardiac arrest. He was subsequently discovered to be potassium deficient. Potassium is required for correct heart function, but it can also be indicated by poor appetite, mental fatigue and apathy, depression and muscle cramps. One American track coach monitored his team over a season and noted a monthly decline in potassium and performance. One of the best sources of potassium is pure orange juice.

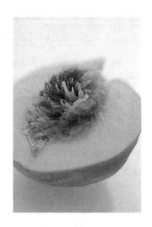

Zinc

Over 2 500 learned papers have been written on the subject of zinc deficiency, which has been linked to a multitude of problems from dandruff, M.E. (Yuppie Flu), to delayed healing, hair loss and even impotence. Surprisingly, it has been estimated that only one in 1 000 coaches is aware of the value of zinc or its influence on performance.

Poor zinc absorption and loss is associated with those on high-bran diets, strict vegetarians, penicillin takers, those suffering from chronic blood loss or taking drugs to release water retention, and those who sweat profusely. Zinc is found in egg yolks, split peas, nuts, oats, parsley, garlic, whole-wheat bread and potatoes.

Zinc and vitamin C, in combination, is believed to be one of the best treatments for the common cold. My own experience both during a three-year stint in (flu-ridden) Scotland, and in South Africa, suggests that a regular intake of this, significantly reduces the risk of such infection. Furthermore, studies show that if zinc and vitamin C lozenges are sucked every hour at the first sign of flu and a sore throat, they can shorten the length of the virus by around four days.

AMINO ACIDS

The controversy around amino acids is still relatively new. Amino acids are the building blocks of protein; there are about 23 different types, of which some people consider 12 to be essential, but even this is under discussion, as some are thought to be 'conditionally essential', dependent on other factors. Generally, it is agreed that at least ten are essential, including the three-branched chain amino acids (BCAA) valine, leucine and isoleucine. The difference between essential and non-essential amino acids is that the former cannot be manufactured by the body and must therefore be supplied through food intake or supplementation.

Because of their 'rebuilding' characteristics, amino acids are seen by some people to be a natural alternative to 'anabolic steroids'. Studies have shown that some of them are responsible for increased circulation of the human growth hormone, or free fatty acids.

The theory is that if you supplement with certain amino acids, you will derive specific benefits. Thus by increasing arginine you 'can' increase the free fatty acids in your blood and thus make it a higher percentage of your energy supply at the start of a marathon, thereby saving some of your glycogen stores until later in the race. L-glutamine is said to assist in the release of testosterone, and improve the immune system. Glutamine is a very dominant nutrient in muscles, and supplementation has been used in hospitals, for burn victims and other patients with severe injuries.

Similarly, claims are made for other specific amino acids, which when taken on an empty stomach at night will increase the growth hormone and thus assist in recovery and muscle building. This should allow you to train harder.

From a physiological viewpoint, amino supplementation has much potential. The controversy no longer seems to be about whether or not these effects take place, but rather if the format of supplementation available to sportspeople is capable of being absorbed through the various membranes into the muscles.

I have personally worked with amino supplementation since the late 1980s and can, therefore, only relate my own experience. However, a significant example of this was the use of supplementation that assisted me to overcome the deficits and destructive effects that I experienced after completing the 254-km Spartathlon ultramarathon from Athens to Sparta in 1992. No doubt, the fact that I tended towards a vegetarian diet made the benefits of the amino supplementation far more noticeable, because taking in sufficient quality protein on such a diet tends to be more difficult.

In ultramarathons, the combination of the three-branched chain amino acids, leucine, isoleucine and valine undoubtedly assist in combating fatigue, when a 0.7% mixture is added to your energy drink. For further information, you would be well advised to read the research undertaken by Dr Eric Newsholme in the UK.

EVALUATING SUPPLEMENTATION

The real problem in evaluating the power of various supplements is that no-one can tell you if the supplementation is working or whether you benefit because you THINK it is working. Ultimately, I don't mind which it is. If it makes me feel better and puts me in a better condition to train, that's fine.

The regime you need to follow is one that only you can develop for yourself, although a good sports nutritionist can assist considerably in this task. He will analyse your food intake over a period of 3–6 days and identify vitamins or other constituents that are missing from or possibly even oversaturating your system. Your needs may change at different times of training, in different weather conditions and when your lifestyle changes, therefore a reassessment once every 12–18 months is recommended.

There is definitely a place for supplementation, but it will vary from person to person, even if the benefit is purely psychological.

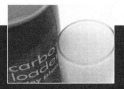

CREATINE

There has been much hype over the use of creatine by top sportsmen and women. South African swimmer Penny Heynes is quoted as attributing her multiworld record performance at the 1999 Pan Pacific Games down to 'God, hard training and creatine'. Many of the 1999 World Cup Rugby players claimed improved performance and strength, and the world of sprinting has seen radical improvement in times from 100 m to 400 m since the inception of 'creatine loading' in the early 1990s.

What is the 'magical substance' that can apparently transform the 'meek and mild' into world-beaters? Perhaps it's best to start with what it is not! Creatine is not a 'drug' or banned substance, nor is it a 'fix-all'.

Creatine is a natural substance found in the body, which plays an important role in the production of energy. Meat is a common source of creatine, which in essence is a particular form of protein. More technically, amino acids are the building blocks of protein, and creatine is a combination of three amino acids – arginine, glycine and methionine. The use of creatine as a supplement has also been used in hospitals in the treatment of heart patients, so there may be additional benefits.

The natural production of energy relies on the Krebs Cycle (citric acid cycle), and creatine is an essential ingredient of that process, which provides the muscle cells with the energy they need to perform their primary contraction function. Without creatine your muscles simply run out of energy. Creatine phosphate is the format used in the Krebs Cycle (see also chapter 22 on energy sources).

Although creatine was first identified in the 1800s, its use in sport only became popular in the early 1990s. It has been found that by increasing the intake of creatine in the form of creatine monohydrate, it is possible to increase the stores of creatine in the muscle. This increase allows the energy production to become more 'efficient' and thereby improve performance. In terms of a vehicle, improving creatine stores provides 'more kilometres per litre'.

It is of particular benefit in exercise that lasts between 10–50 seconds, thus the initial interest by power lifters, bodybuilders, short-course swimmers and sprinters. By increasing energy, these sportspeople can handle a greater training workload, permitting greater progression. This combines the three key elements: effective training, effective recovery and an adequate creatine supply. Without one, the others become less effective and efficient.

Benefit for endurance athletes

The use of creatine by endurance athletes is not as well researched, but many have reported faster recovery times after hard training or competition – particularly true of interval sessions, where they have an ability to handle more intense training, more regularly.

Others who could benefit from creatine are those who tend towards a vegetarian, or low-protein diet. For many years it has been recognised that sportspeople need energy to compete, and therefore the pendulum of nutrition has focused on carbohydrate intake.

Organisations such as the Heart Foundation and Weigh-Less have also promoted a healthy diet built around a food intake that provides about 65% carbohydrate, which has resulted in many sportspeople, particularly those in endurance events, moving away from high-meat diets. Although figures are not available, it may be that this swing has caused some hard-training 'athletes' to have a less than optimal intake of protein-building blocks and may be one reason for endurance athletes reporting improved recovery with creatine use.

Training is a process of adaptation that involves breaking down muscles, causing micromuscle tears, and it is the 'repair' during the recovery period that prompts the muscle to grow stronger and bigger (more muscle strands) than before training. If the time of the repair cycle can be reduced, the training can become more frequent or intense, leading to greater improvements.

Use creatine during periods of high distance or quality training and competition. Creatine should not be continued for longer than 4–6 weeks if you used the loading option of increasing the stores. If you follow a more gradual 'endurance' approach to creatine use, this period can be extended to about 10–12 weeks. Do not try to maintain this regime throughout the year.

Two types of loading

When creatine is first introduced, athletes commence a five-day 'loading programme', taking around 20 g of creatine per day (the exact amount is dependent on body weight – or more correctly, lean muscle mass), moving to a maintenance dose of 5-10 g per day (bodybuilders and explosive athletes use around 10 g). The best absorption is achieved when creatine is taken with ample supplies of fluid and some carbohydrate.

Because carbohydrate and water are essential to the storage of creatine, there is an initial increase in weight and bulk. However, when combined with the more effective and efficient training that creatine allows, the result is an increase in muscle mass.

For the endurance athlete, increases in weight are less desirable, and recent work has seen an alternative approach successfully adopted by some athletes. Instead of a loading phase, athletes take 1.5–5 g of creatine (most runners need only 1.5–3 g) in a daily carbohydrate drink. After 30 days, the levels of creatine in the muscle are found to be comparable to those in people who use the loading option.

Balance or abuse?

Clearly, it's a case of reaching a balance, and perhaps this is where much of the negative publicity that surrounds creatine originates. The ambitious athlete, or naive youngster, with the focus and drive to achieve a particular goal, often overlooks such balance. He might believe that if one dosage is good, then more must be better. Such assumptions are false. As with any overdosage, this can lead to negative side effects, such as muscle cramps. The prime problem is either 'abuse and misuse', or a lack of product knowledge and education.

When and how

Loading and maintenance must only be undertaken during times of intense training or peak competition. Creatine exists naturally in the body; it's not illegal and it is possible to 'load' using meat, a good source of creatine, but the bulk and high protein, and fat content are counterproductive. The best way to take creatine is to mix it with carbohydrates as this improves absorption. You can either add creatine monohydrate to your carbohydrate or protein supplements, or make use of one of the combinations that already contain creatine. Either way, carbohydrate is required and a ratio of 20 g of carbohydrate with 2–5 g of creatine, in a 250-ml drink would be a good mix with which to start. Recent research suggests that magnesium chelate and taurine may further improve the uptake of creatine.

Creatine and caffeine don't work

Some researchers have found examples of athletes who have experienced no benefit from creatine loading – initially appearing to be quite a high proportion. More recently though, it has been suggested that many of the cases where creatine has seemingly gave poor results, the athletes took it with coffee or other caffeine products. Caffeine has been shown to impair the uptake of creatine in muscles.

Creatine is not for youngsters

Creatine works but it should definitely not be used by young people. It is impossible to give a magical 'age of consent' as each person matures through the growth spurt at different levels. By developing stronger muscles, the young trainer will put an additional load onto a joint not yet developed to take that load. To exacerbate the situation, the bones of a teenager during puberty are constantly extending and the increased load applied at the end of a greater bone length adds even more load to the joint, through lever action.

Peer, coach and even parental pressure can be extreme for sports-orientated youth, but it must be controlled. Many of the world's best sportspeople only became top class after they matured, so take the years of change carefully and protect the growing body. Don't allow the pressure to make early gains override long-term health.

A final reminder: it is important to increase your fluid intake when using creatine. With mixes that include carbohydrate, this is of even greater importance, and is one reason why you will experience an almost immediate increase in weight.

PYRUVATE, CARNITINE AND PHOSPHATES

The success of creatine has prompted many supplement companies and researchers to look at other constituents of the energy system to see if supplementation or loading might bring additional benefits. The dream would be to find a supplement or combination that could improve endurance, or provide the ability to withstand intense exercise, e.g. something to decrease the level of lactic acid for a given level of intensity (lactic acid buffering), raise the effective Vo_2 Max of an athlete, improve the efficiency of energy systems and/or provide a greater source of energy.

Research has focused on naturally occurring components and some success has been recorded with three such constituents in particular.

Phosphates

Initial research into phosphates appeared to indicate that supplementation was unnecessary. Tests undertaken on athletes showed that blood levels of phosphate, a key component of the energy cycle, were significantly higher than those of the sedentary population. However, tests also noted low levels of blood phosphate after endurance events, as well as a correlation between poor performance and low phosphate levels in athletes prior to competitions.

We rely on diet for phosphate, as the body cannot manufacture it. Studies on phosphate supplementation claim: a buffering effect for muscle acidity, raised levels of the enzyme involved in supplying oxygen to muscles, and, through enzyme action, an improved storage and usage of muscle glycogen.

In the research trials, trained runners and cyclists took 4 g of sodium phosphate daily for three days. In tests to exhaustion, on either a treadmill or bicycle, runners lasted up to nine minutes longer and showed a 6–12% increase in Vo_2 Max, whereas cyclists cut 3–5 minutes from their 40-km time. They showed a similar 11% increase in Vo_2 Max. Benefits were indicated for both aerobic and anaerobic exercise, with a 17% increase in power output during anaerobic work.

Pyruvate

Pyruvate, the product of glycogen metabolism, has been found to be an effective anti-oxidant that prevents the formation of free radicals. It has also been shown to increase the amount of energy used in mitochondria, promoting the burning of fat, which will no doubt increase its popularity with the 'weight loss' brigade.

Of prime interest to runners is pyruvate's ability to enhance the stores of glycogen in the muscles. By 'pulling' glycogen from the blood into the muscles, the amount of 'high-grade' fuel available for exercise increases, thereby improving performance. Pyruvate works during exercise and rest periods. In recent years, some manufacturers have produced creatine pyruvate as an alternative to creatine monohydrate and it has had some positive feedback.

L-carnitine

The third component of the trio is L-carnitine, the subject of much research over the years, with views for and against supplementation. Quality carnitine is expensive, which is why many products that list it have only trace quantities, in comparison to the 2–4 g that is recommended. Minute quantities have little, if any, benefit.

Carnitine is a key component in the mobilisation of fats and the oxidation of branched chain amino acids and pyruvate. Although the body can manufacture carnitine, exercise requirements are such, that demand can easily exceed supply. Supplementation is thought to reduce the drop in levels of free carnitine during intense or extended exercise. Lower levels of acidity have been recorded during intense exercise.

Supplementation with a combination of phosphate, pyruvate and carnitine has gained positive reports from athletes in search of a greater intensity of training or greater stamina, both of which allow an athlete to train more effectively. It is thought that such advantage will be reflected in the competitive performance. Loading is most appropriately used during the build-up to competition or the intense training phase. After a three-day loading phase, phosphates remain in the system for about ten days of normal training.

Because many of the benefits to be gained from phosphate, pyruvate and carnitine involve the production of energy and storage of glycogen, an effective loading method is to take them with a carbohydrate drink, in order to maximise storage. Take about 1 400 mg of calcium pyruvate, 1 400 mg of L-carnitine and 1 400 mg of a mix of potassium phosphate, sodium phosphate and magnesium phosphate per day, for seven days before a major competition. About half this dose can be used for the period of intense training.

HMB – REDUCE THE DAMAGE

A metabolite of the branched chain amino acid leucine, HMB – short for ß-hydroxy-ß-methylbutyrate (beta-hyroxy-beta-methylbutyrate) – is thought to reduce recovery time and offer a number of potential benefits for athletes. Leucine is found in all dietary protein and is one of the essential amino acids, i.e. the body cannot produce it. A natural product found and used throughout the body, leucine assists in regulating the breakdown and synthesis of protein. It is also in a number of foods, including breast milk.

There have been a number of research studies using HMB both on cattle and latterly on trained and untrained humans. **Some of the benefits claimed out of the research are:**

> ▸ a decrease in LDL cholesterol.
> ▸ increased immune function.
> ▸ a reduction in subcutaneous fat.
> ▸ a reduction in catabolic effect during training.
> ▸ enhanced gains in strength and mass in the cases of trained and untrained weightlifters.
> ▸ a 50% improvement anabolic effect of resistance training.

These are fairly dramatic claims, mostly based on results gained from weight training. However, they have persuaded a number of athletes to subscribe to the supplement. With continued use, distance athletes are claiming that it reduces the catabolic effect of distance training, and at least one of the recent World Cup rugby teams made use of it to reduce the muscle damage in both training and competition.

If HMB reduces the muscle breakdown and increases the anabolic effect, it will provide a double-action mechanism for reducing the recovery time between training bouts, therefore allowing more intense and effective training to be undertaken. However, as with all other dietary supplements, HMB is not a quick fix – regular supplements must be taken for a minimum of 14–21 days before you are likely to see any benefits.

From the research, it would appear that a daily dosage of about 3 g is the ideal amount. A number of quality meal replacement supplements contain added HMB, which is probably the optimum method of taking the correct dosage, although it is possible to buy HMB as a separate item.

GLUTAMINE – PREVENTING ILLNESS

Sports science tells us that a runner who covers 100 km per week is about twice as likely to suffer from colds and flu as a runner who covers 30 km per week. One suggested reason for this is that the immune system is depressed by exercise. Testing in research noted that levels of glutamine are also lowered by exercise and when runners show symptoms of overtraining.

Glutamine is one of the most abundant free-amino acids (thought that free form acids circulate well and easily absorbed) in both the blood and muscle. The interest in glutamine took hold in the 1980s when it was found that it is essential for cell growth in three areas: it can reduce muscle breakdown; it is key to protein synthesis; and it has a big impact on muscle growth. By 1990, it was recognised that exercise produces large quantities of the amino acids glutamine and alanine, which are used and then excreted from the body, leaving a shortfall after exercise.

Blood glutamine

Blood glutamine levels have also been observed to be low when patients suffer from burns, infection, serious injury and stress, or during surgery. Early research on glutamine supplementation found that recovery rates of a patient improved when glutamine or branched chain amino acids (BCAA) were given. This seemed to support the theory that glutamine is beneficial and that the body can also manufacture it from leucine, valine and isoleucine.

Of greater interest to runners is that glutamine levels are found to drop following a hard training session or a marathon. If athletes supplement with glutamine, their blood levels maintain normal levels. An Oxford University research programme found that glutamine supplementation reduced the risk of post-exhaustive exercise illness. In a controlled test of rowers, middle-distance athletes, marathoners and ultramarathoners, only 19% of the participants became ill if they used glutamine supplementation after the exercise, whereas 51% of those taking a placebo became ill in the first seven days following identical exercise, therefore some quality supplements include added glutamine in their drinks and mixes. It also appears to reduce blood sugar level spikes. Interestingly, the frequency of infection was greatest in marathoners and ultramarathoners. Glutamine supplementation may be a good way to boost the immune system and to enhance recovery dramatically.

A 1992 study matched 40 international-calibre athletes who were experiencing overtraining symptoms, with a similar control group. The glutamine levels in the control group were 9% higher, than the 'overtrained' athletes.

Predict overtraining

Can low glutamine levels predict overtraining? This is by no means conclusive, but what does appear to be true is that the risk of infection is higher when glutamine levels are low and that glutamine supplementation can reduce the risk of infection.

There are, however, problems with relying on foods for glutamine. The digestive enterocytes can eat up the glutamine long before it is absorbed into the system. Plain glutamine supplementation may result in only a 40% absorption rate, and it is therefore important to find a more efficient method of supplementing glutamine in athletes.

Research proves that supplementation with BCAA is one way to boost absorption and resynthesis of glutamine. In addition, it has also been shown that a different form of glutamine – ornithine alpha-ketoglutarate (OKG) – is even more readily absorbed than plain glutamine. So successful is OKG, that it has replaced anabolic steroids for the treatment of burn patients, in helping them to recover from trauma and to prevent muscle wasting.

It appears then that glutamine and BCAA supplementation can help you to avoid overtraining, maintain lean muscle, improve recovery and boost your immune system and wellbeing, yet prevent illness during periods of very intense training.

RIBOSE

D-ribose is a naturally occurring sugar, which cells need in order to resynthesise the energy molecule ATP. Just as ATP is the primary energy source for muscles, ribose is also key to most regenerative functions in the body, from cells to hormones.

Throughout the nutrition section, I have indicated the importance of carbohydrates as a means of improving absorption of the various building blocks and nutrients. Ribose is very new to the supplement market, but may well be one of most efficient 'transporters' of nutrients into the muscle because of its deep-rooted and direct involvement in so many of the body's functions. There are no known food sources that supply sufficient quantities of ribose to be metabolically significant, and it is an expensive supplement. At present, few South African sports supplements contain ribose, but some imported meal replacement or protein drinks do contain small quantities. Locally, you will more than likely have to purchase it as a separate supplement and add it to your chosen drink.

A daily dose of 3–5 g should be sufficient to ensure full recovery of ATP stores. I have been particularly impressed by the use of ribose, but must admit that it is anecdotal evidence at this stage. However, don't be surprised if you hear a lot more about it in the future.

CLA – WEIGHT LOSS AND FAT BURNING?

Conjugated linoleic acid (CLA) has become popular in the fight against flab. Studies have shown that it helps to maintain a good balance between stored fat and muscle. Formerly we were able to absorb relatively large quantities of it from milk, meat and cheese, but changes in farming methods and cattle rearing, as well as the move to low-fat products, have seen a significant drop off in consumption. Scandinavian studies, in particular, have shown a loss of body fat by people with a normal metabolism and even greater losses amongst those who exercise.

There are two benefits of CLA of particular potential for runners: it reduces the breakdown of muscle during weight loss, and it assists in the burning of stored fat. There is speculation (research is currently underway) that CLA may assist in events that require an athlete to rely on high percentages of blood fat for energy as it may make the system more efficient.

Some aspects that runners who try CLA supplementation should be aware of is that it may contribute to a rise in metabolic rate (and resting heart rate), and that to be effective, a daily dose of around 3 g is required. This may be reduced after 10–12 weeks. A prime source of CLA supplementation is saffron thistle oil, which is used in SA Natural Products.

MSM

Sulphur is a mineral critical to the formation of protein and connective tissue, and is one of the most common minerals in the body, yet it has largely been overlooked as a supplement. Many of the prime sources of sulphur are vegetables e.g. garlic, onions and cabbage (foods linked with smells). Sulphur also has a long history in medicine as a 'healer'. Methylsulphonylmethane (MSM) is primarily sulphur in a form acceptable to the body and is a derivative of DMSO, which for years has been used around the world as an anti-inflammatory agent for many years.

Although not a 'cure', MSM, has been shown to relieve symptoms in a wide variety of illnesses, including osteoarthritis, and **offers the following wide-ranging attributes that have seen runners benefiting from it as a regular supplement:**

> - ▸ as an analgesic it relieves pain.
> - ▸ reduces inflammation.
> - ▸ can pass through cell membranes.
> - ▸ dilates blood vessels and increases blood flow.
> - ▸ assists in the passage of nerve impulses between cells.
> - ▸ can reduce muscle spasm.
> - ▸ has some antiparasitic qualities to assist against some causes of diarrhoea.
> - ▸ can assist in the normalisation of the immune system.

Moreover, MSM's anti-inflammatory and analgesic properties may give it potential as a prophylactic against muscle soreness and stiffness after racing and training.

My personal experience of MSM is impressive. For a number of months I was involved in a heavy seminar and work-related schedule. Although a welcome point of relief, my running was being squeezed in, between meetings and obligations, and not surprisingly I found it difficult to benefit fully from the exercise. I was also frustrated at the limited time I was able to devote to family life and myself. During a discussion, Estie Schreiber from SA Natural Products lent me a 200-page book that solely discussed the merits and background to MSM.

The information was logical and intriguing, and I can recommend this book, *The Miracle of MSM – The natural solution to pain* by S Jacob, M.D.; R Lawrence M.D.; and M Zucker. Approximately a week later, I experienced a complete rejuvenation of energy – within four days of commencing this supplement. I had changed nothing else in my life at that time, so I do attribute this turnaround to MSM, but remember, it is an experience of one. However, I should also add that, due to the lack of other illness such as the annual cold or flu, my immune system appeared to be better after use of MSM.

00:00:32
SORTING OUT THE QUALITY SUPPLEMENTS

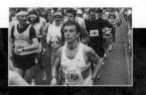

Without doubt, there are companies who are simply in the market to make as much money out of supplements as possible. Some appear to have no scruples and are probably making illegal claims. Although it is impossible to provide a list of products or companies that I would advise against using, there are guidelines that you can use in sifting through the confusion of this market.

It must be appreciated that the market in South Africa for quality sports products is actually very small. Of a population of 42 million, only about a sixth has a reasonable amount of disposable income that would allow them to spend money on supplements, above the basic priorities of eating and accommodation. If you consider the 'serious' sports participation market (running, cycling, canoeing, swimming, triathlon, rugby and soccer), you will be surprised to discover that there are probably only about 200 000 consumers who participate in the sports supplementation market. Other than the market-promoted awareness of carbohydrate, there are many sports that have had little or any exposure to detailed sports nutrition.

The leaders in the sports nutrition field are the endurance sports of running, cycling, triathlons and bodybuilding. Many other sports, including soccer and boxing, have had little exposure, and most of the boxers at the Commonwealth Games in Manchester 2002 achieved their medals purely on talent. Imagine what they might be able to achieve with the resources for better preparation. (Enough general enthusiasm was expressed in exploring this aspect, but if organisers constantly have to find ways of transporting boxers 35 km to a ring for practice, there are obviously more pressing priorities for whatever preparation funds are available. (It's a great pity that corporate South Africa is not as quick to support the country's teams, as the public and media are to fire coaches for the poor performance of teams!)

The point is that South Africa has a small market and a large number of suppliers, many of whom entered the market looking to capitalise on what they thought was a money spinner. You only have to look at the companies that have come and gone from 1999 to 2002 to see the truth of this statement.

Another problem is that many of the technical constituents are sourced from overseas (e.g. creatine has tended to originate from one factory in Germany) and are very susceptible to foreign exchange rates. While supplements in Europe and the USA may be realistically priced compared to their income standards, similar supplements locally are unable to make use of the same pricing structure. Following in the wake of the rand's depreciation, many imported supplements disappeared from the South African market. Furthermore, the size of the local market does not warrant local manufacture of truly hi-tech supplements, therefore we generally have to compromise in comparison with our international peers.

Fierce local competition is good as it ensures that prices are lean, but unfortunately it also tempts companies to make claims about ingredients in their products that, based on their cost and retail prices, couldn't possible be present in any significant quantity. It is legal to put minuscule amounts of L-carnitine in a product and list it on your label in the full knowledge that there are insufficient amounts to attract the benefits implied by its inclusion.

Firstly, make sure that you pick products that provide guides as to the quantities of all ingredients, particularly all active ingredients. Next, consider the flavourings, preservatives, gums and fillers used. To some extent we have ourselves as consumers to blame. In the face of a confusing market, we often select on taste and texture (as well as cost), rather than performance. As a result, manufacturers add significant amounts of flavouring and gums to achieve the right taste and texture profile demanded by the market. This aspect of food technology is often much more expensive than the actual performance of a product, and guess who pays for it? We do, both for the 'research' and in the reduced percentage of 'performance' constituents.

In selecting products, look for the best performance supplements first, then consider taste. Tablets and pills represent an interesting area. The vast majority of tablets are formed by compression, which requires some form of binder. If you clasp a handful of powder together, what holds it together? Inert binders obviously take up some space within the pill and so reduce the active constituents. Many pills have a total weight of under 1 g, and while this may work for nutrients that are required in microquantities, it makes no sense for 'energy' tablets. For instance, we know that we want approximately 25 g of carbohydrate energy per 30 minutes. If each tablet weighs about 1.5 g, we would need eight tablets per half-hour. But remember to factor out the talc or other binder, and this number may easily double. In addition, you are forced to take unnecessary constituents simply to allow the manufacturer to package the supplement the way he chooses (normally based on price). Gel or similar capsules are more efficient and the fact that the constituents may be left in a powdered form means that absorption is more efficient. As a general rule, tablets should not be the first choice of presentation, unless they include a 'time-release' benefit.

Also consider the type of manufacturer and the 'message' he portrays. Be suspicious of labels awash with hype and claims. It's also worth noting that in many cases, packaging costs are a major percentage or even outweigh the cost of the product, so even a manufacturer who provides a quality product may compromise on labelling and packaging to compete in terms of pricing.

Read the information given. Is it designed to help and educate you, or is it there to create hype or confusion? Are there follow-up references for more information, is the manufacturer's contact address and number clearly provided or is he 'hiding' behind agencies or institutions? Be particularly aware of addresses that include tertiary or scientific agencies and seem to imply that these organisations have manufactured the product. While that may be true, it is also possible that the only connection between the product and the organisation is a mailbox or rented space, and nothing more. If a company is willing to mislead you with a link, what other misleading information will it provide?

Quality companies will invite you to contact them; in fact, their whole approach will be one of 'recruiting' the consumer to form a relationship. They will not be afraid of discussing the basic ingredients and reasoning behind the constituents, and indeed, your biggest problem will be to prevent them from communicating with you. The majority of good manufacturers in the local sports supplement industry is passionate about its products, and nothing encourages these people more than the opportunity to communicate with other like-minded ambitious sportspeople. The profit angle is often almost a necessary evil to allow them to continue with their passion. By reading the literature provided with the product, you will understand what the manufacturer intends.

Remember that the market is small and advertising in South African magazines and journals (compared with overseas, and with promotional budgets) is very expensive. Although local magazine readerships are small, production costs are similar to those overseas. Companies who produce for mass markets, have large turnovers and healthy budgets with which to promote their products, which are usually not aimed at the specialist sportsperson. The 'serious' sports supplement market is small with turnovers to match, and because the market competition is fierce, mark-ups are low (assuming you are buying what you think you are). This means that the marketing budgets are also small, so don't expect the quality manufacturers to have adverts blazoned all over magazines or to be major sponsors. Many major sports sponsorships are collared by the federations, clubs, event promoters or other agencies, but this does not mean that all, or indeed any, of the players within that team or sport actually use those products. Sometimes they simply buy TV airtime and coverage, with the implication of use.

It is a minefield out there and it has even been suggested that much of the confusion is deliberately created to assist in the promotion of certain products. The best way to find quality products is to look for the performance constituents, check the honesty and integrity of the labels, understand the restrictions of the marketplace, where possible talk to the manufacturers (particularly those who try to help and educate), and only then to select on taste. Taste doesn't make a winner, performance does.

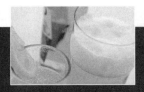

Some runners have experimented with drugs as performance enhancers, and no doubt many of them have won and walked away with the prize money, undetected. This practice should be stopped, but the problem is that it can only be deterred through thorough testing procedures. The UK was at the forefront of the battle against drugs with its random testing programme, and recent IAAF legislation (Edmonton, Canada, 2001) saw stiffer rules in place, whereby athletes away from their 'home' base for longer than two days, must inform their federations of their travel details so that they can be subjected to random drug testing. It is only to be hoped that countries will adopt strict testing programmes, in addition to the measures initiated by the IAAF.

The move to include blood testing in addition to urine testing is a welcome measure that will hopefully reduce the number of abusers of EPO (erythropoietin) and other drugs designed to increase the amount of oxygen-carrying cells.

There still seems to be a perception that the drug problem only relates to top sportspeople. I am not so sure. In South Africa it is likely that the greatest abuse is actually in school rugby teams, where parental, peer and teacher pressure is such that to make the top team would drive many to chemical assistance.

I have presented seminars to many sportspeople, from school to international level, and the number of competitors who have little knowledge of the type and number of items on the banned list never ceases to amaze me. Without doubt though, the greatest 'abusers' are school players; a good percentage of them always admit to having used banned products before and during sport, once I have explained what is and isn't legal. In addition, questions at the end typically centre on what may be used to improve performance.

The use of a small drug awareness card and other communication means needs to be instigated to ensure that every sportsperson, parent, teacher and pharmacist becomes more aware of all the items that are on the banned list. Only then will people truly realise how easy it is to fall foul of the laws, as many of the over-the-counter cold, cough and flu remedies contain substances that are banned. A list of all banned products is available from the Sports Institute in South Africa or sports councils in most countries. The World Wide Web is an excellent source to find lists that reflect the latest products. The list of medicines and remedies change monthly in each country so you need to keep up to date (and is why I have not included a list here – it would be out of date before long). Before accepting any remedy (prescription or over the counter) from a pharmacist or doctor, check it against the current list.

It is a pity that the IAAF reduced the penalty for being found guilty of drug abuse some years ago. However, it is understandable that with the advent of professional athletes, the IAAF is not in a position to defend too many legal battles in cases where athletes claim that their right to work has been compromised. This has made the whole drugs issue that much more difficult to enforce.

Whilst most of the attention seems to concentrate on athletes, I feel that greater worldwide attention should be paid to the suppliers, as well as those who prescribe these drugs. After all, it is necessary to treat both the symptom and the source of a problem.

I sincerely hope my desire for a drug-free sport is clear from all of the above. However, I also believe that it is important that only guilty athletes are punished, and though I feel far more could be done to catch those using drugs, I think there is a specific set of circumstances that has resulted in some sportspeople incorrectly being branded cheats. I am focusing on this because it should also be seen as a possible indication of how far sports supplementation has moved in recent years. I think that many of the cases cited in the following chapter had more do to with more effective supplementation than drug abuse.

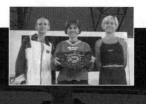

Let me state quite clearly that I do not have a medical qualification (only a sports medicine module as part of a diploma course), and that this book is written from over 30 years of practical experience in many sports, at extremes from rugby to 1 000-km racing, and from competition to coaching. I like to think that you come to know your body and how it reacts when you extend it to those extremes. However, I have reiterated my background so that there can be no misunderstanding about the origins of this chapter.

Since 1999 I have become very concerned about the apparent dramatic increase in positive tests for the steroid, nandrolone. It has been particularly prevalent in the northern hemisphere and has found its way into African sport; the case regarding a Springbok rugby prop was one of the first and most prominent. I try to keep abreast of such situations and from my reading on various cases, I sense that something is wrong. **There is a need for closer investigation if you consider the following:**

> ▸ The number of nandrolone-positive results has escalated dramatically over the past 5–6 years; it was indicated in one media report on the subject that 343 sportspeople tested positive for nandrolone in 1999. In 2000 up to August (with the Olympic Games still to come), 296 cases were recorded.
> ▸ Virtually all the athletes claimed innocence, including some that have publicly supported the antidrugs campaign for their countries.
> ▸ Nandrolone was one of the first anabolic steroids, and remains one of the easiest to detect.
> ▸ Positive tests of nandrolone hit major 'media' athletes before the 2000 Olympics (e.g. Linford Christie, Merlene Ottey, Dieter Baumann) and thus received mega-media coverage.

Why would anyone use this particular drug if they wanted to cheat? There is surely a better explanation for this phenomenon. Athletes continue to be 'banned' and branded as cheats, when they MAY, in fact, be innocent. This situation could be depriving the sport of its true heroes, who deserve the recognition and income. Not that ALL are innocent – I am sure there are deliberate cheats who have capitalised on the confusion, but there are too many unanswered questions for so many to be guilty.

Moreover, a number of official positions have, in fact, shifted. Nandrolone, or its metabolites, was initially thought not to occur naturally in the body and if an athlete was found to have nandrolone metabolites in his urine, the IOC and IAAF deemed him to be 'positive' and he was banned from participation.

Research conducted by I Bjorkeim and A Keiman in 1982 and 1988 respectively, proved that nandrolone and its metabolites are naturally present as intermediates during the production of estrogenic compounds. Given the progress and improvement in tolerances of testing procedures, it is not surprising that metabolite levels are now more easily detected. Despite this, a 1999 study by B Le Bizec showed that 50% of subjects in a test (all of whom were known to be drug-free) proved positive for nandrolone metabolites in their urine samples.

It appears that the IOC has acknowledged this, because in August 1999, the IOC committee sent a memo to heads of all testing laboratories, indicating that only samples greater than 2 ng/ml (men) and 5 ng/ml (women) should be considered as proof of doping. There was no apparent reason for the choice of these levels, and research by R Debruyckere presented at a symposium in 1990 showed that 11% of those tested (known not to have been using drugs) had metabolite levels in excess of the 2-ng/ml limit. One even had 37 ng/ml or 18.5 times the IAAF limit. Le Bizec's research in 1999 showed that exercise prior to testing also had an effect on levels, with some around four times the non-exercise level.

It is important to note that the testing procedure is given as ng/ml i.e. there is no reference to urine concentration or the hydration of an athlete. For instance, a dehydrated athlete (even caused by coffee or training) will have a greater concentration of metabolites than if he was well hydrated before testing. It would seem, therefore, that a test showing high nandrolone metabolite levels should possibly be investigated further before announcing a positive test.

In August 1998 an IOC memo on anabolic steroids apparently recommended that an adjustment to levels be made if the specific gravity of a sample exceeds a value of 1.020, which is an indication of dehydration.

The IOC arbitration board acknowledged this recommendation in June 2000 when it lifted the ban on Merlene Ottey, effectively allowing this crowd-pulling and financially marketable athlete to compete in the Sydney Games. Her original test showed levels of 14–15 ng/ml, however, she had competed in a 100 m and 200 m within 90 minutes in 25–28 °C and therefore her sample showed evidence of dehydration. The panel recalculated her levels in a way that it felt accounted for this and came up with a level of 4.53 ng/ml, which is nominally below the IOC-suggested reporting threshold of 5 ng/ml. We can only speculate at the litigation for loss of earnings that may have followed had Ottey been banned from the Olympics and later found to have been innocent.

Just before the start of the Olympics, Norwegian superheavyweight lifter Stian Grimseth was sent home for testing positive for nandrolone. Anecdotal reports say he was 'three times the near zero levels' prohibited by testing, which suggests a level of 6 ng/ml. Although he wasn't the only athlete sent home from Sydney, what singles him out is that he was the Norwegian Olympic Development Centre's front man in its anti-doping campaign. Prior to the games, Grimseth even went as far as publicly asking to be tested every month to prove that it is possible to reach the top as a clean athlete. It appears that his measured level was well within the range indicated by research that is to be expected when exercise precedes testing. Supposing that further investigation and research proves his innocence, how has his reputation been damaged? What about loss of earnings if he had won a medal, or had excelled sufficiently to earn a sponsorship or endorsement?

Various British athletes have tested positive for nandrolone, including Gary Cadogan (400-m hurdler): 10.6 ng/ml; Dougie Walker (European 200-m champion): 12.59 ng/ml on 1 December 1998; Linford Christie: 200 ng/ml on 13 February 1999; and Mark Richardson. With Ottey recording a level of 14–15 ng/ml and then exonerated, it casts doubt over at least two of these tests. Were dehydration and the research findings taken into account? How has it affected the career of the previously little-known Walker, who immediately after hitting the headlines was removed from the sport?

Christie's case is also interesting. He had already retired after the Atlanta Olympics and only some three years later returned to competition in a German meeting where he was placed fourth. Why would an athlete of his calibre, who had already won at the highest level and was competing at a relatively nominal level in retirement, use a substance known to be one of the easiest to detect?

In the case of Mark Richardson, he tested positive for nandrolone in October 1999. Mainly because there was no other explanation, there was a suggestion that it resulted from some sports supplements he had been taking. However, samples from the same batches that he had used were analysed by two independent laboratories and NO traces of nandrolone or its precursors were found.

Ironically, the IAAF reinstated Richardson after arbitration and he subsequently joined its programme to promote the message that you don't need sports supplementation to become an elite athlete – an interesting switch in sentiment.

However, the disgraced UK athletes had some support from UK Athletics, which prompted a study (under the auspices of, and apparently funded by the IAAF council) by the highly respected Professor Ron Maughan of Aberdeen University, a world-recognised expert on sports drinks.

Professor Maughan studied the levels in those athletes taking dietary supplements. He concluded that such supplements 'could when combined with vigorous exercise, stress and dehydration, result in production of higher concentrations of nandrolone metabolites in the athletes' body fluids'. Professor Maughan also found that there was sufficient reason to consider raising the current threshold five or more times.

In principle, this might have exonerated a number of the athletes, but the IAAF arbitration panel report cited **the following reasons for not adopting the recommendations:**

> ▸The subjects were not accommodated in a controlled, 24-hour supervised environment.
> ▸The number of subjects in the study was not large enough to produce a reliable result.
> ▸Failure to test all supplements for prohibited substances.

> ▸ The supplements in the study were not all identical to those given in the form submitted by the athletes when tested.
>
> ▸ Not all of the Aberdeen researchers were experienced in steroid analysis.
>
> ▸ Not all samples were collected (two of seven samples from one athlete were not collected during a rest day).
>
> ▸ Professor Maughan's study could not be considered independent, as he was part of the UK Disciplinary Committee for the consideration of the cases of Walker, Cadogan and Christie. The IAAF council claimed that this was even more significant, because the study had been conducted before the disciplinary meeting.

In the light of the IAAF's funding of the study, this latter statement is particularly odd, and presumably it was aware of Professor Maughan's status at UK Athletics prior to approving the funding for the investigation.

It could be argued that Maughan would have been more inclined to bias if he conducted the research after the disciplinary meeting, as he might have felt pressured to vindicate his decision.

The IAAF newsletter (August 2000) made the following closing statement, 'The arbitrators' decision in the cases of Cadogan, Walker and Christie was not made to defend the current system. It was made to respect and apply the current rules.'

All of the above leads me back to the question, 'Why would anyone make use of nandrolone if they deliberately wanted to use drugs?' Surely there are no top-level athletes still unaware of the recent spate of positive nandrolone test results?

Some people use the fact that second test samples substantiate the positive first test, as convincing argument for a guilty verdict. I am not sure how much should be read into the present second test process.

As I understand it, the second test is performed at the same laboratory that conducted the first test, and that there has never been a case where a second test has disproved the findings of an initial test. I believe that if there were discrepancies, questions would be raised as to the suitability of a laboratory. Given the financial implication of losing a validation licence, independent assessment would be more appropriate.

Something is amiss. Science has indicated at least sufficient potential for doubt. In most countries, innocence is presumed until guilt is proven. Shouldn't a moratorium, therefore, be declared while further investigations and reviews are completed by science and administration, or could the potential for litigation by athletes who perhaps have been innocently banned and branded, be clouding the issue?

It would certainly be difficult (and expensive?) for administration and sport in general, if it is proved that some banned athletes have been deprived of the opportunity to greatness, and the resultant earnings. This would be further exacerbated if administrators are shown to have been tardy in overlooking steps that would have resolved so many of the arbitration hearings.

If there is any chance that a natural process is responsible for these nandrolone levels, more athletes will fall foul of the rules as they currently stand, and with each banning, the number of potential litigation cases increases. The figures involved will not be small and may have a major impact on the finances of some sports bodies.

COULD SPORTS SUPPLEMENTATION BE RESPONSIBLE?

Is there a natural reason or logic for these results? Although I have limited formal medical training, my training as a structural and civil engineer, and experience as a coach and athlete, have lead me to search for a logical explanation. Based on this, I submit the following layman's hypothesis, which although may not be absolutely correct, will have a degree of potential for more qualified people to investigate.

THE FOLLOWING ARE KNOWN FACTS AND/OR CONCEPTS:

1. The whole basis of training relates to the **body's ability to adapt**. When exercising with a certain workload, there is a breakdown and a recovery process, which increases the body's resistance to the initial workload.
2. **When we train, we break down muscle.** It is not the training but the repair of the muscle that provides the improvement/growth. The greater the training load, the greater the damage and the greater the repair that is required.

3. Growth only occurs when **the correct building blocks and nutrients** (a combination of protein amino acids, vitamins, carbohydrates and essential fatty acids), all in the correct proportions, **trigger the hormonal and recovery systems.**

4. (Following research conducted from 1982 onwards) **nandrolone plays a natural role in the repair process.**

5. As a result of such research, many **full-time or professional athletes not only train at greater intensities,** but more efficiently than their predecessors because they have more time and better knowledge on how to train and recover.

6. The **quality of sports supplements**, and the **education on their use**, is greater now than previously. (For example, an egg was previously thought to be the most complete protein and was ranked with a biological value of 100. Using the same ranking system, some protein sports supplements now rank at 159 or more i.e. a 60% increase in efficiency.) It is not unreasonable to assume that higher quality 'nutrients' could lead to more efficient recovery.

7. Significant advances have been made in the selection of **'transporters'** to assist in the absorption of **'building/repairing'** components. Such improved absorption may, in fact, be the key.

8. When we eat sugar our blood sugar rises, activating an insulin reaction to take the blood sugar NOT back to normal, but initially lower, then gradually back to normal. It works in a 'pendulum' fashion: **the higher the blood sugar, the greater the insulin reaction**, which leads to lower blood sugar levels before returning to 'normal'. It is the insulin reaction that assists the absorption of 'nutrients' into the muscle for rebuilding. Hence a more efficient transporter could, logically, be responsible for more effective recovery.

Given the above, could the following be possible?

- With athletes inducing greater breakdown, and more efficient supply and/or absorption of 'raw' but essential recovery nutrients, will the recovery systems of athletes become more efficient and hence stimulate greater recovery processes?

  This ties in well with the principle of adaptation and the 'pendulum' concept discussed earlier.

- It has been shown that some individuals have a naturally raised level of nandrolone metabolites, and that dehydration raises them even further. Could training and excellent nutrition be responsible for developing a more efficient but natural system?

- If so, could it also be possible that the more efficient the system becomes, the greater the results, and hence the more intense the training that can be sustained? This, in turn, leads to greater muscle breakdown in future training periods, which stimulates a greater response from the natural recovery system.

This hypothesis appears to agree with the reported results of Professor Maughan's study. Furthermore, the South African rugby prop that was found guilty of high levels of nandrolone was suffering from a broken wrist. Anyone who has experienced a broken bone knows that the natural desire is simply to lie down – it is part of the body's way of prompting recovery. Could the trauma of the broken wrist, plus the quality of the sports supplements he was taking have prompted a greater production of nandrolone? It is not clear, but there was sufficient doubt in the case for him to be reinstated after an appeal.

However, it still leaves a question mark over the extremely high values recorded in cases such as Christie at 200 ng/ml and CJ Hunter, reportedly 1 000 times the 'legal' level, which appears to be outside the realms of reason. Obviously, there have been cases of deliberate drug use, but if the above hypothesis is correct, is it also possible that the reaction/stimulation of the recovery system that produces nandrolone is related to the amount of 'damage/breakdown' to muscle? If that were true, an athlete with high muscle mass who has substantial breakdown following intense and thorough training, would stimulate a greater quantity of nandrolone. Christie and Hunter are not small men. Both had been in intensive training and competition for many years. Could their systems have been 'tuned' into greater efficiency over a period of time?

I believe that there is an urgent need to review nandrolone testing. Although my hypothesis may not provide the full answer, it has solicited some consensus from international authorities that have been asked for comment on it, that there are sufficient grounds for investigation. For those who would like to explore this controversial subject further, **I suggest consulting the following references:**

> ▶ Davis, Dr Simon, 'A brief review of nandrolone doping control procedures', Lawrence Berkeley National Laboratories; with sub-references to
>> ▶ Bjorkeim I, et al (1982), *Journal of Steroid Biochemistry*, 17
>> ▶ Debruyckere R, et al (1990), 'Proceedings of 4th Symposium on the Analysis of Steroids', Gorog S (ed.)
>> ▶ Keiman A, et al (1988), *Journal of Pharm Biomed Analysis*, 6
>> ▶ Le Bizec B, et al (1999), J *Chromatogr B Biomed Science Applied*, 723 (1–2)
> ▶ IAAF Newsletter, July 2000, 'Statement following arbitration panel for Merlene Ottey'
> ▶ IAAF Newsletter, August 2000, 'Results of arbitration panel on cases of Christie, Walker and Cadogan'
> ▶ 'List of drug cases linked to Sydney Games', news article on official Sydney Olympic website, 30 September 2000
> ▶ Report on positive test on Stian Grimseth (Norway), Stephen Seiler PhD, Assistant Professor, Institute for Sport, Agder University College, Norway

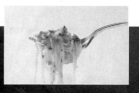

00:00:35
WEIGHT LOSS

HEALTHY EATING LEADS TO BETTER TRAINING AND WEIGHT LOSS

'You are a machine.' Many runners and cyclists might welcome such a remark as a compliment on their sporting prowess, but it is also relevant to a discussion on healthy eating for sport.

The amount of energy you take in (eat) should match the amount of energy you expend in a day, if you are to maintain the same body weight (energy in = energy out). If you eat more than you use, you will gain weight and if you eat less than you expend, you will lose weight.

Unlike machines, humans are more complicated if you consider the composition of the 'fuel' used to power the body. As discussed previously, the purpose of training is to inflict microscopic damage to muscles, which triggers growth and results in stronger muscles. While carbohydrate provides energy for training, protein repairs and builds muscles; both are important.

Recapping on a healthy diet

The amount of protein required varies with the extent and intensity of the exercise, because it will impact on the amount of muscle damage inflicted. For instance, a person who doesn't train needs only a nominal amount of protein to maintain lean body mass (about 0.75 g per kilogram of body weight, which for a 70-kg couch potato means around 53 g per day). However, if that same person decides to take up a reasonable level of training, his protein requirement can increase to 1.2–1.6 g per kg, i.e. a daily total of 85–105 g. If he tackled the Tour de France, it would climb further to around 130 g per day.

What happens if you don't supply the protein needs? Quite simply the muscle cannot be repaired and any subsequent training will inflict further damage on already-damaged muscles. Not only does this inhibit the desired muscle growth, but also results in a catabolic condition and the onset of overtraining.

Carbohydrate meets a number of needs: it provides the energy source needed to power the muscles, but just as importantly, the initial intake of carbohydrate stimulates an insulin reaction, which is required to assist with the absorption of proteins in the body.

In endurance sports such as cycling and running, carbohydrates fuel the muscles for training, which means that your diet should be about 60% carbohydrate. This is quite a task as most carbohydrates are bulky and it is difficult to eat enough each day. For example, running and cycling use 350–800 kcal per hour, over and above the basic energy requirement simply to maintain daily activity in a 'normal' lifestyle. It is not unreasonable for a club 'athlete' to require around 2 500 kcal per day. Ideally, 60% of this will come from carbohydrates (1 500 kcal). Each gram of carbohydrate provides 4 kcal, therefore 375 g of carbohydrate provides 1 500 kcal. A 100-g baked potato only provides 19 g of carbohydrate, so it would take 19 baked potatoes a day to meet the carbohydrate requirements. It should be obvious why carbohydrate supplements form an essential part of an athlete's daily diet and are not merely a pre-event consideration.

Similarly, an 'athlete' might require around 100 g of protein to ensure muscle repair to benefit from training. Each gram of protein also provides 4 kcal, which means that a further 400 kcal needs to be provided by protein. In total, this provides approximately 1 900 kcal and only another 600 g required from fat.

Contrary to 'popular' belief, fat is an essential part of our diet, providing 9 kcal per gram. Fat, or at least certain types, are essential components in the process of hormone production, which is key to recovery.

Avoid saturated fats, opting rather for essential fats often identified as Omega 3 and Omega 6. However, the remaining 600 kcal in our sample case only requires 65 g of fat per day. If you put that into perspective, a simple 100-g bar of chocolate provides over 23 g of fat, and a teaspoon of margarine on toast soon fulfils the daily requirement.

The really tough bit is that fat is integral to the 'taste' in most food, making it difficult to cut levels down to the correct amounts. Moreover, ensuring the right amount of kilocalories is easy enough, but ensuring that the amounts of carbohydrate and protein are correct, becomes challenging.

Reducing kilocalorie intake

For many the concept of losing weight simply means cutting down the total kilocalories, but by now it should be obvious that such an approach is incorrect. Many personal trainers and books promote a simple approach to weight loss that revolves around a restricted-kilocalorie diet and easy, low intensity exercise. Not surprisingly, many of their clients never achieve their goals and are still gyrating around their 'worst fears' two years on! The best way to lose weight is to maintain the same proportions of food, together with intense training.

To lose weight you must expend more energy than you take in, and in this way you will burn off the extra energy your body has stored. By raising your metabolic rate, i.e. the amount of energy burnt per minute, you will increase the amount of energy used in a day. There are basically two ways of doing this: with exercise and by taking diet supplements.

Exercise

Exercise intensity determines the prime source of energy used to support the effort. At very intense speed (exercise of up to three minutes duration), you almost exclusively use glycogen as an energy source. If you go flat out for longer, you start to use a percentage of blood fatty acids. Exercising for even longer increases the percentage of energy from blood fatty acids further. Of course, the longer the duration of the exercise, the lower the percentage of maximum heart rate that can be maintained for that full period of time.

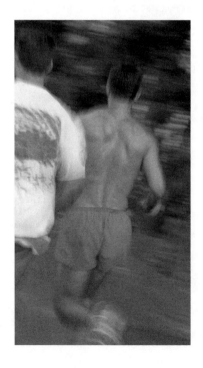

RIGHT *Running in the 'fat-burning zone' is not particularly effective in weight control/loss*

From the above, it is clear why a 'fat-burning' zone has been indicated in terms of heart-rate level. Although running, cycling and other endurance activities do make use of energy from fat burning in this low-intensity zone, many personal trainers or manuals fail to cover the second half of this equation, i.e. 1 kg of fat can be equated to 9 000 kcal and to burn this off it would be necessary to exercise at this low 'fat-burning' intensity for around 15 hours! Another problem with such low levels of exercise is that once you stop exercising, your heart and metabolic rates drop straight back to normal levels.

Conversely, with high-intensity exercise you raise your heart and metabolic rates to much higher levels and it takes considerably longer for the heart rate to return to 'normal' – evidenced by a heart-rate monitor at the end of your exercise. During the post-exercise period, the increased metabolic rate means you are burning energy. As high-intensity exercise burns glycogen (stored carbohydrate), these first-choice energy stores are depleted during the exercise, and assuming that no carbohydrate drink had been taken after exercise, the next option is to burn fat stores.

Exercising at high intensity not only burns more energy per minute, but also has a 'post-exercise' burn that can last for hours, eating away at fat stores as you sit at work or conduct other normal duties in the day. Whereas the personal trainer who encourages his client to go for a one-hour easy run or cycle in the 'fat-burning' zone will promote a total kilocalorie expenditure of perhaps 600 kcal, a wiser option is to indulge in a session of high-intensity intervals for half that time, which can result in a burn-off of more than 900 kcal. In addition, interval work will have a more dramatic effect on your overall race fitness.

Diet pills

This subject is covered in chapter 25 – it is essential that you read it. Please remember, because of the **dangers that diet pills represent,** they should be considered a last option.

The weight-loss prescription

To lose weight, look to a combination of a minor reduction of kilocalories in your normal balanced eating habits, and alternating days of high-intensity intervals (or similar heart-rate-raising exercise) and easy recovery. Don't forget that an increase in lean muscle mass requires an increase in energy to retain that muscle mass. As a result, strength training that increases the muscle mass of the major muscle groups will concomitantly require an increase in energy (as well as the proportion of dietary protein) to allow for further weight loss.

Weight loss is such a 'fashionable' attribute that many people and companies have 'evolved' quick fixes, which have been heavily marketed. However, keeping to a more scientific and long-term approach will provide more meaningful results, without the expense of diet pills. Rather use those funds to ensure the correct balance in your diet.

PART 5:

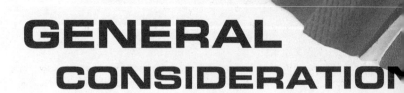

GENERAL
CONSIDERATION

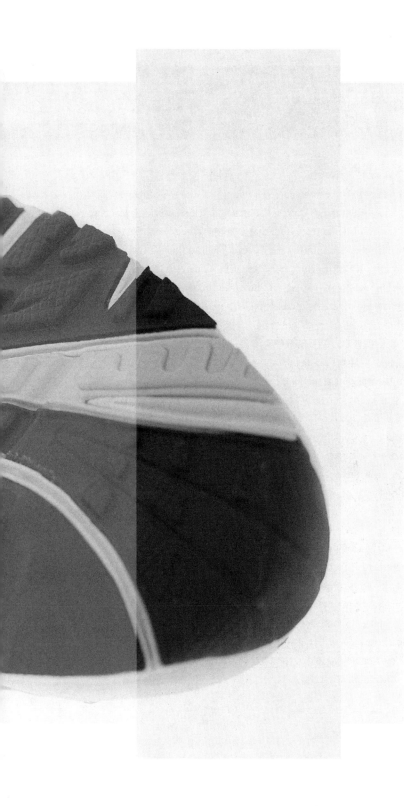

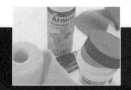

No matter how much reading you do, or how many people you listen to, there will be times when things don't go as planned. It's all very well planning your training, but it's a lot harder to ensure that everything is perfect, than it is to do too much or to do things incorrectly. A universal failing of human nature is to think that the principles we have learnt don't apply to ourselves. We spot overtraining in other runners, but think that we are 'invincible'. Overtraining is the root cause of most injuries and illnesses... and it's the easiest thing to do.

IT'S EASY TO OVERTRAIN

A question that I am regularly asked by novice runners or non-runners is, 'what is the hardest part of running long races such as marathons and ultras?' The answer is simple: the period of heavy training that must be completed before your chosen major race is actually harder than the race. For ultrarunners it is the period of 'endurance training' in the final 6–8 weeks, for a marathoner it's the 'endurance' followed by speed improvement.

At such times in particular, strict discipline is needed and life often seems to consist only of work and running. Any extra time is automatically split up between family and rest, and frequently both of these aspects appear to be neglected. Indeed the support and understanding of your family and friends can be as important as the training. George Sheehan, the American running doctor, summed it up quite aptly, 'It is not the 32-km training run that causes me to be overtrained, but the stress from the argument with my wife when I get back.' He was right; 'damage' from emotional stress can be far more onerous than the physical fatigue of running. In fact, the easy runs are to a large extent stress relieving, if run at the correct pace. But it's impossible to spend every waking minute in running, as overtraining would result. Training is only as good as the rest and recovery that accompanies it.

The trick is to find the balance between the physical exertion of the training, the physical and mental stress of your career, and the combination of a good diet and the amount of recovery time. This was highlighted by the great Wally Hayward who, when given time off to train for the 1952 Helsinki Olympics, was asked how much more running this would allow him to do, answered that having more time would allow him to recover better so that he could train at a higher level. The same approach was mirrored by nine-times Comrades winner Bruce Fordyce, who reduced his speaking engagements and appearances during the final build-up to Comrades, in order to rest more.

Obviously, for a runner with the restriction of full-time employment, the support and backing of family and friends is a critical factor. Generally, it will be met with understanding provided it is for a short period only. But even the best-laid plans often go wrong. A crisis at work, or a family problem or illness, can upset the fine balance. Our natural urge is to battle through and to keep to the training schedule. This is a mistake. A schedule must be flexible to allow for unforeseen stress. Failure to do so will set us back in training and may even result in injury or illness.

While we may be forgiven for not cutting the grass for a month during peak training, failing to meet a work deadline or family commitments will not bring favour! Finding this balance is probably the hardest part of training, especially if the streets are crowded with runners, and the 'word' at weekly club meetings is how much training distance this or that one is putting in for the same race you're intending to run. The tendency is to start worrying that you are undertrained for the upcoming race. However, this is the time to adopt a DON'T WORRY... BE HAPPY approach, safe in the knowledge that you have the flexibility to match your training to your stress capacity and available recovery. With such an approach there is every likelihood that you will pass those 'mega-distance' runners when it really matters ... IN THE RACE!

IS IT INJURY OR ILLNESS?

There are two 'swear' words in a runner's dictionary, which, when spoken, elicit an instantaneous reaction. The first is 'injury', and the reaction is one of sympathy and advice, normally followed by a litany of the 'advisor's' own injury history, as if to let the unfortunate runner know that he is not alone in his misery. The second word is

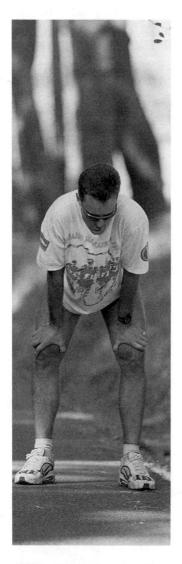

'illness', and the novice runner soon learns the signs that indicate that this second, and more serious, 'profanity' has been uttered. The behaviour is obvious, if not slightly embarrassed, as the afflicted individual is increasingly avoided by others in the group.

These words tend to be used in epidemic proportions in the *eight 'high-stress' weeks* prior to major events such as Comrades and Two Oceans.

Injuries

As opposed to sports such as rugby or football, running injuries are, in general, self inflicted by your desire to run, i.e. most will go away if you stop running. Naturally, that is not to your liking, as it **is your desire to run**, but the onset of an injury is normally a sign that you have overstressed your body in some way. Perhaps you have increased your distance too much over a short period, or have started hill work or speed sessions without proper adaptation. Alternatively, your favourite pair of shoes may have 'given up the ghost' or you may have problems with the selection of new shoes. In most cases, an injury has a fairly simple solution and often involves a period of 'running rest'.

There is a fairly quick decline in VO_2 when we take time off. VO_2 can be described as a measure of the ability to

ABOVE *Sometimes there is no point in 'pushing through' – caution, as well as a conservative approach is the best way forward*

transfer oxygen within the body and in general, the higher the VO_2, the better. This sharp decline during 'off periods' has been a concern for some time, but recent research shows that the biggest portion of this is attributable to loss of blood volume when training stops. Trained runners have a greater blood volume than the average person and therefore more red blood corpuscles, which transfer more oxygen and create a larger VO_2. The challenge is to maintain this volume during enforced running rest.

In times of injury this is relatively easy if you are willing to modify your training. It has been shown that two speed sessions per week will greatly assist in maintaining this volume. Provided you are able to run a session of 4 x 400 m at best 1 500-m pace with as much rest as you wish, your 'fitness' can be largely maintained. Of course, most injuries prohibit running and alternatives have to be found, but the same principles apply. Two hard cycle sessions, which will raise your pulse to anaerobic levels for 2–3 minutes at a time or a twice-weekly session of running in water will maintain the pulse and blood volume. There are many ways to mitigate the 'devastation' of an injury.

Determining the problem

I can't remember how many times I have wished that a physiotherapist or doctor could pull aside the skin to see 'exactly' where and what my soft tissue injury was. Sometimes we have an injury where we can put our hand on the general area, but not the exact spot. If it is a deep injury below layers of other muscles, the matter is worse. Even if we can identify the location it is not easy to see the extent or type of injury. To this extent physiotherapists are working in the dark, using the 'feel' of a muscle, the differences between left and right, and heat as a method of diagnosis. It can be very frustrating for all concerned, and can delay the correct treatment by days. One option is to have an MRI (magnetic resonance image) scan, but it is very expensive for a small injury and generally impractical.

Diagnostic ultrasound has recently come to the fore, which is basically an extension of a system developed in the 1970s to enable doctors to 'see' the foetus in the womb. It was developed commercially in Edinburgh, Scotland, and I am proud to say that my brother, Vernon, was part of the team working on that project. Now it has been expanded to allow a view of the soft tissue in a limb, showing the location of muscle tears, bleeding and other forms of damage and growth. The scan can be completed in less than ten minutes and a photograph and report provided to the physiotherapist or doctor for the relevant treatment to be undertaken. The cost of this scan is in the region of a normal physiotherapy treatment and is an excellent first step in the treatment of an injury.

Anti-inflammatory drugs and alternatives

There is often a drive to use anti-inflammatory drugs in the treatment of injuries, but I recommend that you avoid these wherever possible. The problem with many anti-inflammatories is that they have a negative effect on the 'cox 2' prostaglandin around the injured area and also affect the 'cox 1' in the stomach. A prime objective of the anti-inflammatory is to inhibit the production of 'cox 2' because it induces swelling and pain. However, 'cox 1' is a vital protection to the stomach lining and when it is destroyed, there is a significant increase in stomach ulcers, etc. The long-term use of anti-inflammatories, typically 'non-steroidal anti-inflammatory drugs' (NSAIDs), results in the hospitalisation of 270 000 Americans annually, and of that 16 000 die from the side effects. For this reason, such drugs should always be taken on a full stomach. It also highlights the reason why taking such medication before a race should be a last resort.

Another word of caution relates to the use by children under 16 of aspirin, Disprin or combinations containing these. Studies in the UK have shown that, particularly if taken after a flu infection, these can cause degradation of the liver and swelling in the brain. It is, therefore, important for children not to use them. However, I prefer to use a Disprin as a final 'emergency' measure as an anti-inflammatory if I develop a problem in a race. This is limited to one tablet every fours hours and is only taken if dissolved in water and after eating something, even if it is only a slice of bread. The use of stronger painkillers or drugs is not warranted in most sport situations – the race will still be there in future years, make sure you are!

There are alternatives to NSAIDs to consider. In 2000, new 'cox-2 inhibitor' drugs came on to the market. They are selective in only inhibiting the cox 2 and not the cox 1. This is welcome progress, although there are anecdotal reports of some side effects at present.

Another useful and well-researched alternative is the use of a ginger compound of two species of ginger, extracted from the plants in extremely high concentrations and found to act as a good anti-inflammatory by inhibiting the production of the precursors to pain and inflammation. Studies and research over nine years have proven this to be as effective as ibuprofen and it has been used in the treatment of arthritis. In 1999 I met Olympian Carl Lewis, who also shared his very positive experiences with this remedy. The only drawback is that it must be taken for 3–4 weeks before any effects are felt, so it is certainly appropriate for chronic pains. An additional positive appears to be its ability to reduce the effects of muscle damage and DOMS in training and racing, although this has only been based on anecdotal reports. The product name changes from country to country but in the UK, USA and South Africa it is known as Zinaxin.

Homoeopathic remedies

There is no doubt that more attention is being paid to homoeopathic remedies, and scientists and doctors are beginning to understand and accept their role in medication. Homoeopathic remedies have been around for years in Europe and, indeed, started in Germany in the 1700s. The basic principle is to treat 'like with like' – the same principle used, for instance, with the antiflu injection. There are many homoeopathic remedies, including for flu and cold, which deserve to be tried, and it is highly likely that they will gain a greater place in sport. Apart from the benefits of fewer, or no, side effects, homoeopathic remedies do not fall foul of the banned drugs listing. These products are now stocked by many pharmacies and are losing their 'witches brew' label.

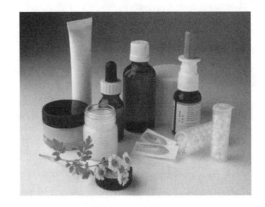

One reason why many doubt the efficacy of homoeopathy is that most of the solutions are very dilute and, theoretically, they don't have even one molecule of the original substance left in the solution. However, the more dilute the solution, the stronger it is considered. Anyone unfamiliar with homoeopathic remedies will find this bewildering, but despite this, electroscopic analysis of a solution shows levels of activity that don't show up in water put through the same production process. Quite simply, when the solution is made, it is vigorously shaken, then diluted again. The process is repeated until the required level is reached, and it appears that this shaking alters the molecular state and activity.

Apart from the use of arnica and arnica products (see under prevention and also under homeopathic anti-inflammatory drugs), since 1990 I have experienced great benefit from **a number of remedies:**

> ▸ Combinations that promote 'calming' to aid sleep the night before an event
> ▸ Echinacea for boosting the immune system
> ▸ Combinations that provide a general system boost during recovery periods.

Homoeopathic acceptance in sport is still growing and only in 2002 did some South African sports bodies acknowledge the possibilities of homoeopathic remedies and combinations. Research has been instigated to see what benefits may be obtained through the regular use of 'system boosters' during preparation and competition periods.

While not wishing to give the impression that I am against orthodox medicine, all athletes owe it to themselves to search for alternatives to allopathic drugs and/or products that can provide an edge, while not contravening the drugs laws, or risking damage to processes or organs in the body.

Acupuncture

The Chinese have used acupuncture for centuries, and although it is hard to explain, I can testify to its success. Orthodox western medicine has tended to steer clear of the so-called 'complementary' medicines. Even chiropractors are still relatively new in their acceptance in many countries. Perhaps the diversity of South African culture, which has required various medical bodies to give more credence to traditional healers, has worked in favour of some of the other medical arms. I have benefited from acupuncture and electro-acupuncture machines in particular. These are usually small, handheld battery-operated devices that are used on the point of injury and on various 'node' points on the body.

Basically, the practising acupuncturist believes that the body has a number of lines, called meridians, connecting joints, points and organs. Sometimes these lines of communication are blocked or jammed, which results in injury or illness. By stimulating these lines at node points, they break down the blockage and revitalise the lines. This can be done with needles, or with a very mild electrostimulus. In electro-acupuncture, holding a machine in one hand, and a terminal on the relevant points with the other, creates a circuit. Each of the designated points is stimulated for 40 seconds, and there are normally 4–6 points associated with each diagnosis.

Does it work? I believe it does, and offer this experience as testimony. My father-in-law, Jan Strydom, is a medical doctor with over 45 years' experience, and has been involved in, and been a follower of, sports medicine for years. He has an open mind to finding new and relevant solutions, but is also a committed member of the Dutch Reformed Church, which as a denomination, does not accept acupuncture as a medical solution. When he stayed with us in the UK in 1997, he aggravated an old lower back injury by carrying suitcases.

One night, when all the orthodox medical solutions had failed, and the pain persisted, I convinced him to try a small electro-acupuncture machine. By the following day, the relief was significant enough to have this erstwhile 'doubting Thomas' on a programme of regular use, and even contemplating the purchase of one for himself. His views on acupuncture had changed, and that included an alteration in religious viewpoint.

I can relate many more examples, but the point is that acupuncture is well worth consideration by the injured or ill athlete as it has no side effects and can speed up the return to running.

Balance and bite can improve your health and performance

Most athletes and coaches would agree that the more technically correct sportspeople tend to be the most successful in their chosen sport. It is unusual to see a hunched athlete dominate a middle-distance track race. Indeed, the commentary in media coverage of the African domination of athletics, be it marathons, track or cross-country, often alludes to the easy, relaxed manner and grace of the athletes' loping style. The same principles apply to most sports.

Correcting your body's imbalances and adopting mechanically efficient styles can assist you to achieve your true potential in sport. More importantly, it can contribute to your overall health and welfare.

Incorrect posture or an unbalanced style often leads to injury as forces are then transferred to other muscles or joints, which become overloaded. The first reaction is to treat the point of injury, but this effectively only treats the symptom, not the cause. In more recent years, runners have begun to accept that looking for problems with their shoes is the first step in treating many injuries. Worn-out shoes or ones that give no support (or conversely, insufficient flexibility) are often at the root of their injury problems.

This works on the principle that each person is individual and that shoes are selected to 'correct' the natural imbalances of the ankle/foot mechanism. Treating or 'correcting' postural imbalances, to provide a more efficient 'base' structure extends this logic further. Possible sources and methods of such 'balancing' may be surprising, but the results can be dramatic. The muscles, bones and membranes of the body are totally interrelated. Movement or disposition of one part has a reciprocal effect on other areas. Tension in the neck or back, can affect the rotation of the pelvis and hence leg length, which in turn affects the foot plant during running. The change in strike and push-off adds load onto different muscles to those previously trained and can result in calf or hamstring injuries. Whereas initial treatment will focus on the injury, the only way to solve the problem is to identify and treat the chain of causes. This highlights the concept that a 'rough' day sitting in front of the computer can end up as a lower leg injury during that night's training.

Balance from the foundation up

Applied kinesiology analyses body movements, strengths and weaknesses in both an insular and holistic approach to bring the whole body back into balance. Balancing the body's structure has been used to great effect by a number of top sportspeople, including many UK and SA sportspeople. In the mid '80s there was much media hype surrounding the diminutive running sensation Zola Budd and her world conquering times. Budd experienced a dramatic fall-off in performance through chronic hip and leg injury. Despite attention from physiotherapists, doctors and sport science assessment, there seemed to be no return to previous form. In South Africa she consulted Ron Holder, an applied kinesiologist, known to many South African ultrarunners as the 'guru', who was able to 'treat' her problem by balancing her body structure. Holder released areas of muscle tension and provided various wedges (made from *Yellow Pages* telephone directories) to distribute the loads more evenly. In doing so, it strengthened the weaker muscles and the wedges were gradually reduced in size. Now a veteran athlete, Zola continues to make regular visits to Ron Holder to maintain her running.

The basic principles of the analysis are to test muscle strength and movement as the athlete's body is gradually put into a balanced position. The greatest strength exists when 'balance' is achieved. Assessment often begins with 'rubbings'. These break down adhesions and release various membranes around the body, allowing them to 'reset' when put into the position of balance. A torturous combination of tickling and irritation, these momentary rubs provide vivid memories for patients, who frequently twist and gyrate under Holder's elbow or thumb, but the benefits outweigh the ordeal. Wedges are constructed to keep the runner in a balanced position, while final tests determine the thickness of wedges to an unbelievable one-page accuracy. Although runner's wedges fit under the innersole of the shoe, canoeists sit on their wedges.

Ron Holder has used this protocol to assist a number of top sportspeople, from Johnny Halberstadt and Mark Plaatjes in the 1980s, to the South African 1995 World Cup Rugby team, and Britain's longtime 400-m champion of the 1990s, Roger Black, who is quoted as saying he would never have been able to continue his career without Ron's assistance. When completed, the runner's stride-length becomes equal and this 'balance' can be heard in the even, rhythmical sound of shoes touching the ground. Shoe wear will often reduce as well. Similarly, simple resistance tests are undertaken to identify a lack of protein or minerals such as iron in the body.

I was fortunate to meet Ron in 1985 and his treatments have allowed me to run thousands of injury-free miles. On a most memorable occasion, I took one of my athletes, who had recently competed in a national cross-country competition and subsequently sustained a sciatic nerve injury, which virtually prevented any walking or prolonged sitting. In a single half-hour, Holder produced a 'Yellow Pages' heel wedge that had the athlete walking smoothly, attending social functions at night, and running, albeit a short distance, the following day!

Incidentally, as long ago as 1985, Ron and I shared a belief in the need for protein in Comrades and longer events, and he provided a mix he jokingly called 'whale sperm', which consisted mainly of liquid amino acids (see supplementation chapter). He is a man of vision and someone I am grateful to have as a friend.

Balance is in the mouth

Studies have also shown reason to balance the body from the top down. The average person's head weighs approximately 6 kg, one of the heaviest parts of the structure. If the head is held out of alignment, the remainder of the body needs to adjust to compensate and maintain an upright position. Every 25 mm the head is held forward increases the strain threefold. Part of the head, the jaw, performs regular and relatively large movements, thereby altering the balance. When the alignment of teeth is incorrect, the muscles in the jaw compensate by applying a torque to bring the teeth together, causing muscles to be overworked, and a chain reaction of load transfer begins.

There are 68 pairs of muscles above and below the jaw that determine the head, cervical, shoulder and jaw posture. Over 50 years ago, Penfield and Rasmussen, demonstrated that almost half of both the sensory and motor aspects of the brain are devoted to the dental area, therefore half the brain's 'programming' comes from the dental system. The key to this is the correct positioning of the temporomandibular joints (TMJ), two joints that connect the jaw to the skull. When correctly aligned the vertical axis should pass through the foremost part of the ear and C1 to C4 vertebrae of the spine. The horizontal axis aligns with the underside of the upper teeth. Poor dental closure can cause malposturing of C1 and C2, which in turn can show as 'hump back', side sway of the spine, rotation of the pelvis and uneven shoulder height or leg length.

The body follows the head and you can realign your entire body by moving your head backwards or forwards. Such movement can reduce your vital lung capacity by up to 30%, which would have a devastating effect on any endurance sport. While we are primarily interested in the potential improvements for sport, it is worth noting that over the past 30 years, an increasing body of evidence has been amassed showing that corrections to dental structures can provide a remedy for a wide number of chronic ailments. Perhaps it is more correct to say that many chronic symptoms are a result of dental dysfunction. Recent media coverage has even highlighted health improvements that follow the removal of metal fillings from teeth, underlining the connection of teeth to other body functions. Those with a basic knowledge of acupuncture and reflexology will know that there are points in the soles of your feet that relate to organs around the body. Similarly, each tooth has a relationship with joints and organs, e.g. a painful knee can relate to a tooth abscess.

The main objective in correcting the dental closure is to build up the rear molar teeth in such a way that they are first to close. This can be done temporarily using an orthotic that adds height to the rear teeth, or more permanently by building directly onto the rear molars. Considering that we swallow twice per minute while awake, and once per minute during asleep, even with a small 1-kg force applied to the teeth with each swallow, the total daily load on muscles is substantial. It is not surprising that a correct bite is important.

A simple test to reveal a malposition of the head is to stand in front of a mirror with arms outstretched to your sides. Close your eyes and move your head from side to side. Keeping your eyes closed, move your head to the point at which you feel you are looking straight ahead. Bring both arms and hands together in front of you. Are you looking directly at your hands or slightly to the left or right? Ideally you should be looking directly down the line of your arms. As an athlete, the bottom line is whether balancing works. What are the benefits? There can be no doubt that better posture will help you perform at a higher level and reduce the risk of injury. Top performances derive from periods of consistent training, which can only be achieved if you remain without injury.

If these methods are so wonderful, why haven't you heard about them before? Both applied kinesiology and TMJ work have been around for years, but have often been overlooked as they do not fall into the preconceived ideas of current norms, and are not fully understood. No matter what the level of your performance, it is worthwhile having your posture and bite assessed. Even if it only improves your results by a few places, it could well improve your overall health and lifestyle.

A CHECKLIST FOR THINGS TO DO WHEN INJURED

1. As soon as you feel the initial twinge or hint of an injury, **ice the offending area immediately** after each training session.

2. If discomfort persists, use the **anti-inflammatory properties of aspirin** (but see section above), but also consider homoeopathic and natural remedies after sessions.

3. f you're convinced it isn't a 'one off' twinge, examine your shoes. The majority of injuries start with these 'foundations', even if it hurts in the knee, hip, or lower back! Check for wear and place them on a level surface to see if the heels have been bent over or they tend to 'fall' to one side. **The only solution for worn shoes is replacement**.

4. If your injury occurred soon after wearing new shoes, your **model selection** was probably wrong. Try to exchange them, or sell them and look for another option (see chapter on equipment).

5. It you are able to run, immediately **reduce distance and effort**. If it is a soft tissue injury, **consult your physiotherapist** and, if possible, someone who can undertake an ultrasound scan to determine the exact location and nature of the injury. DO NOT struggle on by yourself with different remedies unless you are absolutely sure what the problem is and why it occurred. A few days lost in obtaining a diagnosis at the start of an injury can cost weeks of training later.

6. Injuries to **joints and bones** should be referred to orthopaedic specialists.

7. In all cases, select **medical specialists who compete or have competed in athletics**, or have a recognised sports medicine qualification. Their understanding of your needs and problems is usually better than their less active counterparts.

8. Be prepared for a short lay-off from running if prescribed but inquire about **alternative exercises to maintain your fitness level** (see chapter on supplementary exercises).

9. If you have to reduce your exercise level, make a conscious effort to **reduce your total food intake** to compensate. Many runners eat more

during a lay-off simply because they have more time on their hands and also because the body seems to 'overcompensate' (the pendulum syndrome) the appetite during this time.

10. Follow the 'prescription' of treatment or **therapeutic exercise** with the same enthusiasm that you apply to your running. Runners often fail to follow the medical advice given, thereby delaying their recovery and return to training.

11. When you are ready to return to training, do so at approximately **50% of your previous level** (both in terms of distance and speed), and build back over a few weeks. If you fail to do this you will probably suffer a recurring injury.

Tim Noakes' books, *Lore of Running* (OUP) and *Running Injuries* (OUP) (the latter coauthored by Stephen Granger) are excellent sources of advice on specific injuries. They stress the need to consult a specialist doctor, but if you are on the spot or heading for the doctor, they offer advice on some simple things you can do to help.

Illness

Illness is a more serious problem that often strikes when you least expect and frequently after a patch of particularly good running. A runner in peak fitness lives his life on a razor edge – a little too much training can push him over the top and make him susceptible to illness, and there is always a willing flu or cold donor waiting in the wings for such an opportunity to offload his virus!

During your build-up to a peak, it may be worthwhile to have an antiflu jab. The problem is that there are many strains of flu and this will not protect you from the others. However, the more bases covered the better. If having a flu inoculation, train in the morning prior to going to the doctor, have the injection around lunch time, and leave any further training until the evening of the following day. The flu injection contains a small amount of the virus and thus, as in homoeopathy, it is used to stimulate the development of antiflu virus. If you train too soon after the injection, your immune system will be suppressed and you are likely to develop flu.

Similar depression of the immune system in the 2–3 weeks after a major competitive peak results in a high percentage of runners picking up a viral infection. Studies suggest that the immune system also has a 'pendulum' or 'swing' analogy as discussed in previous chapters, with a depression immediately after racing followed by a period of supercompensation. One tip to maintain a high-immune level is to supplement with zinc and vitamin C tablets, which are cheap and readily available in pharmacies.

A further area of high susceptibility is on passenger aircrafts. The cabin pressure equates to an altitude of about 3 000 m, which most people are unaccustomed to, while the air-conditioning uses a relatively closed air circulation.

A recent study suggested that one of the reasons for the increasing incidence of 'air rage' is that a number of airlines have reduced the amount of new air circulated in the cabin. If true, the risk of infection would increase even further as viruses or germs from other passengers are circulated throughout the plane – not the healthiest of situations. Added to this is that exposure to the stress of lower cabin pressure and flying probably reduces our immune systems making us even more susceptible to viruses. Flights are, however, planned events, so it makes sense to boost your immune system through supplementation with vitamins, glutamine and other immune builders such as echinacea (see chapter 30 on supplementation, and below).

If you become ill, seek a diagnosis, advice and treatment as fast as possible. Don't struggle through by yourself for a week, only to have to go to the doctor anyway. Save the initial week and the frustration!

Many illnesses will require a lay-off, which is where you face the biggest problem. Any virus that requires rest will result in a drop in blood volume and hence VO_2. This means that the pace and intensity of training must be severely reduced on your return. Failure to do this will put you into a 'low' again and could result in a recurrence of illness.

Although these are frustrating and depressing times, be grateful if it happens early in your build-up rather than a week or so before an event. There has been some research into the connection between simple flu and colds and those who subsequently suffer a chronic illness or ME. Ensure that you are over the virus before returning to full training or you may pay a heavier price.

Doctors often prescribe antibiotics for illness and it should be noted that this generally means you should stop taking any vitamin supplements during the treatment. Antibiotics unfortunately have a negative effect on certain vitamins and intestinal cultures as part of the treatment. However, it is important to reinstate the vitamins as soon as treatment is complete. Your doctor will be able to give you precise details of your requirements, but the use of vitamin B and a multivitamin is generally a good starting point.

An additional point on the use of antibiotics is that you cannot expect to perform as well if you finished a course of antibiotics within three weeks of your race. The longer the event, the more it impacts on the expected performance, which calls for a reappraisal of both your 'target' time and your pacing.

PREVENTION IS BETTER THAN CURE

This age-old saying has much to recommend it. The easiest prevention for a running injury is not to run, but this doesn't really help. Apart from the recommendations above and elsewhere concerning tapering, rest and recovery, there are a few things you can do in the hope of reducing the likelihood of injury.

Check your shoes

Regular inspection of shoes is vital. In the chapter on shoes, I recommend a shoe glue spread thinly over the sole to reduce wear, yet the shoe retains its mechanical balance. Worn shoes cause a redistribution of stress that can result in injury.

Massage

One of the best preventative measures for the serious trainer, or the runner in heavy training, is massage. A regular weekly or fortnightly massage will ease the tension from muscles, restore an even balance to the structure and highlight any 'hot spots'. Hot spots are areas susceptible to injury. If you go for a long run and something on the run (or even your shoe) causes you to land differently, it is possible that one muscle is being used more than normal and may be tight

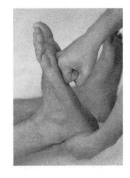

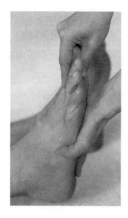

after the run. If on the following day you go for a faster pick-up, because the muscle hasn't eased yet, the additional load of speed may cause a minor tear and the muscle will continue to feel tight until properly rested or relaxed. The tightness will cause you to land differently, throwing more load onto other joints and muscles. A good masseur will detect this and will know how to relax the muscle. Massage also promotes circulation of nutrient-rich blood, which assists in the normal repair of training breakdown, thus speeding recovery.

Homoeopathic anti-inflammatory as a prophylactic

Some of the much-publicised drug abuse, including painkillers, is probably associated with pre-race medication in the hope of delaying certain conditions. Although there is no place in sport for drug abuse, over the years there have been many promoters of vitamins and natural remedies that are supposed to improve performance or have prophylactic benefits. Their use is open to discussion but may warrant your consideration.

For years I had used the homoeopathic remedy, arnica, during long runs as a means of reducing leg pain and inflammation. That and aspirin seemed to be the only legal things that worked for me and I have gone to fairly long lengths to investigate what is available within the IAAF limits. I spent hours with top Durban orthopaedic surgeon, Jack Usdin, searching for medications that do not contravene the drug rulings and are safe to use. Jack was a Comrades and 100-mile runner himself (as well as a graduate of Edinburgh University Medical School) and he could relate to my needs. Strangely, the outcome of our search always brought us back to arnica and aspirin (see also Anti-inflammatories above).

In 1992, an arnica-based homoeopathic combination was introduced to the South African market and it appealed to both Jack (who had worked in a homoeopathic hospital in the UK) and myself. In addition to a large percentage of arnica, it contains 13 other homoeopathic ingredients, and is available in tablet, drop, cream and injection form. I have experimented with this product before and during a number of long runs, and found that it reduces the inevitable leg soreness during and after such events. One of my first attempts was during a 7:39 100-km training event in Gaborone, Botswana, and even three hours after the race I was able to tackle five flights of stairs, two at a time... both up and down!

Following this training race, which was in August, I competed in the 1992 International Spartathlon from Athens to Sparta, a distance of 250 km. This gruelling race, at the end of September, was my major peak for the year and included a 1 200-m high mountain, which had to be climbed on a rock- and shrub-strewn path. As most runners know, it is the 'downs' that cause trouble and there was an equally devastating downhill to be negotiated after reaching the top. This all happened after my legs had been suitably 'softened' up at 155 km. I finished the event in sixth position after 29.5 hours, so the muscle damage does not need much description (consider six back-to-back marathons!).

Having used this arnica combination prior to, and after, the race, I became convinced that my recovery was speedier than usual and/or the damage limited. In an attempt to 'test' this theory, and against all my own advice, I attempted another long run only 13 days later in Port Elizabeth. There, during howling 55-km per hour winds, I completed a 100 km, finishing second. Make no mistake, my legs were sore by the end, but without the benefit of this treatment I doubt I could have completed a marathon distance, let alone a 100 km.

It must be stressed that this was an experiment, and it was done after my peak for the year. **I do not advise such action** by other runners. Some would argue that such benefits are as a result of a placebo effect. I doubt it, but if so, I'll live with it for as long as it works.

Check and recheck what you take!

It's worth noting that South African athletes have the advantage of being able to check the latest edition of *MIMS: Drugs and Sport* (TML), to determine if any medicines are on the banned list. Don't forget that many of the over-the-counter medicines contain banned substances and it is YOUR responsibility to ensure that you are not using these.

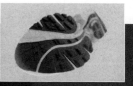

'All you need is a pair of shoes, an old pair of shorts, a T-shirt and socks and you're on your way. That's the beauty of running.'

Strictly speaking, I suppose this often-quoted statement is true. However, this chapter will look at the sport in more detail in terms of the equipment that you will need and may wish to consider using in your training. If nothing else, give this to your nearest and dearest to read and perhaps you will find some of the less essential, but highly desirable items popping up in your Christmas stocking, or as a birthday present!

One thing I would like to clear up right at the start is that, in many cases, I have been lucky enough to be given several pieces of equipment over the years. I have never regularly used anything that I didn't believe was the best available on the market for my purposes at that particular time. There are two 'key' points here. Firstly, that it was the best on the market at the time and, secondly, it was the best for me.

I have written the following section offering 'best advice' on equipment based on the current situation, as I believe it to be. In this manner, you can make up your own mind from what I believe to be available, and what you may find works for you. I would not like this to be construed as a commercial for products with which I may be associated. I hope it will be viewed as an unbiased appraisal, yet giving recommendations where I feel they apply across the board. I hope you appreciate this open approach.

IF THE SHOE FITS

Buying shoes is one of the most important, if not the most important choice that any runner needs to make. Far too many runners leave much of this decision making to chance.

Why is shoe choice so important?

Just as you have a unique fingerprint, you also have a unique running style, which is the result of a combination of many aspects including muscular balance, flexibility, distance run, type of terrain, your weight and a host of others. The question of looks, colour or even brand is of secondary consideration.

Each shoe has certain features, benefits and characteristics. The 'trick' in shoe selection is to balance the 'negative' characteristics of your running style, with the positive characteristics of the shoe you choose.

What happens if you don't wear the correct shoe?

It can be argued that one of the reasons so few people completed Comrades in the early years related to the shoes available. The simple 'tackie' offered very little support, cushioning or protection, so people who were not 'mechanically' perfect ever reached the start line, as injury caught up with them in training. Nowadays, there is a vast array of shoes that caters for a wide variety of runners, and allows many who would not normally be able to 'pound the roads' to attempt anything from recreational running to Comrades.

The wrong choice of shoes usually results in some form of injury. In fact, most sports scientists will tell you that the majority of injuries relate to improper shoes for the distance. Your feet are the contact with the ground and hence the 'foundation' of your running. As with any other lever, any small movement at the point of contact, results in greater movement further up, therefore a small movement at the feet can cause significant movement at the knees, hips and lower back. Often it is this movement that triggers an injury.

Supination and pronation

There are many different problems that can arise from the wrong choice of shoes, but two terms have dominated the shoe industry: pronation and supination. In truth, every runner pronates and supinates; it is part of the natural running style. Problems only commence when either becomes excessive.

When standing behind someone it is fairly easy to spot excessive movements. Pronation is the movement of the foot to roll inwards, whereas supination is the outward roll of the foot. People typically look for this at the heel, but it can occur at any stage during the stride. Quite a few runners have excessive supination off the forefoot as they drive off at the end of their stride. Only excess pronation or supination is a problem and in such cases the idea is to find a shoe that restricts the rolling at that point in the stride, to 'normal' levels.

Runners strike the ground with their heel – don't they?

Another fallacy is that all runners first land using the heel of the foot. It would be a very interesting race if the world's greatest milers all landed on their heels before trying to drive on at sub-2-minute, 30-second kilometre pace!

The faster a runner runs, the further forward is the first point of contact with the ground. Test it for yourself – try sprinting but landing heel first. It's like putting the brakes on with every stride. Even marathoners running just over two hours tend to be forefoot runners rather than heel runners. Ironically, if they have to go slow enough to strike with their heels, some of them may have over-pronation problems that would require additional features in their shoes. However, they often wear light shoes with little protection, as they never have to endure the same forces through the heel when running fast.

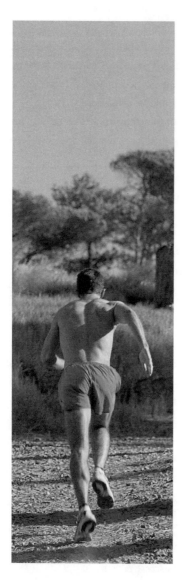

ABOVE *Not every strike starts with a heel – the faster the run, the further forward you tend to land on your shoes*

It's not only the fast runners who strike midfoot. Runners with poor flexibility between the lower leg and ankle are forced into midfoot striking. Typically, they will have large calf muscles, as they work these muscles with every stride. Ironically, this can further reduce the flexibility of the ankle joint making a heel strike even more unnatural to the runner.

If you run up or down many hills, your stride will change, so the terrain and ground surface will also affect your choice of shoes.

How to choose the correct shoe

Firstly, you must know the mechanical strengths and weaknesses of your own running style. The more experienced runner may well have a good feel for this, but be aware that an imbalance in training or change in type or amount of a particular form of training, can result in a change in foot strike.

The way to ascertain the correct information on your stride is for a qualified podiatrist to analyse your running. This is best done on the road and only normally takes about a kilometre, but a treadmill may be used as an alternative. In conjunction with some measurements, this will normally provide a good description of any potential problems with your stride. Armed with this report and recommendations, find a shop with experienced salespeople who not only know the full range of shoes and their features, but also have sufficient experience to work with you in the selection of your shoes.

It is important to differentiate between the 'leisure or fashion' shops and the serious specialist outlet. It is unlikely that you will find the necessary experience in a salesperson that sells shoes to the 'fashion or leisure' market. Find someone who regularly deals with runners and running shoes. It is worth establishing beforehand from other runners just how good they rate the advice given by a particular shop and salesperson. After all, their advice could increase or decrease your chances of injury.

In addition, try to find out whether the salesperson is sponsored by any shoe company, as this may influence his selection of recommended shoes, although I would hope not. You are rarely charged for such expertise, so even if the cost is a few rands more than the 'superstore', rather buy from such shops. In this way we will ensure that such expertise is around in the future.

When you are fitted with the right shoe, your potential stride problems will be much reduced when you run in the shoes. Obviously, the more information you provide the assistant, the more quickly he will direct you to the best option. If you complete the questionnaire at the end of this section, it will help you to focus on what you are looking for and give the assistant a good starting guide.

Another danger is the assistant who changes his recommendation of a shoe because he finds the store doesn't have your size in stock. If the recommendation is truly correct, he will order the shoe for you or even direct you to another store, which has it in stock. This latter attitude is the sign of good advice. In 1984 I had a partnership in a running shop in Durban and I was taken aback at some of the attitudes to buying shoes. Below are some of the more 'popular' ones and my feelings on the subject:

'I'm not a top runner like Gert Thuys, Andrew Kelehe or Elana Meyer, I don't need an expensive running shoe... I want a shoe for R70' (at a time when shoes had an average price of R150).

Most of the top runners are top runners because of their inherited ability and physiological suitability to run. Many could run in any shoe because they don't have mechanical problems or pronate excessively. However, the average runner is not as lucky as that and has mechanical problems with his foot strike, which to some extent probably explains why he is not as fast. It is these 'mechanical problems' that require extra protection in the shoes and this involves more technology, more work and therefore costs more. The chances are that because you are not a top runner, you should actually be paying more for your shoes, not less.

'I don't want to pay much for the shoes. They never last me more than three months then I need a new pair. My dress shoes last me longer and cost less.'

It's interesting how many people compare the lifespan of dress shoes with running shoes, yet they never compare the type of life each has. Dress shoes are worn on special occasions, cleaned afterwards and put away for the next big occasion. If it rained, they are stuffed with paper, allowed to dry, polished and packed away with care.

Many runners have only one pair of running shoes and wear them daily in training. The shoes cover many more miles than the dress shoes and at the end of the run are shoved into a kit bag along with all the other damp, sweaty kit. In some cases, they never see the light of day again until the next morning's training run, while still damp. Such shoes never dry out, are taken on safaris through puddles, mud, gravel, sand, and have Coke and water spilt on them at refreshment stations. Is it any wonder that they don't last as well as the dress shoes? Is it a surprise that the stitching starts to rot after a couple of months?

In truth, every runner should have at least two pairs of good usable training shoes, and there is a good case for increasing that to three so that there is always another pair on hand when one pair wears out. In addition, a runner may opt for a lightweight racing shoe for special races, to add that final edge to the competition. It all sounds expensive, and initially it certainly is, but in the long run it's much cheaper. (Trust me, I'm a Scotsman!)

Each pair is used in rotation and has a chance to dry out thoroughly. This time lag also allows the runner to check the wear on the undersole and ensure that a thin film of shoe glue is spread over the wearing areas – so thin it's like a layer of 'clingfilm' to protect these areas. All you are doing is wearing down the 'clingfilm', not the sole of the shoe. If the sole is allowed to wear down, you totally change the 'foundation' of your footstrike and the shoe can no longer do the job for which you initially bought it. It is important to ensure that your sole is always in good condition. This sort of care will ensure more wear out of your shoes and your initial investment goes much further.

It's also worth buying two different models of shoes for training, especially if you do a lot of distance. This relates to the previous comments on the characteristics of shoes and feet. Every one of us has specific footstrike characteristics, so too each model of shoe. If you continually train in one model of shoe, the 'stress' must be continually loaded on specific sets of foot muscles and ligaments. It makes sense to rotate the stress slightly by changing your shoes. Obviously, both shoe models must be suitable for your style in the first place.

Orthotics

Sometimes it is impossible to find the ideal shoe to suit your running style and foot structure. One way of solving this problem is to place an insert in your shoe that holds your foot in the correct (or neutral) position. Called an orthotic, there are various types and different materials used – it depends on how you run as to which is best. Those who require flexibility around the arch tend towards soft orthotics, whereas an excessive pronation in a heel striker might find a hard orthitic best. Orthotics are tailormade for the individual, but it is important to work with people who have had experience in running and sport, as orthotics are also made for some people for everyday use and the problems of sport can be significantly different.

Modifications

Because the sports shoe market is relatively small in South Africa by world standards, and because the exchange rate is erratic and unfavourable, most manufacturers only make a selection of their full international product range available locally. Naturally, they focus on models that apply to the greatest portion of the market, which means that there will be a market sector that will not necessarily find the ideal shoe. This often affects runners looking for more flexible, but well-cushioned shoes, or shoes with higher or lower heels than normal.

In many cases, it is possible to modify shoes to provide these features. For instance, cutting a slit across the forefoot of the outer sole will provide more forefoot flexibility, or cutting the top of the heel cup can often remove an area that causes chafing of the Achilles' tendon in an otherwise perfect fitting shoe. Differences in leg length can also be compensated for with wedges in the midsole. However, only runners who understand shoe construction and the movement of their foot should attempt such modifications. Cutting into an air, gel or other such shoe technology could be catastrophic, whereas modification of the cell technology is possible if you understand how it works. Modifications can be made to a brand-new shoe to turn it into your ideal shoe. Only a few orthotic and running shoe outlets offer such a service, but they have years of experience and are the only ones to be trusted with such work.

General guides to shoe types

Below are a few 'guides' to assist in the selection of your shoes. For the majority of cases they hold true, but there are exceptions and that is where experienced staff and podiatrists can help:

Curve-lasted shoes (where the outer sole has a definite curved appearance): Runners with a high or pronounced instep arch are usually comfortable with these, as are those who land on their fore to midfoot when running. These shoes are fairly flexible and, typically, this applies to most racing shoes. Such runners also tend to need good forefoot cushioning.

Straight-lasted shoes: These tend to suit runners with flat or lower instep arches. The outer appears straighter and the extra midsole makes the shoe less likely to twist in running, which helps prevent overpronation at the heel. Resistance to twisting has become an overly popular aspect of shoes brought into South Africa, and it should be remembered that they will not suit everybody. If all the features of modern shoes were necessities for everyone, how did Zola Pieterse (Budd) and many others ever run bare foot?

To determine whether a shoe is straight or curve lasted, look at the outersole and draw a straight line from the centre of the heel to the centre of the toe box. If the outersole is 'equal' on either side of this line, the shoe is straight lasted. If the line goes to one side it is curve lasted. In the latter form there will also be a more pronounced cutout in the sole for the arch area. Which do you require? This

SHOES

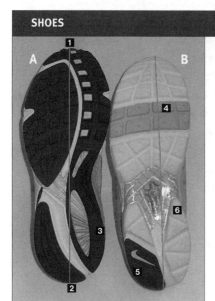

SHOE A
*This is a straight-lasted shoe, so the sole is almost entirely balanced on either side of line **1–2**.*
*There is added reinforcement on the inner side (**3**) at the heel to reduce pronation.*

SHOE B
*This lightweight trainer/racer has a curved last, so there is more 'sole' in the area **6**.*
*Only points **4** and **5** have harder-wearing sections, as these are the contact points. The focus of other areas is flexibility and light weight.*

depends on your foot's mechanics, but as a general rule it is worthwhile doing the 'bathroom test'. With wet feet, stand on a smooth floor and leave two footprints. If your footprints leave arch areas, you have a high instep, if there is less indication (or no indication) of the arches, you have an average or low-arch instep.

Runners with low-instep arches: These runners look for rigid shoes and less cushioning because they tend to have mobile feet that require rigid shoes to achieve the correct 'balance'.

Runners with high-instep arches: Such runners should look for curve-lasted shoes with plenty of cushioning, as they have rigid bone structures and need flexibility and cushioning to absorb impact forces.

Board-lasted shoes: This refers to the method of construction between the upper and the midsole (cushioning) of the shoe. Board lasting is more rigid and also helps to prevent twisting of the shoe, which will appeal to those who pronate or supinate excessively. A disadvantage of board lasting is that it requires longer to 'break in', as the board must be 'taught' to bend where your feet flex. Boards may be made from thick card or a fibrous material.

Slip lasting: Here the upper is constructed almost like a slipper and stuck onto the midsole material. It is much more flexible and allows rotation of the shoe in all directions. Expect a racing shoe to be constructed in this manner.

Combination-lasted shoes: As the name suggests, this shoe is partly board lasted and partly slip lasted, with the purpose of providing rigidity in the heel area and flexibility in the forefoot. Only a very few shoes have board lasting in the forefoot, but it can be useful for the runner who pronates or supinates in the forefoot area.

Midsole: The midsole is the section of the shoe between the upper and the outer wearing sole. Typically, it consists of a 'cushioning material' such as EVA or polyurethane (PU) or a tradename such as Phylon. The prime purpose of a midsole is to cushion the force transmitted from the sole through to the leg. It also provides the 'shape' and height difference between the sole and heel areas. The midsole section may be a combination of different density materials positioned to resist distortion under the action of pronation or supination. These differing densities are normally of different colours, although some may be hidden inside the midsole and there are even examples where PU is mixed with EVA for a combination of benefits.

EVA is a good cushioning substance, but doesn't last as long as PU. However, PU has a weight disadvantage. Many EVAs are treated to improve cushioning and/or lifespan. Puma has recently manufactured shoes from a cellular material that replaces EVA.. This has the advantage of a longer lifespan, but initially provides quite a hard ride. Reebok also experimented with a combination of foam and rubber for its new midsole material, which provides a very light solution with good initial cushioning but perhaps not the resilience of other midsoles – only time will tell.

Nike Air, gel, Hydroflow, torsion and others: Each manufacturer has its own 'technological features' that 'make the shoe'. I do not want to knock or support these as I believe every runner must make up his own mind as to their benefits or not. It is interesting, though, to note some of the conflicts. For instance, the Airsole is something that often runs throughout the sole, to provide extra cushioning. On the other hand, gel pods are usually located in set positions within the shoe – presumably to reduce weight. The most common cushioning systems are Nike Air, Asiacs gel, Adiprene and New Balance Absorb. Air is positioned in the heel and forefoot, or in full-length pockets, but may also be found in the midsole and on the outsole. Gel is placed in heel or forefoot pockets, while Adiprene, a shock-absorbing material, is put in heels or under the forefoot. New Balance Absorb material displaces the energy of impact sideways. An Absorb ball will not bounce when dropped from a height, whereas a normal EVA ball will. Reebok and Puma use honeycomb-shaped membranes for cushioning, which, even if the outer shoe is punctured, continues to provide cushioning. Brooks Hydroflow uses chambers and valves through which fluid is squeezed to dissipate the pressure of the foot.

All these cushioning devices are worthy of consideration, but make sure the cushioning is in the area where you require it and that the overall shoe is stable enough for your running. The most stable shoes are those closest to the ground, therefore a shoe with a large cushioning device in the midsole is more likely to be unstable, which may result in injury.

Heel counter: At the rear of the upper is a heel counter that 'cups' the heel of the foot. In very cheap shoes, this is made out of an easily manipulated card or board material, thus offering little support. In more expensive shoes, a formed plastic heel cup is provided with additional support from 'leather' coverings. Currently, many heel cups have the addition of a plastic band on the outside around the base between the upper and the midsole, all of which prevents the supinator or pronator from bending them over. Generally, racing shoes do not offer much protection in this area, whereas a trainer for the worst pronator will have a very rigid heel cup.

To judge whether you need a good heel counter, place your old shoes on a flat surface and examine them from the rear. Do they lean inwards or outwards? If so, you need a stiffer heel cup than in your previous shoes.

Outsole (wearing surface): As with most things, this is a compromise. The higher the rubber content in the outersole, the longer it will wear, but also the heavier it will be. Blown rubber offers more cushioning but wears much faster. The blown rubber 'vibram' sole used by New Balance in the mid '80s was one of the first to provide good grip, lightness, cushioning and reasonable wear. There are still companies that offer such outersoles for repairing old shoes.

For the best of both worlds, in many shoes a combination is used so that longwearing (carbon rubber) pieces are placed at the points of wear, while lighter, softer rubber is placed in areas not expected to wear. Mizuno was one of the first shoes to have only heel and forefoot rubber sections. The remainder is exposed midsole. This is now fairly common and companies have designed lightweight methods of connecting the heel and sole to provide some rigidity between the two.

Outsole treads vary the amount of grip on various surfaces. Close profile surfaces pick up mud in cross-country events, but flat surfaces offer no grip. Decide how the shoe will perform in the rain. The old Adidas Atlanta was an excellent shoe in many ways as it was light enough for a racer, cushioned for a trainer, offered some support, was hardwearing on the outersole, but caused 'wheelspin' in the wet. A number of shoes need to be slightly worn before they provide good grip on wet tar – due to the smoothness of the rubber from the injection moulding.

Innersoles: Most shoes have a removable innersole; if you take this out, even one that has only done 100 km from new, and inspect the forefoot area, you will find that the toe and ball of the foot areas have lost their cushioning. The 'bounce' at the rear may be better but compared with the rest, the forefoot is 'dead'. Innersoles are probably the most underrated section of the shoe. In my rugby-playing days I discovered Spenco inners and used them in all my shoes until recently. They are lightweight, closed-cell rubber innersoles that seem to last for about ten years. Spenco produce various types of inners, including ones with a basic orthotic bed. I suggest you find the type that suits you best. As further testament to their efficacy, I placed a Spenco inner into a brand-new Nike Duellist two days before the 1989 Comrades. The combination helped me to run 90 km of Comrades in 6:07 without any problems. A Duellist is a racing shoe weighing only 180 g with very little cushioning. I need cushioning, as I am basically a forefoot striker and this proves my point. I have been able to run long distances with lightweight shoes and vary my choice between the flat Spenco inners and those with a semishaped heel made from polyurethane shock-absorbing material. Although slightly heavier, these 'PolySorb' inners were better suited for landing on my heels in longer events. These insoles are imported and expensive compared to foam ones, but their life expectancy justified the expense.

However, an innovative South African design, known as Comfeeze, has taken cushioning to a new level, and offers the product in heel and full-foot options. It consists of a sheet of shaped nodules made out of cushioned rubber 'gel', which replaces or fits under the shoe's own removable inner. Impact compresses the nodules (and entrapped air) to provide cushioning. The Comfeeze are significantly cheaper than the Spenco inners and do not need the depth of material that the PolySorb version does. These inners also have a lengthy lifespan. These inners have also received accreditation from the South African podiatrists.

Lacing features, upper fabrics: There are many other features apparent from an external inspection of a shoe and this is where the 'ideal' list comes into play. Only you know what feels good and works for you. For instance, I like to keep my laces quite tight, so I prefer the plastic D-ring lace holes because they don't pull through as easily. It's all a matter of preference.

The importance of uppers choice was reinforced for me in October 2002, during the Augrabies Extreme 250-km desert, run over seven days. Much of this course is run in soft river-bed sand and though I normally choose an open mesh upper for 'breathability', I wore a Nike Presto racer with all-enclosed tight-fitting Lycra upper for this event. Despite external laces, the Lycra upper has no tongue section through which sand can enter. Moreover, the Lycra catered for foot expansion from heat and distance, while the laces allowed me to keep the shoe comfortably tight. Of the 31 competitors, 12 dropped out with blisters, and only one other runner went through the race without any blisters. Choose the right shoe for the job.

The only modification I had to make was to cut the rear heel counter down after a day of acting as a guide to the blind runner Geoff Hilton-Barber. The reason for this is that when speed-walking, my foot moves through a different range of movements from those of running and the counter irritated my Achilles. A simple modification made the shoe ideal.

Shoe surveys and sponsorships: The problem with most magazine shoe surveys is that they seldom test a shoe fully. A shoe must be given to a runner with the correct running characteristics for that shoe, and then it should be put through some meaningful distance, conditions and terrains. While it's worth reading these articles to see what's available, there is very little to be gained from most of the surveys in terms of the shoe's suitability for you. Because a shoe is popular or has some innovation, it does not mean that it is the shoe you should be wearing. There is no substitute for a correct shoe. Note that I didn't say an 'expensive' shoe.

Some runners watch what the top runners wear and think that because they wear Adidas, Mizuno, Nike or whatever, that must be the 'winning' shoe. That, of course, is not the case, it's merely that a particular model in the manufacturer's range suits the athlete concerned. To be absolutely mercenary about it, in some cases a top athlete may actually wear a shoe purely because of his sponsorship contract.

Do you know what you want?

Complete the following questionnaire to help you and the shop assistant determine the type of shoe you need to consider buying.

What is your **height**? Your **weight**?
How long have you been running? Less than 3 months? 3–12 months? over 12 months?
What shoes are you currently running in? Have you been happy with them? What would you **change** (if anything) in them?
What is your **weekly** distance?
What is your typical **long run**? What is your typical **short run**?
Will you use the shoes for **racing**? Are you likely to use them for **speed quality** training?

Will you use the shoes for **off-road training**? Will you use them for **cross-country** racing?

How many times will you use them per week?

How many other shoes will you use per week?

From the bathroom wet footprint test do you have a '**high**', '**average**' or '**low**' arch?

Do you wear through the **upper** above your toes?

How would you describe your **foot strike**? Heel first? Midfoot strike? Do you run on your toes?

If you place your shoes on a flat surface and look at them from the rear, does the heel on any shoe lean **inwards** or **outwards**? (Circle as appropriate)

  Left shoe: Outward? Inward?

  Right shoe: Outward? Inward?

Do you have a preference for the **material used in the upper**?

  Closed nylon? Open mesh?

  Other (describe) ....

Do you have a preference for the **style of lacing**?

  Normal U shape through material? D ring?

  Velcro closing?

  Other (describe) ....

Do you find that you build up **hard skin on your feet** in any particular areas?

  Left foot: Heel? Under midfoot? Under big toe?

  Under second toe? Outer side of the big toe?

  Right foot: Heel? Under midfoot? Under big toe?

  Under second toe? Outer side of the big toe?

Do you regularly suffer from **blisters**? Yes No

  Where? ....

Do you use **orthotics** or other inserts that you put into your running shoes?

Do you **replace the inners** in your shoes?

Have you had your previous shoes **built up** or altered in any way? Yes No

  If yes, how? ....

Now take your filled questionnaire, old shoes and your typical running socks with you to assist with the correct selection of your new shoes.

Why every runner needs a racing shoe in his cupboard

The role of the racing shoe in South Africa seems to have been forgotten. Much of this stems from one of the greatest fallacies in running – that runners land on their heels first. This 'urban legend' has arguably damaged the depth of knowledge in the sports shoe industry. As a result, the vast majority of shoes on offer are designed for runners who pronate or supinate excessively. Many are also designed for the heavy runner.

Because 50% of runners finish in the last quarter of a race, they represent the biggest market sector. Consequently, the typical shoe has little, if any, midfoot flexibility and many control features to maintain a neutral stride.

To test the heel strike theory, go down to your local soccer or rugby field and try a fast run across it. You do not land on your heels, neither do the galloping Kenyans cruising along a sub-3-minute kilometre. To land on your heel, your stride must either be very short, which means you are running very slow compared to your capacity, or it requires you to straighten your leg out in front of you, which would induce an immediate 'braking' action. In fact, this is what happens when many runners run downhill and suffer from sore quadriceps in the days after a long downhill race.

There are many runners who strike with a mid- or even forefoot in their normal running. Among this group are most sub-3:15 marathoners, and 42-minute 10-km runners, and also runners with poor flexibility at the ankle joint (possibly caused by tight calves).

Midfoot runners find the flexibility of racing shoes beneficial to their stride. But so do runners using speed or quality sessions to improve their running. As we know that the faster we are over the shorter distances, the faster we become at longer distances, it becomes clear that even the most dedicated Comrades 'back marker' could benefit from some faster work. Doing this in inflexible shoes is not only difficult, but also puts stress and load onto joints and muscles in a different way that can lead to overuse and injury, which typically shows up in a calf strain. This is where the role of the racing or the lightweight flexible trainer comes into its own.

No matter how slow a runner, when he runs at his best short time trial or 5-km pace, there is a move to land further forward on the shoe. As discussed in the training chapters, running intervals over 400 m at slightly faster than your 5-km pace should be a regular session. Whether that is on road, grass or track, it is unlikely that your heel will do more than 'clip' the ground as you extend your stride and pick up speed. Imagine trying to do this with a plank of wood strapped to half the length of the sole of your foot. Compare that to the barefoot running of many African runners, in which case the flexibility of the instep is a natural provision.

As a runner, you should include at least one, and up to three quality sessions per week in training. These will not only improve your performance at all distances, but will also take you to a mid- or forefoot landing, and are preferably done in flexible racing shoes.

Just as the features of training shoes differ for lightweight and heavier runners, so too will the requirements for racing shoes. Every runner should have a pair for such sessions. But where do you find them? Thankfully, shoe companies are becoming more enlightened and Adidas, New Balance, Reebok, Nike and Asics all have at least one such shoe in their range. However, the challenge is to find a retailer that stocks them.

If the truth be told, the depth of knowledge in running-shoe retail has dropped since the late 1980s and early to mid '90s. The advent of sports shop chains, as opposed to specialist running outlets, means that the range and advice relating to running shoes has deteriorated. Too many shoes are being sold by sales staff with little experience or understanding of the key principles. That is why the specialist running groups stock racing shoes. They recognise the need for different shoes for different running styles and different training sessions, whereas the staff in many chain or small 'all-sport' shops go no further than size, model popularity and even colour. If you doubt this, try asking such assistants for a detailed breakdown of features and benefits of each model they sell and see how few variations they offer.

The final hurdle is with average runners themselves. They have difficulty in accepting the expense of different shoes for different uses. However, investing in racing or lightweight trainers for quality sessions is not a major expense. Assuming they are only used for the quality session work, they can last for a few years, which is a small investment for having the right equipment – particularly if the wrong shoes can cause injuries that will cost far more in physiotherapy and medical bills. No matter where you rank yourself in the 'running pecking order', acquire some shoes for quality work and seek specialist advice to ensure you use the correct training and racing shoes for your style.

Use of spikes

It is often assumed that road runners and ultrarunners do not spend much time in track training. If you follow the recommendations in this book you will find that there are many reasons for such runners to spend time in track training, and thus to make use of spikes. You may think that this can be done with normal road shoes, but I also believe that if you 'look' the part, you tend to perform better, and having the right equipment definitely helps. Another benefit for me, as an ultrarunner, is that it helps me move back onto my forefoot after the long event or training, which is a more correct style for speed running. Because of the resistance to spikes, our knowledge of the correct type to use is limited. The following details, provided by Adidas a few years ago, will be of assistance to runners as a base from which to experiment. Spikes should also be considered as essential when racing 5 km or less on the track. Finally, bear in mind that one set of spikes will last an average road runner many years and is therefore a relatively cheap investment,

This is not a full dissertation on shoes, but it should provide you with some key issues to consider when buying shoes and will help protect you against disreputable dealers.

CLOTHING

Shorts

Although we are often restricted to club colours, the choice of shorts is second only in importance to your running shoes. Shorts must allow full movement of the legs, be comfortably tight around the waist, and be made of a light, non-absorbent material. Many companies manufacture shorts, but the standards of production and materials vary dramatically, as does the fit. The right feel at the waist is important, particularly in long events where pressure on the stomach can have a detrimental effect. The amount and type of material in between the legs and how low it sits, is relevant to the likelihood of chafing in very humid or wet and cold conditions.

As a guide, I recommend the following materials from least to most desirable: cotton combinations, rip-stop nylons, lightweight microfibres, Dri-Fit.

The need to carry energy gels in racing and training makes the innovative 'Accolade Energy Shorts' a natural choice, and the addition of a drawstring (not normally in shorts), allows for an even more comfortable fit around the waist. In addition these shorts can be custom-made making the fit one of the most comfortable, but it does mean they are harder to find. Obviously more attuned to the needs of the runner, they also have shorts capable of carrying energy gels, or other bits and pieces you may need on the run. I expect this to be the way of the future for other mainstream manufacturers.

Nowadays, most shorts have inners, and this is the area in which most shorts manufacturers fail. The position of the inners, the material and the quality of workmanship often leave much to be desired. For example, leg elastic is frequently the wrong size and first to give, which is why it's often a good idea to buy shorts without inners or remove the ones provided. Advances in material and technology have seen companies like Falke bring out sports underwear in materials that wick away moisture, to provide cooling, comfort and support in all the right places. These proved to be ideal during six days of running, without having to carry several changes of shorts in the Augrabies extreme 250-km marathon, which saw temperatures varying from 7–44 °C.

Vests and tops

These are a matter of personal preference, but look for materials and fits that leave you free to move without chafing, even when wet. Think also of the weather conditions in which you intend to run. If it's hot and humid, wear mesh and lightweight material. Opt for lighter colours as they reflect the heat. In races you are restricted to club colours, which limits your choice, but consider proposing a change in colours if your club uses vast areas of dark colours in a vest or top. This will take time to go through committees and structures, but why handicap runners with colours or materials that attract heat?

Top UK marathoner of the 1970s, Ron Hill, was the first to wear a string vest in heat. Fabric and fibres have advanced significantly and you (and clubs) are well advised to look into the latest materials for warm weather running. In 1991, a change in clothing was noticed on the world track and field circuit, as the ladies opted for 'boob-tube' vests. The 'shorty' vest also made its appearance for males in triathlons. There is much to be said for using such vests in hot and humid climates as the exposure of the midriff allows for better cooling, but it is by no means the ultimate. If you intend running in hot weather, keep looking for new ideas, as the slowing effect of heat is dramatic.

During long events in hot and sunny weather, it is important to wear some cover. In the 2002 Augrabies marathon I also needed to wear a vest or shirt as I was carrying a backpack that would have chafed if no protection was placed between the backpack and my skin. In this instance I opted for white (heat-reflecting) shorts and a long-sleeved Dri-Fit Nike shirt. I found this to be the coolest of options and letting it hang over the shorts assisted in cooling.

By contrast, there are an increasing amount of 'adventure' type events likely to involve cold weather for which you will need warm and rainproof clothing. In my experience the best material is polypropylene, which draws the sweat away from the body. Many companies have brought out similar products, but which are far more expensive. A normal T-shirt maybe fine in mild weather, but keeps the sweat close to the body, which causes chafing and is cold in wind or when you stop.

The key to running in the cold is to layer your clothing. In the coldest weather, start with a polypropylene shirt, short or long sleeves, followed by a cotton long-sleeved shirt, and finally a showerproof jacket. In essence, you create a 'microclimate' inside the jacket. As you run, the heat builds up, sweat is wicked away from the skin to the cotton shirt and condenses on the inside of the jacket. Although it becomes very wet on the inside, it is never cold. The temperature can be controlled using the jacket zip. One thing to bear in mind when wearing this amount of clothing is that you will sweat as much or even more than normal. The importance of replenishing fluids cannot be overstated. With layering, you can always remove a layer if the weather changes or you become too hot.

Rain-/showerproof tops

Every runner needs something for rainy days, although in areas such as Durban a run in the rain without a jacket, can be one of the most refreshing experiences, particularly in the height of the summer heat.

Rainwear is available in a variety of options, from rip-stop nylon pullovers, to the fully rainproof Gore-Tex style. As noted in previous chapters, when running in cool weather, the heat causes a build-up of sweat inside the jacket so the benefit is not in keeping dry, but rather in keeping warm.

Many jackets are claimed to be breathable, but this really only works during walking or very light exercise. Material technology is forever evolving and there are jackets with vents and zips that alleviate this problem to some extent. However, most of the real technological leaders in this field have been developed overseas, making them unrealistically expensive for the uses that most South African runners can expect.

For me, one of the most important features of a jacket is to keep the wind out. Once you are out running in the rain, it doesn't feel too bad. Provided the wind is kept at bay, it can prove enjoyable. For this reason, one of my favourite jackets is a simple rip-stop nylon pullover. It can be crumpled up and put under a hat, or in a pocket during a long run, and if needed, simply pull it out and put it on. If the weather clears, put it back in the pocket.

My other preference is for a Pertex jacket, which is covered in reflective ink. It is relatively waterproof, breathable and can be opened with zips from top or bottom for temperature control. The reflection works extremely well and is ideal for ultra-events at night or in adverse lighting conditions. The headlights of oncoming cars can easily pick it up.

For normal running, I do not think there is a need for rain trousers. If, however, you consider moving up to ultra-events, particularly those longer than 100 km, the length of the run and the lower intensity may justify their use. A full rain suit is useful for warming up and cooling down.

In the case of trousers, try to find a pair with long zips or stud openers on the lower legs and ensure that they are long enough to allow you to remove the bottoms without first having to remove your shoes. In some instances, an additional strap is necessary around the ankle level to prevent the bottom of the leg from flapping, while at the same time allowing a wide enough opening to accommodate a shoe to fit through.

Look for something bright for night running, light for ease of carrying, windproof, and in your price bracket.

Socks

Over the years I have tried most types of socks. When I first began running, I preferred calf-high baseball socks. They were thick and self-supporting, and I even ran my first Comrades in 1981 in these socks. (One of my sporting heroes at that time was the Cuban 400-m and 800-m athlete Alberto Juantorena – who I would later meet in 1997 at the Mallorca Marathon – whose trademark was his calf-high socks, which probably explains this early choice.) Realising how much sweat they could hold, my next choice was to go without socks as the inside of the running shoe seemed extremely comfortable in comparison to the rugby boots to which I was accustomed. Because I perspire a lot, this idea was soon discarded as a result of the smell and slipping. I moved to well-cushioned, tennis-type socks, and eventually to thin cotton socks.

In 1992 I met up with American Roy Pirrung at the Spartathlon. He had developed a pair of socks with a padded sole, and a material that wicks away the sweat from the foot. These were very good and I kept them specifically for longer events. Although they were at the cutting edge at the time, modern technology, fabrics and fibres have changed the whole sock market. Buying a sock now can be as technical as purchasing shoes.

Materials have a far greater ability to provide cushioning and protection at the points of greatest contact. In addition, the use of open weaves on the upper face of the sock combined with wicking materials can not only provide protection, but also provide cooling to the foot.

In years past, running through streams, puddles or even the moisture from heavy sweating could end up with socks becoming waterlogged and moving around in the shoe. The moisture management in socks now quickly wicks fluid away from the foot, keeping the foot dry, and warm in cold conditions. So many advances have been made that it's best to try a variety of high-tech socks to find those best suited to your requirements, but you can safely overlook the basic cotton thins, or tennis 'joggers' of yesteryear.

Falke, who are technology leaders of the sock industry in South Africa, have not only developed right- and left-footed socks to ensure a perfect fit with non-irritating seams, but also a sock that can be used to carry the timing transponders that race organisers frequently use to time runners in today's events. This attention to detail and the needs of sportspeople is reflected in their product range, which also includes running underwear and shorts. I rank the use of Falke's ergonomic runners sock together with Nike's Presto shoe as the prime reason for my being able to run the 250 km in the sand of Augrabies marathon without developing a blister.

We really are all different. Many runners use Vaseline on their toes, but I found this to be the only time I developed blisters! Just as we run with different strides, so too our toes and feet move differently in our shoes, which can impact on your sock requirements. But I am confident that current technology will provide you with socks to suit your needs.

Tights and gloves

When the average South African runners talk of cold weather, particularly those in Durban, they mean that it has dropped to below 10 °C! While on a contract in Scotland in late 1995, I quickly learnt to understand the concept of 10 °C summer mornings, 2 °C spring mornings, and that -20 °C was a typical winter morning! The wind would add, or more correctly subtract, from these temperatures.

As noted previously, it's all a matter of dressing for the occasion and the advent of running tights has gone along way to making this a realistic possibility in these cool temperatures. Made of Lycra, tights are close fitting, flexible and currently fashionable in health clubs. Support underneath can be provided by specialist sports underwear, which has the ability to deflect moisture away, as well as ensure a comfortable run. If it is too cold for nylon tights, opt for the microfibre cotton Lycra-type, many of which also have a wick-dry system. They are thicker than their nylon counterparts, but better quality ones can stretch in a so-called 'four ways' direction (actually vertical and horizontal, as opposed to two-way stretch, which is normally only horizontal).

Some international manufacturers have produced tights with sprinkles of reflective paint for running at night, as legs are one of the first things that car headlights pick up. I first used these in the 1996 Belfast-Dublin 104-mile Peace Run. It was interesting to see how cars on the opposite side of the road slowed down as soon as their headlights caught the tights.

This reflective paint is now also used on T-shirts, jackets and even shorts as well as vests. I can recommend nothing better for any runner who runs in the dark. To increase your safety, add a lightweight, flashing red cycle-type light on your back and a headband light or a small Mag-light to see the road ahead.

Hands are also a sensitive area to cold, although, generally, I dislike covering my fingers. If it is not too cold I wear cotton mittens (gloves with the fingers cut off), but as the chill sets in, I use one of my long-sleeved shirts with integrated gloves. The latter is a 'pocket' sewn onto the outer of the sleeve. When folded back over the hands, it encloses the end of the sleeve, providing glove-like protection, but is convenient because the 'glove' can be folded away when no longer required. For colder weather, a fleece glove is the answer. I'm sure that the average runner doesn't need such a variety of gloves, but my dislike of hot hands has resulted in an armoury to cover the different conditions of ultras.

Ears, head and eyes

My first line of defence for cold ears or head is the hood on my rain jacket, but in cooler weather a 'beanie' does the job well. An additional benefit of this 'woolly' cap is that it provides a receptacle for carrying a thin rain top (see rain-/showerproof tops) or other items 'under your hat' on a long run. I run with glasses and use this convenient storage space when rain makes the use of glasses impossible.

In deepest winter I opt for a Balaclava (a Scottish by-product of the Crimean War), but this is a last resort for me. Similar to the 'beanie', it folds down to cover the face with the exception of the eyes and nose and is the sort of thing favoured by SAS soldiers during a mission. I have sometimes greeted someone in the street while wearing one and needless to say, received no recognition from the other party, but at least I was warm.

It's important to remember that the head is one of the main areas where heat escapes and while it makes sense to trap this heat loss in the cold, it is also essential to ensure that the heat is dissipated in hot conditions.

Until recently, I had been against the use of hats in normal or warm weather, as they simply stored the heat, but there are some very good products available now that wick moisture and heat away. If sweat or moisture can be evaporated from a surface, it will cause a cooling to that surface. Look for mesh hats made from high-quality, light-coloured materials. In Japan I found an excellent hat, which not only offers all the above qualities, but is also silver in colour to 'reflect' the heat and the underside of the peak was designed not to reflect the glare into the eyes. If you can't find a suitable hat (normally from specialist running stores), but need some shade from the sun, foam peaks, which are often handed out as promotional items by manufacturers, are the ideal. The head is left open and the peak provides the shade.

When I first ran in South Africa, people often wondered why I ran with my normal spectacles, and yet they would see me without them at work or at functions. The reason was simple, even though I was short-sighted, I could see far enough ahead to be able to run, but my spectacles were photo-chromatic, i.e. they also protect the eyes from the sun. When running ultra-distances, I was in the sun for extended periods and needed some protection. I held the spectacles in place with a rubber band called a 'croakie', which I bought in Hawaii in 1984. Since 1988 I have worn the now fashionable running and triathlon glasses whenever I run in the sun. They definitely alleviate the stress of eyestrain. Not all manufacturers produce similar products and it's worthwhile taking time to review the range before investing the fairly substantial amount required to purchase them.

Initially, I tried wearing contacts below these glasses, but found that extended periods of running resulted in dry and irritated eyes. Bollé were first to introduce a prescription solution that was suspended off the front of the frame behind the main lens. This worked quite well, but altered the balance of the frame and presented problems if the prescription misted up between the shaded lens and the prescription lens. Oakley brought out quality sports glasses with prescriptions and this was a major step forward.

Now Nike have taken it a stage further with ultra-lightweight frames capable of taking prescription lenses. They are innovatively designed to ensure an airflow that minimises the chances of misting. In addition, the frame is designed so that even when the 'legs' are opened across the forehead, the lens is optically correct throughout the curvature of the spectacles. In one model it is possible to change the colour and density of the lens, which means that I can also use them for cycling or running in low-light conditions. To prove how comfortable they are, I also have a Nike wire frame with clear prescription lenses that I use for normal wear. Moreover, the frame can withstand considerable flexing and 'abuse', which makes it ideal for the rough and tumble of sport.

Incidentally my short-sightedness and Scots accent have led to many a funny situation, such as the early morning greetings exchanged between runners. Often a 'Howzit' and 'Good morning Norrie' have been addressed to me by a runner I was unable to identify. When I replied with a 'Whose that?' in my accent, I received a 'Fine thanks, how are you?' in return. It pays to be able to see, and to all those I don't greet by name, please understand my dilemma and let me know who you are!

WATER CARRIERS

If you have read the chapter on fluid replacement you will know my feelings on carrying bottles and the disadvantage of this. However fluid replacement is a critical feature of running.

In 1986, while involved with the organisation of a triathlon in Newcastle in KwaZulu-Natal, I was told how runners put water bottles behind the kilometre signs on their training route the night before a long run. That is complicated and time consuming. I have yet to discover or hear of a better device than the Tripper which provides water carriers front and back (see 'Carrying gel or goo energy in an event or training' in chapter 27). Over the years I have tried many other types of water carriers for my runs in the mountains and in particular for the Western states 100-miler in USA. There are belts that carry bicycle bottles, tubes of water that fit

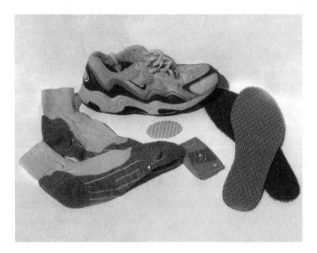

around the waist, and hand bottles made for holding small amounts of water, and so on, but none that match the Tripper at this stage.

However, the situation changes drastically when participating in very long events, where there is additional equipment that needs to be carried. For instance, in the 2002 Augrabies Marathon I certainly experienced the benefit of the Camelbak range of backpacks (see page 384).

HAND AND RUNNING WEIGHTS

Perhaps the place to start is with hand weights as there has been much said in the past about the idea of running with weight in training, thereby developing strength for racing. I believe these alter your running style and are of little benefit. The only possible exception to this is a light hand-weight, which may help improve arm-strength endurance.

In this regard, two types come into mind. Heavy hands are a handgrip onto which weights can be added from 0.5–15 kg. Obviously the 1 kg is ample for running with, anything more is likely to make you look like a Neanderthal man with your knuckles scraping the ground after the first mile. Water-filled hand bottles are another way, which have the benefit of providing liquid on the run. These can hold anything from 150–700 ml, depending on size (each millilitre of water will give a gram of weight) and 500 ml in each hand would be optimal.

Relatively recent research has promoted the use of a weight vest for running. Possibly the best solution is to use the Tripper, which with fluid on board will add 1 kg to your body weight. Using the larger 2-litre model will double that. A major benefit is that it is designed to distribute the weight through the axis of the body and will not affect your running style much.

CREAMS AND RUBS

Walk into any sports changeroom and there is a smell of some rubbing cream. In the old rugby changing rooms the smell of liniment 'clings' to the walls. At the start of major races, the odour of eucalyptus clears the blocked nostrils of runners in a 10-m radius.

Some creams are used almost as a replacement for a warm-up, others as a means of painkiller, or as a method of reducing stiffness – the claims are as bountiful as the preparations on the market (see also chapter on Injuries). I think that some of these have a place in injury recovery. They increase the flow of blood to the injured area and may contain a mild anti-inflammatory or painkiller. However, their use before a run is something I would question. If a runner has that sort of problem should he be racing? I would rather leave these for each runner to establish his own preference. My only advice is to look at the contents of the cream and seek pharmaceutical advice as to the likelihood of it achieving the advertised claims as a solution to your problem.

On the other hand, chafing is a problem that affects most runners. There are two main types of creams: greasy, more accepted ones such as Vaseline, and lesser-known water soluble types such as Sportslube and Elastoplast Anti Chafe. It is a personal choice, but consider some disadvantages of each. What I hate about the greasy type is that it is difficult to clean off your fingers if you put it on during a run. You can hardly stop to wash your hands and it 'contaminates' everything you touch, which I find annoying. I tested the Anti Chafe cream during my record run from Johannesburg to Durban in 1985 and this suited me best. The only drawback is that it does wear off after a while, and must be reapplied during long runs.

RADIOS, WALKMANS AND MUSIC

I find running with music to be a pleasant way of covering a long run, but there are a number of problems. How do you carry them? What products actually work? What models can withstand the sweat and bounce? If you are looking for a radio, cassette or other music player, the prime considerations should be:

Weight: You need the lightest possible; batteries are frequently a large percentage of weight.

Tuning: Radios that use a tuning dial are a waste of time in running because they do not stay on the station. The best option is one that uses digital tuning, particularly if it also has a means of locking the buttons to prevent inadvertent change. There are several imported 'search and tune' button-operated small radios,

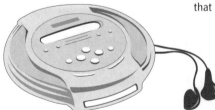

which work quite well. Their main disadvantage is that there is no indication of which station you are on, or where you are in the tuning range. However, they are relatively cheap and extremely light, which may well compensate for their 'failings'.

Waterproof: Be it cold and rainy or hot and sweaty, your radio or player will become wet and, as such, requires additional care after each run. I place mine into a small polythene cellphone bag, before I put it into its carrier. Pay particular attention to the battery area, as this is one of the first areas to let in moisture. Moisture and electronics don't mix well and sweat magnifies the problem. It may well be better to opt for the cheaper models, recognising their limited lifespan, than to spend more on a superior model that will also experience moisture problems. Some are claimed to be water-resistant but to date these seem to be considerably bigger and heavier.

CDs and tapes

Walkmans need to be 'antibounce' otherwise the music simply stops or misplays. There is also a limit to the length of music that can be carried without taking additional tapes or CDs (more weight).

MP3

The latest technology is the MP3 player, which solves the weight and bounce problems. MP3s are digital players that use memory cards or sticks as their music source. The music can be downloaded from the Web, or converted on a computer from CD, and can store approximately two hours of music before you go into repeats. These players are still very expensive so you may not wish to risk the rigours of running and moisture, but given their size, and with care during and after the run, damage can be avoided. This is without doubt the highest quality of sound, and Nike has even produced a watch with an MP3 player in it.

Carrying

Radio headphones as a combined unit are quite a useful solution, but rain or sweat takes its toll, and the weight carried solely on the head can become uncomfortable. When using a more conventional option of radio and headphone, choose the smallest digital radio in your price bracket and carry it in a Tune Belt – a neoprene belt with a pocket to hold the tape, radio or CD player. It stretches to fit around your waist and carries the weight in the small of your back. A small polythene cellphone bag will assist with sweat/rain protection.

A problem with any headphone system is that the cable has a bounce that continually tugs at the connection to the earphones, which eventually causes a loose connection and irritation. I have yet to find a solution to this, so rather buy cheap headsets on a regular basis.

A final point to bear in mind is that from 2002 the IAAF declared these devices an 'assistance' in racing and they may not be used in competition. They remain, however, a great asset in training.

ICEPACKS

I have included this item because I believe that at some time every runner will have the misfortune to suffer some form of injury that needs attention. Without a medical background I am not qualified to say much about injuries, but from personal experience I can say that, for many types of injury, putting ice on as soon as possible is helpful. Blocks of ice from ice trays are not convenient for this, but will do if there is nothing else. The best icepacks I have come across are the 'bag-type' that have a rubberised material and screw top into which you place the blocks. They permit direct contact and some are available with a neoprene 'knee' bandage, used to hold the bag against the injury.

Gel packs are useful, as they can easily be re-used and can be heated as well as cooled, so they are more versatile when alternate heating and cooling is prescribed. Some gel packs come with a 'pocket bandage' to hold them in position. Personally, I don't feel the gel pack keeps the injury as cold as the 'bag' version described above. A cheaper option is a packet of frozen vegetables – but the cook in your home might not be overjoyed!

Although you need specialist advice if you are injured, one of the first things that you should do is to apply ice to the injured area. Where possible, raise the injured part, and take the weight off it. If nothing else, this will help to stop any internal bleeding from the muscle tears, will reduce swelling and may even reduce pain.

One other benefit of ice that may come as a surprise to many is that it helps to relax muscles, and so also improves stretching. Masseurs use ice treatment after an event and before a massage. Place a polystyrene cup full of water into the freezer. When frozen, rip off the top section and hold the underside of the cup, so you can use the ice face for massage. This works really well.

WATCHES

The market for running watches is growing, and has shown dramatic technological advances. Not long ago the only thing available was a simple stopwatch that you started at the beginning of a race and stopped at the end. Knowing your overall time was easy, but working out your time over the last kilometre of the race was a major mathematical feat. Some watches now work this out for you. They also allow you to programme target times, memorise up to 100 laps or kilometre times, and can even be used as a running logbook.

One of latest watches on the market is a model that incorporate GPS and provides pacing, distance and speed. (see chapter 39). Technology is advancing so fast that by the time this book reaches the shelves there will, no doubt, be even more advanced watches. For this reason, I do not intend recommending any particular model.

A watch is a great training and racing aid, so buy one of reputable make that is specifically designed for sport. The corresponding advances in heart-rate monitors now combines all the needs of a runner in a single unit. **Here are a few features that I like in a watch:**

> ‣ stop watch
> ‣ time of day, date, alarm
> ‣ countdown timer with repeat (some will have multiple timers)
> ‣ min. 50 lap and recall
> ‣ good full-face night light
> ‣ 10 preprogrammable target times
> ‣ easy-to-use start/stop/lap buttons
> ‣ the display of laps and running time must be clear for use during the event
> ‣ waterproof for swimming
> ‣ not too big
> ‣ heart-rate features
> ‣ suitability for everyday use

BACKPACKS

It may seem strange to include these, but many runners run to and from work if they are to put in all the training they need, and backpacks have a place here.

The major problem with most of the backpacks currently on the market is that they are not designed for runners. Additional weight carried during a run tends to change running style, and a runner needs a pack that will distribute the weight equally about the body. I initially solved the problem by taking the bags out of my largest Tripper and using it as a sort of front-and-back pack for carrying kit to and from work.

For carrying small or very lightweight amounts, a runner pack on the back is fine. These normally have both a waist and a chest strap, which ideally should be elasticised to allow for comfortable breathing. It's better to have a number of small, rather than large, pockets as it help to prevent things from shifting about with the running action.

There is an art to packing these bags. Heavy items such as shoes should lie as close to the body as possible, to reduce bounce. Unfortunately, they are usually the hardest and most uncomfortable to have close to the body, so a compromise must be reached. Another problem with packs is that their straps cut into you, particularly if you wear them very tight to eliminate bounce. To solve the problem I developed a design in conjunction with a local manufacturer that allowed me to breathe, even with tight straps. It is a loop of elastic attached to straps so that they extend with breathing. No matter what they're made of, backpacks absorb perspiration. The easiest solution is to put your clothes in a plastic bag before packing them in the backpack – also helpful if it rains.

Remember, for daily use over small distances, small is beautiful. A small pack keeps the weight close to the body and makes running more comfortable.

For longer events, as with the new trend in adventure racing, you need to be able to carry, not only a few clothes, but also food, other kit and fluid. This is where the Camelbak backpacks come into their own. Most incorporate a fluid bladder that is built into the back of the backpack. A tube is fitted through the straps so that hydration can continue as you run. The padded waist and chest straps, as well as straps to consolidate the backpack, all assist in minimising content bounce. The Camelbak range covers a diversity of sizes to cater for short and long treks, and most are available directly from Cape Cycles in South Africa, while some require a special order through the agents. Before purchasing one, seek professional advice from other adventure racers to ensure you buy the right size. However, like shoes be prepared to make modifications for greater comfort. For instance, I prefer to incorporate an elastic chest strap for freedom of movement in breathing. Because the ideal backpack will distribute weight through the centre of gravity to maintain a normal running style, also look at incorporating a front section to assist in balancing the weight.

A FINAL WORD

Other items to consider buying (or putting on a list for friends at birthday time) include a sports bag, a tracksuit, lace locks for holding laces in position without actually being tied, a reflector belt for night running, and a wrist wallet for carrying money and/or keys. Another way to carry a single key is to tie it into shoelaces and then tuck it under the other lacing lower down the shoe, or with one of the Falke pocket socks.

If you enjoy gadgets, the best way to see what is available is to look at the November and December issues of running magazines; they nearly always feature a comprehensive list of 'things to get the runner for Christmas'. But everything you carry adds to the weight you have to take with you every step of every kilometre!

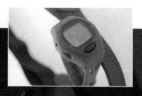

00:00:38
HEART-RATE MONITORS
AND MONITORING

It is speculated that some sportspeople, including runners, use drugs in an attempt to improve their performance. Many could achieve this through bettering their basic fitness rather than any benefits derived from drug abuse.

Resorting to 'chemical manipulation' is often seen as a shortcut to peak performance. In truth, many people put in a substantial number of hours training without considering how much of that time represents effective training? Far better and safer than drugs, is the efficient use of training time. Until the late 1980s/early '90s, the ability to monitor the body to ensure training efficiency was restricted to a privileged few top sportsmen under the guidance of sports scientists.

The advent of accurate personal heart-rate monitors has changed all that and opens the door to 'athletes' in all sports, despite their differing needs. Personal heart-rate monitors provide an efficient and effective aid to training.

BENEFITS

Although heart-rate monitors are alluded to throughout the book, the benefits are summarised here. Performance in any sport relies on the efficient generation of energy to 'power' the muscles. Think of it as four basic energy systems; depending on the speed and duration of the event, energy will come from one or a combination of different systems. The runner needs to train the energy systems that he will require in competition in order to improve the efficiency of each system.

For each individual, performance within these systems can be related to a particular level of heart rate. By accurate and constant monitoring of the heart rate during training, athletes can ensure that they train effectively on every occasion. The energy systems and training of sprinters differ from those of distance and marathon runners. By using heart-rate monitoring, training may be tailored to the specific requirements of an event, and the correct proportion of time spent on each energy system. Many runners fail to reach their potential by pushing too hard in all their training sessions, and just as many don't train hard enough at the correct times.

The pulse is a good measure of recovery – the faster it returns to normal at the end of exercise, the fitter you are. For years this was used as a way of determining fitness, but because it was necessary to stop in the midst of exercise, which resulted in a fast drop in pulse rate, it made the method of counting a pulse over a ten-second period and multiplying by six, quite inaccurate for exercise monitoring.

Likewise, a rise in an athlete's waking pulse, while still in bed, is an indication of poor recovery from the previous day's training, or the onset of an infection. Thus, keeping a record of early morning pulse can ensure that training is not overdone. But the benefits are not restricted to the competitive sportsperson. Recreational runners, cyclists, walkers and even those just wanting to commence an exercise programme can benefit substantially from pulse monitoring.

Such are the benefits of heart-rate monitoring that one American sports body even considered banning the monitors in races after a runner, Andy Jones, set a new American record in a 50-mile race. They felt it could be regarded as 'unfair technological assistance'. This is surely a testament to their effectiveness. A meeting of the IAAF in the second half of 1992, however, determined that the use of heart-rate monitors in competition was legal. Interestingly though, the rule change in 2002 (IAAF rule 144) now lists 'any kind of technical device' as assistance, which is not permissible, therefore this decision may have been changed for racing.

Either way, athletes dabbling with syringes would be better off investing in heart-rate monitors.

Heart rate vs pulse

What is the difference between pulse and heart-rate monitoring? Your pulse is taken at the wrist or neck, and is a 'reflection' of the pulse of blood being pumped from the heart. Heart rate is measured as the contraction of the heart muscle, and is recorded by an electronic heart-rate monitor.

SETTING RANGES – A RULE OF THUMB

If you want to improve your cardiovascular condition, exercise within a set range of your maximum heart rate. Theoretically, as you age your maximum heart rate drops by approximately one beat per year. The rule of thumb to determine maximum pulse is to subtract your age from 220. It has recently been suggested that a more accurate formula for maximum heart rate might be 214-0.8 x age (for men) and 207-0.7 x age (for women). These formulae are thought to be more appropriate to people who have exercised.

However, the best way to ascertain a true maximum heart rate is to run 800 m flat out, take 30 seconds recovery and repeat another 800 m. You will reach your maximum heart rate in the second 800 m. Alternatively, use two 300-m sprints up a steep hill with about 20 seconds recovery. You will need a 600-m-high hill, so that the recovery is kept to a minimum. In both cases, a heart-rate monitor that memorises either maximum heart rate or records heart rates at five-second intervals, will give the best results.

You could also use the heart-rate monitor in the treadmill test discussed on page 107 on measuring progress. This will allow you to reach maximum heart rate during the final two-minute session on the treadmill.

The next figure you require is your waking pulse (or heart rate), which is best taken before rising in the morning. Keep your movements to a minimum and count the pulse over a full minute. Alternatively, put on the heart-rate chest strap and relax for about two minutes.

The combination of minimum (resting) and maximum heart rates allows you to calculate a heart-rate range through which you can exercise. From this, various levels of exertion can be calculated as percentages of your full range. For example a 30-year-old with a waking pulse of 60 would have a maximum of 220-30 = 190, and a range of 190-60 = 130. Thus 65% effort would be 130 x 0.65 + 60 = 144.5.

USING A HEART-RATE MONITOR

Because the energy systems that you use at differing speeds can be related to your heart rate, it may also be used as a guide to the level of exertion of your training. All that is required is an initial laboratory test to determine your heart-rate levels at various speeds, as well as lactate and energy levels.

Thereafter you can set various heart rates for each type of training session in the confidence that you will make the most efficient use of the time you spend in training (see also chapter 8).

At this stage, it is worthwhile looking at lactate, a substance that has caused runners much confusion. It is a chemical produced by muscles during exercise. The amount of lactate in the exercising muscles gives an indication of the intensity of the exercise. When these levels become excessive, they prevent the same intensity of exercise being maintained as a safety system to prevent the muscles from being damaged. However, lactate is not responsible for sore muscles. When exercise recommences at low intensities the excess lactate will be used as a source of energy – a good reason for cooling down after races.

The most commonly used 'training zones' are given below, and an explanation of the energy systems they relate to is given in chapter 22 on energy replacement. A sample training schedule for a 10-km race is provided at the back of the book.

TRAINING ZONES	
Zone A	55–65% long slow distance or recovery runs
Zone B	65–80% medium distance steady/runs
Zone C	85% time trial or threshold training
Zone D	85–90% interval sessions longer than 400 m
Zone E	90–95% quality work of 400 m or less

For each zone the formula is:
heart rate = working range x (required %) + minimum heart rate

Example: Consider a runner with maximum of 190 and resting (minimum) of 50 beats per minute. Working range = max - min = 190-50 = 140 beats.

Zone B 80% effort = working range x (required %) + minimum heart rate = 140 x (0.8) + 50 = 162.
Thus Zone B 65% = 140 x (0.65) + 50 = 141.

The amount of time you spend per week in each 'level' or 'zone' will vary with the distance of the race for which you are training, i.e. a track athlete will spend far more time in the 'ATP+creatine phosphate' energy levels than an ultrarunner concentrating his efforts in the 'fat-burning' energy level. This will also change at different stages of training throughout your build-up period.

One of the first things that many runners will note when using this sophisticated device is that they have been training too hard during 'easy' days and too easy during 'hard' days. This is an unfortunate side effect of the marathon boom of the 1970s and '80s, and the desire for fast improvement in fitness.

MONITORING PROGRESS

An improvement in fitness will result in a decrease in waking pulse over a few months. The heart-rate monitor can be used variously to monitor your training progress. One method is to set a standard running route, such as a 5-km time trial, to be undertaken once every 6–8 weeks. As fitness improves, the heart rate required for the 5 km will decrease. Thus, if one month you run for 20 minutes on a flat course with a heart rate of 140 beats to cover the 5 km, using the same distance and heart rate you may take 19 minutes, 30 seconds the following month. It is easier and less destructive to use this sort of measure than to try the flat-out exertion of seeing how fast you can cover 5 km on each occasion, which is basically a race condition and requires recovery before any training can be resumed. Alternatively, you can run the same time trial distance at the same pace, and see what your maximum and average heart rate is. As you improve, your heart rate will reduce.

Another indication of improved fitness is your recovery heart rate. If you record the length of time it takes to drop back to normal levels, it will take less time as your fitness improves. This is easily monitored after a variety of sessions.

Heart-rate monitoring is also a useful addition to the treadmill progression discussed on page 107 on training, and keeping track of your waking pulse has already been identified as a method of ensuring that full recovery is achieved.

TYPES OF MONITORS

Over the years many commercial pulse monitors have been produced but few have ever proved accurate unless their source of detection was directly to electrodes on the chest. These, however, are bulky, expensive and inappropriate for use during exercise. Earlobe- and finger-monitoring pickups have failed for most people during exercise as a consequence of the inconvenience, as well as sweat disturbance of the reading.

Recognising the advantages of such monitoring, I tried almost everything on the market over the years but failed to find anything remotely accurate during exercise, that is, until I acquired my first wireless heart-rate monitor in 1989. Technological advances and micro-computing now allow a simple elasticised chest band to hold electrodes against the chest while a transmitter sends pulse readings to a receiver in a watch strap. Monitoring your heart rate is literally at the flick of a wrist.

This technology has resulted in a whole range of alternatives, from a simple digital pulse reading to sophisticated range alarms and memory (for storing heart rate taken on a run and downloading or recall later). At the top end it is even possible for a record of the pulse to be kept at five-second intervals throughout exercise and then to be

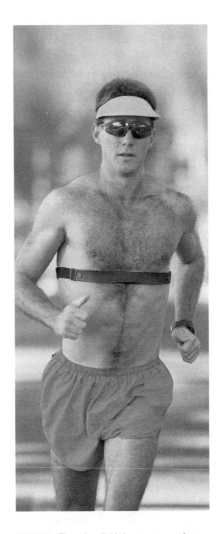

ABOVE *The only reliable heart-rate monitors are those that monitor electro-activity directly from the chest and feed this, normally by radio signal, to a watch or other display. A distinct advantage is that you may replace batteries yourself in many of the straps and watches*

downloaded to a computer for graphing and analysis. After 18 months' use, I was so convinced of the benefits of these monitors that I moved up to a model that downloads directly. It allows close monitoring of my own training, and is also an excellent way for me to gauge the condition of runners and sportsmen I coach.

If you are considering investing in a heart-rate monitor, go in at the highest end of the range that you can afford, rather than the low end only to find that you require more features.

When a wired heart-rate monitor is more appropriate

In a seeming contradiction of the above, I had the opportunity of trying out a wired heart-rate monitor in 1997 – the Cardio Sport Heartspeak 20. While it took years for manufacturers to create wireless heart-rate monitors, wires are one of the keys to the success of the Heartspeak.20. It consists of the same chest belt, which is connected to a matchbox-sized processing box by a wire with two terminals. A second wire leads to an earphone with a comfortable behind-the-ear hook to hold it in position. A simple in-line control adjusts volume. Plugging both wires into the unit starts the monitoring period. A voice reports the heart rate at 20-second intervals and the elapsed time every ten minutes. The benefits derive both from the simplicity and the audio feedback.

The wires ensure that there is no interference when used on a treadmill or other gym equipment, which makes it ideal for testing of runners while the coach wears the earpiece to monitor the heart rate at 20-second intervals. This prevents an athlete from being psychologically affected from an awareness of the heart rate. Because the feedback is audio, the coach's hands are free to take lactate samples or do other work. Connecting the unit to a tape recorder provides a record of the heart-rate tests.

And the benefits don't stop there. Arm movement makes it difficult to read a heart-rate monitor while running long intervals or fartlek sessions. With the Heartspeak 20, if hard efforts are two minutes long, it's simply a case of listening for seven announcements of heart rate. (i.e. six-number, 20-second intervals). It can also be used as a tool to assist in relaxation before visualisation and to mentally prepare for competition. In such a case, the objective is for the biofeedback to reduce the resting heart rate (see chapter 18 on mental preparation).

SAMPLE TRAINING SCHEDULE FOR 10 KM USING HEART-RATE MONITORING

	Zone type	Example
week 1		
Day 1	E	rest
2	D	(1 x 200, rest 30 sec, 1 x 400, jog 400 or rest 2.5 mins) x 3–4
3	A	5 km easy
4	B	8 km moderate
5	C	3–4 km steady steady (10 km pace) (keep constant pace)
6		12 km moderate
7	D	4 x 800, rest 2.5–3 min
		Total 52 km
week 2		
Day 1	A	5 km easy
2	C	2 x 2500 (10 km pace), 2 km jog between
3	B	8–10 km moderate
4	D	(2 x 400, rest 2.5) x 4
5	A	5 km easy
6		1 x 200, rest 30 sec, 1 x 400, rest 1 min, 1 x 600
7	E	rest
		Total 53 km
week 3		
Day 1	B	12 km moderate
2	C	4 km (10 km pace; same pulse as week 1)
3	A	5 km easy
4	D	(1 X 200, rest 30 sec, 1 x 400, jog 400 or rest 2.5 min) x 4
5	B	12–14 km moderate
6	D	3 x 800, rest 2.5 min
7	A	5 km easy
		Total 65 km

Zone types:

A Fat-burning/ recovery (55–65% max heart rate)

B Endurance (65–85% max heart rate)

C 'Threshold' (85–90% max heart rate)

D Anaerobic (90% and above max heart rate)

E Rest

	Session type	Example
week 4		
Day 1		3 x 2000 at 10 km pace, jog 5 min (or 5 km race at 90%)
2	B	8–10 km moderate
3	D	2 x (1 x 200, rest 30 sec, 1 x 400, rest 1 min, 1 x 600, rest 1.5 min, 1 x 400, rest 1 min, 1 x 200)
4	A	5–6 km easy
5	C	2 x 1500 at 10 km pace, rest 2.5 min)
6	E	rest
7	B	12–15 km moderate
		Total 64 km
week 5		
Day 1	B	8–10 km
2	D	6 x 800, rest 2.5–3 min
3	A	5 km easy
4	B	15–18 km moderate
5	D	(1 x 400, rest 1 min, 1 x 200) x 4, rest 3 min
6	A	5 km easy
7	C	8 km time-trial (10–15 km race pace), keep to set pulse
		Total 73 km
week 6		
Day 1	E	rest
2	B	8–10 km
3	C	3 x 2000 at 10 km pace
4	A	5 km easy
5	D	(2 x 400, rest 45) x 5, rest 2.5 min
6	B	15–18 km moderate
7	D	4 x 800, rest 2.5–3 min
		Total 52 km

	Session type	Example
week 7		
Day 1	A	5 km easy
2	C	4 km at 10 km pace (use same pulse as weeks 1 and 3 – corporate time
3	E	rest
4	D	1 x 800, rest 3 min, 1 x 600, rest 2 min, 1 x 400, rest 1 min, 1 x 300, 1 x 200
5	B	8 km moderate
6	C	1 x 3000, rest 5 min, 1 x 2000, rest 2 min, 1 x 1500 at 10 km pace
7	B	12–18 km moderate
		Total 46.8 km
week 8		
Day 1	T	5 x 400
2	A	4 x 400
3	P	3 x 400
4	E	2 x 400
5	R	rest
6		rest or 1 x 400 at 1500 pace
7		race 10 km race
		Total 16 km
week 9 (recovery week – your target starts here)		
Day 1	E	rest
2	A	3–5 km easy
3	B/A	6–8 km easy/moderate
4	E	rest
5	A	5 km easy
6	B/A	6–8 km easy/moderate
7	E	rest
		Total 26 km

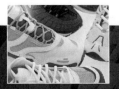

00:00:39
KEEPING PACE WITH TECHNOLOGY

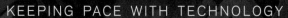

Judging how much effort you are putting into training is one of your greatest challenges as a runner. Many methods have been used to monitor this.

Initially, we used perceived effort, which employed a scale of 1–10 or 1–20, depending on the version you chose: 1 was easy and 10 (or 20) maximum effort. Each level had a description relating to mental perception or the ability to talk. This gave the athlete a measure of easy and hard paces, the objective being to ensure sufficient easy sessions between the hard training, and to ensure that hard sessions were effective. However, this relied purely on an athlete's judgement, which is difficult for the competitive runner.

The next stage reached by technology was that of heart-rate monitors, which are more scientific as they monitor the body's reaction to stress. By relating training pace to heart rates, they purport to determine paces during training, but the drawback is that they try to mix two different training aspects – the cardio-vascular/energy response and the muscular/neural need to train at different paces (see heart-rate monitors in chapter 38).

While the cardiovascular aspect can be trained by pushing the heart rate to specific levels, the ability to use muscles at race pace (or faster or slower) requires a specific movement, but there are many variables affecting heart rates, blocking a direct relationship with running pace. Pre-race apprehension, a poor night's sleep, heat, humidity, hydration level, wind, fatigue, and even the food or liquid taken prior to training or a race can completely change the heart rate for a target race pace. So although heart rate provides a valid means of expressing 'stress', it is a poor pace monitor.

Pace is important and in order to progress, previous race performances determine the necessary training paces. Direct relationships exist between performances over a flat-out six-minutes, 5 km, 10 km, marathon and ultramarathon, while abilities at set times and distances relate to physiological parameters. Training at these 'paces' will result in progress but the problem is to maintain a consistent pace. Although tracks are useful, their hard surfaces and corners can increase the risk of injury, but it is a more accurate method than heart-rate monitoring or perceived effort in judging pace.

In combination with a heart-rate monitor, the latest GPS (global positioning system) monitoring technology, provides detailed feedback for effective training. Using satellites and trigonometry, GPS calculates and tracks the movement of the monitor to show not only how far we have run, but also (at any stage) exactly what pace we are running in kilometres (or miles) per hour, or in minutes and seconds per kilometre (or mile). This removes the doubt on pace. Marathon and ultrarunners, in particular, will immediately see that much of their easy running is at too fast a pace. It is this constant drive to push too hard that causes many runners to arrive at an event overtrained, and with damaged muscles.

No matter if your goal is 10 km or Comrades, a key session is to train at race pace, and GPS makes it easy to monitor. Previously we had to use road distance marks and adjust the pace as we passed each one, but corners and hills always skewed the calculation. Now the effects of hills can be seen immediately and a runner can work on 'even effort' or 'even pace' as changes in pace are revealed.

Lactate sessions, criss-crossing between 10-km and marathon pace, become more accurate and hence more effective. With distance, pace and time you effectively have a training track anywhere you need it – even on a hill! At last, perhaps, time trials will become what they should be – sessions to monitor training progress whereby you can run at a consistent pace, over a set distance and monitor your heart rate. Repeating this on a six-weekly basis will give more precise feedback on your progress, and, hopefully, stop you from 'racing' time trials to 'set PBs'. Your training sessions should be more specific, effective and productive.

Manufactured as a collaboration between Timex and Garmin, the first GPS watches became available in mid 2002. Rather than providing information on location, they provide details of speed, pace and distance, all linked to a wide variety of sports timing functions including stopwatch, countdown timer, laps and recall options. Initially there were 50- and 100-lap options, with the latter sporting a very useful feature of an alarm that can be set to warn if the pace or speed moves out of a set zone.

I discovered these units in the UK at the Manchester Commonwealth Games, where I assisted a fellow IAAF A-grade measurer, Hugh Jones, to do the final set-out of the marathon, race walks, and triathlon courses. Courses are normally measured using a bicycle with a counter system on the wheel. This digital counter increases 20 'clicks' for every turn of the wheel and is calibrated against a standard distance of 300-1 000 m. It provides an accurate method of measurement, which picks up changes in temperature, surface roughness, and is the only protocol accepted by the IAAF. During our work in Manchester, I undertook several trials to determine the accuracy of the GPS, by comparing it to the same calibration distance and parts of the courses used in the Commonwealth Games.

Generally, it seemed to be correct to within 4 m per kilometre. Back in Durban for three days, I tried the GPS during a basic track session and found a similar accuracy. However, this also emphasised the importance of where the monitor is carried, as it is the line of the monitor that is measured not the runner. Wearing it on the left arm on the track, it measures the inside lane, on the right arm it measures further than you run.

A few days later I used the GPS unit in the Business Trust 1 000 Mile Relay World Record attempt, which involved ten of South Africa's top distance runners sharing the running from Cape Town to Johannesburg, with some laps at the end to take them up to the full 1 000 miles. The GPS was the preferred method of measurement (over vehicle odometers), and I first calibrated the GPS against a standard calibration distance at Green Point in Cape Town, then against each vehicle and also against a Clain Jones counter on a bicycle – creating a full set of comparisons. By the end of the run, which saw the runners set a world record time of 99:03:27, the GPS showed a difference of over 30 km less than the readings of the seconding vehicles, but good comparisons with the bicycle-measured distances at various venues from start to finish.

There are, however, a few points to bear in mind when using the GPS:

> ‣ Switch it on about 5–10 minutes prior to using it, as it takes time to 'log and locate' the satellites.

> ▸ The unit must be within 1.5 m of the watch receiver and it is best worn on the same arm as the watch.
>
> ▸ The unit needs a clear view of the sky – going through tunnels, bridges or even heavily treed roads can disrupt the measurement.
>
> ▸ Always ensure that the batteries are above the final quarter level before setting out.

Throughout these tests, the GPS has performed quite impressively and in late 2002, I used it to measure a 250-km six-stage 'off-road' event in the Augrabies National Park, South Africa, as a preliminary step to having the process registered as the official international protocol (to be recognised by the Association of International Marathons (AIM)), for measurement at such events. The Augrabies involved terrain where it is impossible to measure by bicycle or even a vehicle.

This technology advance (by late 2002) is probably one of the great advancements in training and racing equipment in the last decade. The potential to use GPS in racing could change the way people run races, particularly at marathon level and beyond. It can be conservatively estimated that 75% of runners start Comrades far faster than they should. Imagine if they could see what pace they were running from the first 100 m and for every stride thereafter? With even a modicum of discipline, they could keep much closer to their 'realistic' racing pace and would be more likely to reach their training potential.

The potential also exists for measuring swim, surf-ski, climbing and canoeing distances, which would mean that triathlon and other multisport disciplines would become more comparable. More importantly from that comes the opportunity to make such training more scientific as you no longer have to estimate training pace in canoeing or similar sports.

When heart-rate monitors first came onto the market, a Canadian ultrarunner set a new North American 50-mile record using one of them. The use of the monitor in racing was initially questioned by USA Athletics authorities and then at international level, but was later approved, and I foresee a similar pattern for the use of GPS. It is certainly equipment worth acquiring for training and racing.

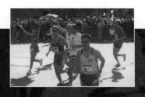

00:00:40
THE PROBLEMS OF BEING
A WORLD-CLASS ATHLETE

It is very easy to recommend a certain approach to training, racing and preparation in athletics. It is even possible to do some of this without ever having participated in the sport, and indeed there are some coaches who fall into this category. The truth of the matter is, that the recommendations for race preparation contained in this book are only the starting point, from which you must develop your own approach to cover your own particular needs. Preparation is everything... the outcome of the race is in many ways predetermined and your participation becomes the fulfilment of your preparation. This was well illustrated in an interview and discussion I had with world record-holder Sebastian Coe in 1991, on the 'simple' matter of flying.

FLYING WITH SEBASTIAN COE

As more and more opportunities arise for athletes to compete internationally, and as more events are held outside a simple two- or three-hour flight from home, we are entitled to ask, 'Do the athletes really know what they are letting themselves in for... even before they reach the stadium?' This was a particularly relevant question for South Africans in 1992 when the international sporting ban was lifted, and sportsmen and -women began the return to international participation.

To Sebastian Coe, one of the world's greatest athletes, flying was something that had to be managed to ensure that the effect on performance was minimal. Whereas the average traveller views flying as something between an exciting experience and a relaxing means of moving around the world, the same journey to Coe was something that required considerable planning.

Living in a world where performances and records are measured in 1/100 of a second, the results of 'rocketing the human body' across time zones – no matter how comfortably – could destroy a goal he had worked towards for over four years.

A case in point was the 1984 Olympics, where Coe faced a seemingly easy flight, along with the rest of the British team, from London directly to California on the west coast of the USA.

In all, the journey involved a relatively minor eight-hour time change, which many business and vacation travellers regularly handle with ease. To the dedicated athlete in search of Olympic titles in the cut-throat battleground of the 800-m and 1 500-m track championships, a more scientifically analysed regime is required. The flight had to be broken down into smaller more manageable sections by stopping over in the north-eastern city of Chicago. Only after four weeks of full acclimatisation and training, could the shorter 'hop' to Los Angeles be tackled, which still left a further two weeks for recovery before taking on the best the world could throw at him. It is history now that such an approach helped Coe become the first man ever to retain the Olympic Gold in the 1 500 m. There is little doubt that a similar approach to competition helped him set four world records within a space of 41 days.

Having retired from international athletics, the rigours of such preparation are things of the past. However, the softly spoken Englishman has since embarked on a political career and continues to fly as much, if not more, than during those memorable days of the 1970s and '80s when he captured not only world records and gold medals, but also the imagination of millions. Coe became the hero of a nation, kept school children up late, and was every mother's ideal son-in-law, as he 'flew' victoriously around the tracks of the world with the apparent ease of a walk to the shops. In truth, though, the attention to detail that preceded such travel is awesome, leading to his involvement in the research of Dr David Martin in Atlanta, on the hormonal changes of flying. Martin discovered, for instance, that there were minor changes in the hormone balance of long-haul travellers, which could last up to six weeks. This is of no consequence to the average passenger, but to an athlete in search of the slightest edge on the competition, such facts must be taken into account.

Whereas most passengers are in search of sleep, Coe was at pains to stay awake throughout a flight in order to make acclimatisation easier at his destination. Even the quantity and timing of meals had to be considered. A preference for soft drinks and water as opposed to the pleasures of wines and other alcoholic beverages became important to ensure that the dehydrating effect of flying was minimised.

Such details can now be left to impulse for the busy executive, who is involved in a few business ventures, over and above his political ambitions. The resultant change in emphasis and attitude are obvious. His basic requirements of air travel are still the same, he says with typical British humour, 'The first priority is that it must stay up!' Such repartee is not surprising from a man who grew up through the Monty Python era of British comedy. Obviously he is now able to take a more relaxed view of flying, but, like most of us, he finds it intriguing when passengers are ushered aboard a flight at scheduled take-off time and promptly told that there will be a 50-minute delay. Why can't they leave the passengers relaxing in the airport lounge, as such annoying delays can totally upset preparations?

In competitive years, his preferred flight was London to Atlanta, which also provided an opportunity to meet with David Martin to gain deeper knowledge of the effects of flying. Totally at home with flying, Coe remains puzzled by the universally uttered, 'Enjoy your flight,' prior to each take-off. 'What does it mean?' he muses, with a glint in his eye and a straight face. 'I understand, "Hope you had a good flight," and "We trust that you had a comfortable flight," but "Enjoy your flight?"' There is no answer from the man who has obviously come to terms with spending many hours in the sky.

CHILDREN'S DEVELOPMENT AND DISTANCE RUNNING

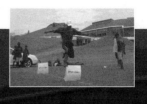

The role of children and teenagers in distance running is a controversial subject with a number of anomalies. Kenyan runners dominate many of the world's cross-country, track and road events, and an inspection of the activities in the Rift Valley reveals children running 10 km and further every day. It has been suggested that this is the secret to probably the most successful distance-running nation to date.

In South Africa, the history of moving poorer communities to outlying areas, as well as the limited provision of facilities, has resulted in a similar situation whereby it is the norm for children to jog-trot prodigious distances to and from schools, towns, or even water points on a daily basis.

By comparison, primarily medically-based recommendations from Europe are that children should not be exposed to the high impact of distance running until they have passed through puberty. A key aspect of concern is that during growth spurts, the bones in the legs are susceptible to damage as they are 'soft' and have weak joints. This certainly has a logical basis, but does it mean that 'rural' African children must cease to go to school or fetch the daily water supply during this period? Clearly not. So why is it acceptable and possible for a rural child to run these distances, but his urban counterpart is 'protected' by the rules of the sport?

In 2002, the South African domestic addendum to the IAAF rules prevented any athlete under the age of 16 from competing in any of the ASA Senior Championships (normally 10 km, 21 km and marathon) and they had to be over 20 to compete in the marathon or longer. Yet in many recreational 10-km events, which are supported by rural communities, it is often young girls of 12 years of age who rocket into the top positions in times that leave their urban counterparts standing.

Closer examination of the differing situations may give an indication of different approaches, which may account for some of the apparent anomalies. In most rural cases, initial exposure to longer running is as the sole means of transport and is undertaken at a pace that allows sufficient time to arrive at the destination with enough energy for the task ahead, after which there is a return journey later in the day. There is no emphasis on speed, but adequate time is allocated to handle the distance comfortably. Energy is conserved because there will always be another kilometre to cover. This is reflected in the training of older, more established athletes. If you see a culturally mixed group of runners in a long run, it is not unusual to see black runners towards the rear of the group, loping along at an easy pace, while others keep their heart-rate 'revs' up towards the front. Ironically, the roles are completely reversed in races, which highlights the role of the pendulum discussed in the training chapters. Only by going easy in appropriate training sessions does it allow the energy and strength to go fast in others and in races.

Urban children have many transport options. Running (or walking for that matter) to and from venues is not the fashionable or selected mode of transport. Cars and 'mum's taxi' even count way above the use of a bicycle. When children are exposed to running, it derives from family or school for 'competitive' reasons, e.g. team/sports training, and is not only an exception to their basic lifestyle, but is also 'pressurised by the clock'. If the child shows some ability in this field, the pressure intensifies from school, a coach (even the introduction of a coach is a statement of pressure), parents and even peers, particularly during the hormone-raging period of puberty.

The objectives of the two situations are opposite, but consider which one creates a more successful athlete in the longer term. Certainly not the pressured situation, which yields only a short-term return at a level that brings little recognition or tangible reward for the child. It is obvious why the medical 'dangers' are of greater concern to the urban child than his rural counterpart whose body has 'adapted' from a young age, in a non-pressured environment, to the rigorous distance. This principle of gradual adaptation has been well documented throughout the book.

Compare this to the way we learn to read: we start with the alphabet, learn to string individual letters into words, and then join words into sentences. Many children's first exposure to sport is when they are lined up at school to play soccer, rugby or cricket, picked on size, height or some other physical 'attribute', placed into a particular position on the field, a ball is thrown into the pitch and they are told to 'play'. Only when the technique/skill errors are identified, is there an attempt to sort them out, but this tends to be by command rather than focusing on the skill.

In the mid 1990s I expanded on some of the concepts initiated by George Bunner in the UK, to evolve a development programme for children in South Africa. The programme is called Papadi Ya Bana, and targets youngsters of all backgrounds from 7–14/15 years of age. The objective is simply to use fun exercises that develop the alphabet of sport – running, jumping, hitting, kicking, catching, throwing and balance. These skills effectively form the basis of all land sports, and the impact of initiating them in children not only reduces the need for each sport to provide a development programme in that age group, but also allows them the opportunity to explore and develop each of the skills, which will help them to identify the sport they are good at or in which they desire to achieve.

Running, too, can benefit from the greater agility of jumping and balancing skills; after all, running is simply a series of jumps (bounds) forward from one foot to the other, and landing on one foot requires a degree of balance. The impact of 'more rounded' sports development will assist at all levels in the future, right up to international level. How often have we lamented that a particular soccer player has a particular skill but lacks ability in another, or a rugby player is a great scrummer and tackler, but lacks ball skills?

Another benefit of the Papadi Ya Bana (which means 'street play' in Sotho) is that it comprises low-cost formal kit that can handle up to 100 children at a time, with the potential to improvise each piece of equipment from normal recyclable and waste material. Cardboard boxes are easily turned into hurdles, goals, bats and jumping objects. The infamous plastic shopping bags, become balls, shot putts, start and finish lines, and even measuring tapes. Cardboard cups, bottles and empty household containers become markers and cones. The programme is accessible to every sector of South African society and it requires very little supervision and minimal training from an organiser.

In conjunction with Pick 'n Pay, a pilot programme was initiated in five regions of South Africa, alongside the Comrades Marathon roadshows of 2002. It was presented at the finish of Comrades with the assistance of the Starfish Charity using older children from a local orphanage as 'leaders'. Papadi Ya Bana is set to expand further and already Isilulu Security runs a weekly session with street children in Durban (for more information on Papadi Ya Bana, see website **www.coachnorrie.co.za**).

There is a perception by many in South Africa that 'development' is something only for rural areas, involving a restricted section of the country. This is false, as is the notion that it is a South African idea. Development is simply the gaining of knowledge or experience, and involves us all. It happens at the highest levels as teams are prepared for the Olympics, world championships or other major events, and it should be provided to all sportspeople, officials, coaches, administrators, spectators, the public at large and the media. There are many cases of misplaced reporting because a reporter has not been 'developed' to understand the intricacies of the game. For this reason it is necessary to select focal aspects of development.

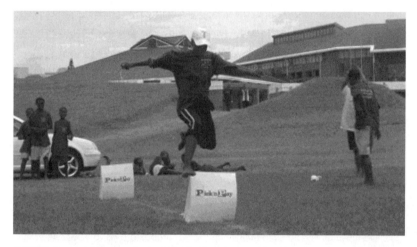

ABOVE *Street children from Durban's Thuthu Kani Shelter enjoy a Papadi Ya Bana session – the natural athletic talent is obvious*

In South Africa our socio-economic and cultural past requires us to identify the following groups: children/youth; those who previously have not had the 'opportunity/exposure'; women; disabled or handicapped; elite e.g. ambassadors, role models of and to the country. Realistically this will result in development focusing on people of colour, but it should also be seen that at its basic level, it is not an issue of colour, but rather an issue of 'opportunity', and building the future.

By comparison, the focal points in UK are listed as: children; women; disabled or handicapped; senior citizens; elite. The similarity is clear, and the addition of senior citizen is necessary to address the socio-economic problems of the UK, where there is an increasing number of people retiring, and living longer.

Ultimately, development is something we all need to be involved in and gain from, and as coaches, parents, teachers, and simply South Africans, we all need to have an influence on that growth. As far as it affects children's development and distance running, **I suggest the following:**

> ▸ It is not distance running *per se* that is the problem, but the manner in which it is introduced and the reason for going the distance.
>
> ▸ That there is definite potential for damage to a child if long distances are undertaken either in a 'sudden' load, or under pressure. The risks involved will be exacerbated during a child's growth spurts.
>
> ▸ There are wide variations in ages when individual children experience puberty and a rigid application of age groups and restrictions is probably an inappropriate, but practical option for sports bodies to shoulder these responsibilities to the protection of the child.
>
> ▸ It is clear that teachers and parents are the prime people to burden the responsibility of restricting children's involvement in sport, but, where necessary, this should be to further restrict the rules applied by the governing body of the sport, not to try and circumvent them.
>
> ▸ The benefits of a child's involvement in distance running at a young age must be questioned, in comparison to a broader development of skills, and what the longer-term benefits would be.
>
> ▸ In conjunction with the above, you will find numerous references in this book and others to the fact that a child's ability (and an adult's) to go faster over a shorter distance, or jump further/higher, or any other explosive elastic strength, is the best indication of his ability over the longer distance in later years. For that reason it makes sense for a child to be focusing on short distances and multiskills, rather than long distance.

Is it any wonder that the Kenyans may dominate the long distances, but have little impact in the sprint or team-sport arena where short and explosive power is 'king'. No doubt someone will point to the agility and domination of the Kenyans in the steeplechase, which further supports the above argument, as this skill has been developed from a young age by bounding over fences and rocks in their runs. The focus on agility is what makes their running balanced and fluid, and hence more efficient. I suspect the influence of altitude is less of a physiological factor than we believe, but it is an 'easy out' for people who enjoy the comforts of life more than their ambition to duplicate the rigours of those long, slow jog-trots from the day they start walking.

Most of you will be long past the age when this chapter applies to you, but you will be in a position where the impact and concepts may have a wide influence on your own or other people's children. I urge you to consider playing your part in the development of the future stars.

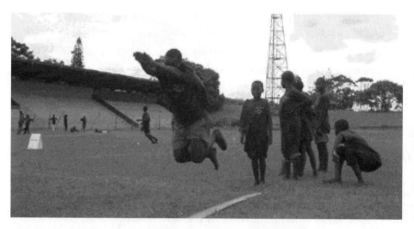

ABOVE *A standing long jump of over 2 metres! Imagine the potential of these street kids*

00:00:42
THE SPORT EVOLVES

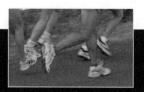

Humans are inquisitive and explorers by nature. However, most of the world has been explored and there are few areas left to be 'discovered' by the man in the street. Exploring the universe, or deeper understanding of science, now usually requires million- if not billion-dollar technology. Even within sport the evolution of records has reached the stage where massive investments are required to shave off fractions of a second or advance them by a millimetre in length. Our need to 'explore' is left largely unfulfilled so perhaps we tend to explore our own limitations to a greater extent.

It was arguably this that created the marathon boom of the 1970s, when average people did the 'seemingly impossible or improbable' by completing a 42-km run. Even this frontier has been conquered as the field in City marathons now exceeds 35 000, while in South Africa 24 000 athletes line up for a double marathon. The practical limitations of time make efforts at longer distances more of a restriction, but the search for excitement and exploration is helping to evolve a number of other events.

It is no coincidence that the range and diversity of attempts to gain recognition in the *Guinness Book of Records* has reached extremes. This is reflected in a similar diversity for the couch potato with the evolution of 'reality' TV covering the obscure and absurd to see how others react in certain situations. In the endurance sector, there have been moves towards adventure racing, eco challenges, triathlons and multiday survival events.

Such events are set to increase, and the correct preparation will be a major aspect in any competitor's success. However, the method of preparation will not differ in principle to what has been discussed in this book, although some additional aspects will have to be considered. The basic method of preparation may be summarised as follows:

THE BASIC METHOD OF PREPARATION FOR ENDURANCE EVENTS

1. Analyse the event in terms of energy expenditure each day: is it over a short period of time, or endurance over a large percentage of the day, with little recovery before the next task, or is it continuous?

2. The prime consideration of your physical training should be a mix of fast and short for all events, after which you must only do the minimum amount of long training necessary.

3. From the event analysis, identify your weaknesses and strengths. Identify what time and effort it takes to minimise your weakness and what impact that amount of time would have on your strengths. Find the optimum balance for maximum gain.

4. Calculate your energy expenditure and ensure that you follow the nutritional rules to gain recovery not only for energy, but also to promote repair of damage throughout an event. You cannot run/perform for six days on carbohydrates alone and, indeed, the need for fat and protein will be a key issue.

5. Work out how you will access the food along the way. If you have to carry it, calculate the optimum kilocalorie to gram ratio of the foods/supplements you carry. Anything above 3.5 kcal per gram (15 kj per gram) is worth considering. Find out what sources of water will be available as many items are produced in dehydrated form and therefore weigh less. In the 250-km Augrabies Extreme desert run, American Bob Sitler introduced me to the delights of dehydrated ice cream and powdered Coca-Cola – just add water!

6. Minimise the weight of everything, cut off anything unnecessary. Extra weight has a dramatic effect on energy expended and attainable speed.

7. Whatever you do carry, balance them in such as way that your natural running style is maintained. Train with the equipment in several different environments to identify problems, then review, amend and try again.

8. Plan your eating, drinking and sleep breaks – ensure that they are spaced at regular intervals. Don't miss the early breaks. It is easy to leave one out if things are going well towards the end of an event, but you put yourself under pressure if you have to include one that wasn't in your original schedule.

9. Plan a simple recovery/sleep routine so that you know exactly what must be done at each stage break or point. Don't waste time by developing these things during the event.

10. Plan and book all travel and logistics arrangements around the event.

11. The planning may take months or years, but restrict your training to no more than 10–12 weeks and keep it realistic and conservative. In most endurance events it is better to enter slightly undertrained and sharpen up along the way, than to arrive on (or over) the fitness knife edge and sustain an injury/illness.

12. Spend time dreaming and visualising the event – look at good and bad scenarios, and imagine what a 'win' will mean to you.

13. Do it – but remember it is not what you do in the beginning that counts but what you don't do that allows you to have the energy, strength and calmness to achieve your goals in the finish.

These races are set to expand in the future and will become more accessible to more people. With that will come a major move in technology as people push to be faster, or go longer. Either way, the above will be a useful checklist to plan and prepare for endurance events.

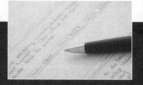

THE COMRADES TRAINING SCHEDULES

These day-by-day training schedules are designed to assist entrants to reach their full potential within the limits of time and current ability.

While elite runners 'go for gold', most entrants have restrictions of family, work, etc, that limit their training. By selecting the appropriate section, you can maximise the effectiveness of your training time, to reach your best within these limitations.

Base your choice of the three schedules on:

> ▸ your natural ability.
> ▸ Your priority for running.
> ▸ Your available training time from January to June.
> ▸ Your running experience and current personal bests.

Comrades seeding

Since 2000, Comrades has used seeding – based on your qualifying time – as a mechanism to ensure that each runner has a smooth and safe get-away at the start. You need only run in the 'band' of time that will give you your best seeding. If you want to be part of group C, run only just within the time limit for that band, even if you can run faster – why 'damage' your body by doing 5 or 10 minutes faster when the outcome will be the same as doing the slowest time for the category.

In 2003 the ability to upgrade your seeding was introduced, but there is no point in doing this unless you are sure that another race will take you into a new category. You also have to balance a slight improvement in time gained at the start, with the muscle damage inflicted by an extra race. Your focus should be on doing well in ONE race – Comrades in June – everything else should add to that.

Remember:

The KEY principle in training prior to March is to improve speed over the shorter distance, and not to become too involved in long distance. Your optimum performance in Comrades can only be achieved with a restricted racing programme from January to June. Time trials and races from 5–21 km can be accommodated in the schedule.

If weekly races are used for 'training' runs, these must be at your slow, easy pace that requires willpower and discipline, which only a few runners have.

Choose either a qualifying marathon or a 56 km as your one significant effort prior to Comrades. All other long events should be 'dry runs' at Comrades pace.

SCHEDULE A

YOU:

1. **Are a Comrades novice** – without a distance background.
2. Can run **50–85 km per week** in peak training.
3. Can only train **5 days per week.**
4. **Personal bests around:**
   10 km slower than 51:15 minutes
   21.1 km over two hours
   42.2 km over four hours
5. Have covered **25–40 km per week** in December.

This schedule will result in a Comrades time of **10–11 hours.**

SCHEDULE B

YOU:

1. Can train **6 days a week.**
2. Can run **70–100 km per week.**
3. Have **not done track training** in recent months.
4. **Personal bests around:**

    10 km between 1:40 and 2:00

    42.2km between 3:40 and 4:00

    you are looking to improve on previous Comrades time.

This schedule will result in an 8:50–10-hour Comrades.

SCHEDULE C (The Bill Rowan Medal)

YOU:

1. Train **6 days,** occasionally with 2 sessions in peak training.
2. Have run for **at least a year.**
3. Can run a **maximum** of about **120 km per week.**
4. Have some recent **track training experience.**
5. **Personal bests around:**

    10 km between 40–45 minutes

    21.1 km between 1:25–1:40

    42.2 km between 3:10–3:30

You have a desire to finish Comrades in 7:30–9 hours (a silver/bronze medal).

Silver medal

If you qualify with a sub-3:05 marathon (or a 38–40 minute, 10 km in mid May), you are a borderline silver medallist, and can modify schedule C to break the 7:30-hour silver medal barrier.

Most runners will benefit from using heart-rate monitoring principles. Heart-rate zones provide a more accurate measure of training intensity as it reflects the body's reaction to training, poor sleep or a hard day's work.

Where a single zone letter (e.g. B) is listed, it applies to all three schedules. When three letters are shown, (e.g. B/A/E), they apply to each of the three schedules in order. Use a quality heart-rate monitor such as the Cardiosport, Reebok or Impulse ranges that have an elastic chest strap and a watch receiver.

INSTRUCTIONS AND FEATURES OF THE SCHEDULE:

A typical week comprises:

- At least one 'quality' session.
- A medium length mid-week run.
- A weekend long run (or back-to-back long runs).
- Recovery/easy running on other days.
- Hard days (distance and/or quality are hard!) are followed by easy days.
- Weekend long runs alternate in length (again hard and easy principle).
- When two medium length runs are placed back-to-back, they develop the necessary endurance but without requiring the same amount of recovery. This is the preferred method of building endurance – many long runs drain and fatigue the muscles.

Learn to run and walk

While 10 km, 21.1 km and to a lesser extent the marathon are intense 'races', ultras and Comrades require a more relaxed 'journey approach'. Running five seconds per kilometre faster in Comrades will only reduce your time by 7.5 minutes! The concentration required to maintain this extra intensity when running for seven, eight or even 11 hours, takes a punishing toll on the majority of runners. Running the whole way is only appropriate for the top 70 or so runners going for a gold medal, as they are able to train to peaks of 180–200 km per week. Few runners achieve above 80–120 km per week. In daily training, we 'stop' regularly to have a drink of water – so how can we run 90 km without stopping in Comrades?

Most runners will achieve PBs by mixing running and walking in the longer runs. Train and run longer races in this manner throughout the schedules. As a start, try about 8 km runs with three-minute walks, right from the start of the session. You will soon find that what you do then allows you to have more energy at the end!

Fartlek

Speed is an essential element of training. Running everything at a long, slow speed develops a long, slow runner. All schedules use fartlek for this reason.

Each session involves:

> ‣ Jogging an easy 2–3 km warm-up.
> ‣ Some basic stretching.
> ‣ Alternate the next few kilometres with faster and easy periods until the required session is completed.
>   **Example:** Fartlek 8 km 5 x 1H 3E. **means:-**
> ‣ 2–3 km warm-up.
> ‣ 5 faster runs of one minute each (ie 1H).
> ‣ Followed by 3 minutes easy running (ie 3E).
> ‣ Finished with 2–3 km easy running.
> ‣ The fast sections are about your best 5-km race pace.

Hills

Hill sessions are excellent for introducing runners to track sessions, improving leg strength and hill running style. Two types of hill are used:

Short steep hills

> ▸ Concentrate on strength.
>
> **Example:** 3 x 4 x 35 seconds.
>
> ▸ Run hard uphill for 35 seconds.
>
> ▸ Jog down.
>
> ▸ Repeat 4 times – then walk down.
>
> ▸ Repeat the second and third sets of 4 hard runs.
>
> ▸ Longer shallower 400-m hills: 8–10% gradient.
>
> ▸ Develop muscle endurance, and hill running style.
>
> ▸ These are run about 10 seconds per kilometre faster than 5-km race pace.

Track
Track sessions: (not in schedule A)

> As a guide, the speed of the track sessions (unless shown otherwise) are:
>
> ▸ 1-km repeats – about your best 10km pace.
>
> ▸ 400-m repeats: 5–10 seconds per kilometre faster than your 5-km race pace.
>
> ▸ Keep moving (walking/jogging) during recovery periods.
>
> ▸ warm up and cool down before/after the session
>
> ▸ Do NOT try to run as fast as possible – keep to given pace.
>
> ▸ Improve, by reducing the recovery NOT increasing speed.
>
> **Example:** Track 8 km 10 x 400 m 1R **means:**
>
> ▸ The total session including warm-up and cool-down is about 8 km long.
>
> ▸ Run a 400-m run about 5 km race pace.
>
> ▸ Recover for 1 minute.
>
> ▸ Repeat until 10 x 400-m have been run, then cool down.

Weight training

Ideally, some specific strength work, particularly for the 'down run', should be included once or twice a week. This should not replace running, but should augment the schedule. Weights are an ideal part of the injury rehabilitation process, and your medical adviser should be able to provide you with guidance on suitable types of exercise.

> ▶ Use the step or toning circuits, aiming for 15–20 repetitions during each work period.
> ▶ Include leg extensions once per week – concentrate on lowering slowly.
> ▶ Reduce to one session per week in heavy training, and stop completely by the end of May.
> ▶ Possible weight days are marked 'W' – choose one or two per week for your sessions.

YEAR PLANNER FOR DOUBLE 'PEAK' IN MARATHON DISTANCE
(FIRST PEAK COULD BE USED FOR 50–56-KM EVENTS SUCH AS TWO OCEANS)

Jan	Feb	Mar	April	May	June	July	Aug	Sept	Oct	Nov	Dec
3 week festive break	Jan 26th–20 April marathon buildup	Marathon on 20th	Recovery to 18 May	X-C and speed training events	1 July–28 Sept marathon buildup				Recovery to 28 Oct	5- and 10-km sp improvement	
		Goal 2						Goal 1	Recovery	incl – two 5- and 10-km races	

YEAR PLANNER FOCUS ON COMRADES MARATHON – WITH QUALIFIER FOR THE FOLLOWING YEAR

Jan	Feb	Mar	April	May	June	July	Aug	Sept	Oct	Nov	Dec
Holiday	Gradually increase distance – keep quality aim for best 15–21-km race	Active Recovery	Specific training 10–12% increase per week	Peak Distance	taper	Rest and Recovery period	Regain 'speed' – lower dist	Rebuild on back of Comrades training for Qualifier	Taper and marathon	Recovery Period	Drop Dist. Focus on quality and race at 5–10-km events

TRAINING SCHEDULE FOR 10 KM IN 55 MINUTE TARGET – 6-WEEK PLAN

DAY	TRAINING	AM HEART-RATE	ACTUAL TRAINING	PERCEIVED EFFORT (1 = EASY 10 = VERY HARD) OR HEART RATE	COMMENTS AND ROUTE DETAILS
1	Rest				
2	7 km fartklek with 4 x 45 sec hard 3 min easy				
3	4–6 km easy @ 6:30 per km				
4	5–7 km easy @ 6:30 per km				
5	Rest				
6	8 km fartlek with 3 x 90 sec hard 6 min easy				
7	8–9 km easy @ 6:30 per km				
total	36 km	weight			
1	Rest				
2	7 km fartklek with 6 x 1 min hard 4 mins easy				
3	5–7 km easy @ 6:30 per km				
4	Track 4 x 200 m in 62 sec with 2 min recovery				
5	Rest				
6	6 km fartlek with 6 x 30 sec hard 3 min easy				
7	8–10 km easy @ 6:30 per km				
total	36 km	weight			

If time allows repeat these blocks 2 to 3 times

DAY	TRAINING	AM HEART-RATE	ACTUAL TRAINING	PERCEIVED EFFORT (1 = EASY 10 = VERY HARD) OR HEART RATE	COMMENTS AND ROUTE DETAILS
1	Rest				
2	Track 4 x 400 m in 2:13 with 2 min recovery				
3	easy 6 km @ 6:00 per km				
4	5–7 km fartlek with 6 x 30 sec with 3 min recovery				
5	Rest				
6	Road 2–3 x 1000 m in 5:25 with 3 min recovery				
7	9–10 km easy @ 6:30 per km				
total	38 km	weight			
1	Rest				
2	easy 5–6 km @ 6:00 per km				
3	3 x 1000 in 5:10 with 3 min recovery				
4	Rest				
5	easy 7 km @ 6:30 per km				
6	5 x 200 in 59 sec with 2 min recovery				
7	12–13 km easy @ 6:30				
total	39 –40 km	weight			

If time permits repeat this after following week

DAY	TRAINING	AM HEARTRATE	ACTUAL TRAINING	PERCEIVED EFFORT (1 = EASY 10 = VERY HARD) OR HEART RATE	COMMENTS AND ROUTE DETAILS
1	Rest				
2	5–6 x 400 m in 2:05 with 2 min recovery				
3	easy 6–8 km @ 6:30 per km				
4	4 x 100 in 5:25 per km with 3 min recovery				
5	Rest				
6	7–8 x 200 m in 59 sec with 2 min recovery				
7	9–10 km easy @ 6:30 per km				
total	42 km	weight			
1	Rest				
2	4 x 400 m in 2:13 with 2 min recovery				
3	3 km fartlek with 3 x 30 sec hard 3 min easy				
4	easy 3–4 km @ 6:00 per km				
5	Rest				
6	easy 1–2 km then 3 x 200 in 66 seconds (this is race pace) as much recovery as wanted				
7	10 km race				
total	28 km				

COMRADES TRAINING REQUIREMENTS AND PACES

Best 10-km time	33.00	37.25	41.40	45.50	50.00	54.30	58.20	60.20
Best 42.2 km time	2 hr 35 min	2 hr 55 min	3 hr 15 min	3hr 35 min	3 hr 55 min	4 hr 15 min	4 hr 35 min	4 hr 44 min
Best Comrades	6 hr 5 min	6 hr 50 min	7 hr 35 min	8 hr 20 min	9 hr 5 min	9 hr 50 min	10 hr 30 min	10 hr 57 min
Worst Comrades	7 hr 45 min	8 hr 40 min	9 hr 30 min	10 hr 20 min	11 hr	11 hr	11 hr	11 hr
Least distance Jan to June	900 km	900 km	900 km	900 km	1 000 km	1 150 km	1 370 km	1 450 km
Max distance Jan to June	2 500 km	2 250 km	2 100 km	1 860 km	1 720 km	1 590 km	1 500 km	1 450 km
400-m Intervals (per lap)	1 min 12 sec	1 min 22 sec	1 min 31 sec	1 min 42 sec	1 min 52 sec	2 min 2 sec	2 min 13 secs	2 min 17 sec
1 000-m intervals Per km	3 min 8 sec	3 min 33 sec	3 min 55 sec	4 min 20 sec	4 min 50 sec	5 min 20 sec	5 min 45 sec	5 min 55 sec
Mod 8-12 km run per km	3 min 45 sec	4 min 12 sec	4 min 22 sec	5 min	5 min 30 sec	5 min 55 sec	6 min 20 sec	6 min 35 sec
Training 35-45 km per km	4 min	4 min 30 sec	4 min 44 sec	5 min 25 sec	6 min	6 min 30 sec	7 min	7 min 15 sec

NOTE: 1) Doing more than maximum is likely to result in overtraining **2)** Peak training is based on 10–12 hours per week training. Doing more is unlikely to allow sufficient time for recovery unless you are a full-time athlete **3)** Realistically, the slowest qualifying marathon time required to finish Comrades in 11 hours is 4:32 minutes! **4)** Keep easy runs easy and quality work in 400 m and 1 000 m at suggested pace **5)** If training in a race – keep it easy. Fordyce could run 2:17 for a marathon but often trained at 2:59 min – slower than his Comrades pace.

RCH	Dist	Dist B	Dist C	Schedule A	Schedule B	Bill Rowan Schedule	Heart-rate
		8	8	Rest	easy 8 km	easy 8 km	A/E/E
	8	32	36	8 km fartlek with 3 x 2 min H 5 min easy	am 20 km easy pm 12 km easy	am 18 km pm 18 km all at comrades pace	
	20	15	15	25 km LSD (ideally split 15 km in morning 10 km night)	am 15 km easy with 30 sec pick up every 5 km	15 km comrades pace with 1 min @ 10-km pace every 3 km	
ek 1							
n				Rest	Rest	Rest	A
s	5	8	8	5 km fartlek with 5 x 30 sec hard easy 3 min	Fartlek 3 x 2 min hard 5 min easy	Track 4 x 1000 @ 10 km pace with 3 min recovery	C/C/D
d	8	8	10	8 km easy	8 km easy	8–10 km easy	A
rs	10	15	15	10 km	12–15 km easy	15 km	B/A/A
		8	8	Rest W	Hills 4 x 200m walk back	Hills 5 x 200 m jog back recovery	-/D/D
	10	10	12	10 km with 3 x 200 m hills walk back	10 km W	10–12 km W	C/B/D
n	22	22	25	20–22 km LSD	20–22 km LSD	20–25 km LSD	A
ek 2							
n				Rest W	Rest	Rest	
s	8	12	12	Hills 6 x 100m walk back	12 km including 5 km time trial	12 km including 5 km time trial	D
d	12	10	20	10–12 km easy W	8–10 km easy W	18–20 km	A
rs	8	17	10	Fartlek 4 x 1 min hard 3 min easy	17–20 km	10 km W	D/A/B
		8	8	Rest	8 km easy	am 8 km easy pm Hills 6 x 400 m	-/A/E
	25	10	15	25 km LSD	Hills 7 x 400 m walk back recovery	10–15 km W	A/D/A
n	21	35	40	18–21 km LSD	35 km LSD	38–40 km LSD	A
				This should be run at Comrades pace – NOT FASTER			

MARCH	Dist	Dist B	Dist C	Schedule A	Schedule B	Bill Rowan Schedule	He rat
week 3							
Mon				Rest W	Rest W	Rest W	
Tues	10	8	18	10 km easy	Hills 2 x 5 x 35 sec walk back rec	am 8 km easy PM Track 10 x 400 m @ 10-km pace rest 1 min	A/D
Wed	18	16	25	15–18 km LSD	16 km	20–25 km	A
Thurs	8	8	8	8km W	8 km easy W	8 km W	B/A
Fri	6	10	16	Fartlek 4 x 1 min hard 3 min easy	Fartlek 3 x 2 min hard 5 min easy	am 8 km easy pm Hills 2 x 6 x 35 sec jog back	D/D
Sat		10	15	rest	8–10 km easy or rest	10–15 km easy	-/A/
Sun	10	15	20	10-km Race	15 km @ half-marathon pace	20 km with 2 x 4 km @ 10-km pace	D/B
week 4							
Mon				Rest	Rest	Rest W	
Tues	8	8	10	8 km easy	Fartlek 4 x 1 min hard 2 min easy	Track 4 x 400 m @ 3 000-m pace rest 3 min	A/D
Wed		10	15	Rest	10 km easy	15 km easy	A
Thurs	5	8	8	3–5 km easy	Fartlek 6 x 30 sec hard 2 min easy	track 6 x 400 m @ 10-km pace rest 2 min	A/D
Fri		5	8	Rest	3 km easy or rest if Sunday race	8 km easy or rest if Sunday race	
Sat	56	60	60	50–60 km short ultra at Comrades pace (see table 1) or 3 km easy if Sunday race	50–60 km short ultra at Comrades pace (see table 1) or 3 km easy if Sunday race	50–60 km short ultra at Comrades pace (see table 1) or 8 km easy if Sunday race	
Sun				50–60 km short ultra at Comrades pace (see table 1) or swim or cycle if Saturday race	50–60 km short ultra at Comrades pace (see table 1) or swim or cycle if Saturday race	50–60 km short ultra at Comrades pace (see table 1) or 5–8 km easy if Saturday race	
				Use this event as a dry run to test out your Comrades schedule, kit, and drinks – don't race. Aim for finish of 1.5 x marathon time not faster.			

APRIL	Dist	Dist B	Dist C	Schedule A	Schedule B	Bill Rowan Schedule	Heart-rate
Week 5							
Mon				Rest	Rest	Rest or 5 km easy	A
Tues	5	8	8	5 km easy or rest	8 km easy or rest	5–8 km easy W	A
Wed	8		10	8 km easy or rest	8 km easy	8–10 km easy	A
Thurs	10	15	18	10 km	12–15 km easy	15–18 km	B/A/B
		8	8	Rest W	Hills 4 x 200 m walk back	Hills 5 x 200 m jog back recovery	-/D/D
Sat	10	10	12	10 km with 3 x 200 m hills walk back	10 km W	10–12 km W	C/B/D
Sun	22	22	25	20–22 km LSD	20–22 km LSD	20–25 km LSD	A
Week 6							
Mon				Rest	Rest	Rest W	A
Tues	8	10	10	Hills 6–7 x 100 m walk back	6–10 km easy	Track 3 x 800 m @ 10-km pace 1 ½ min rec	D/A/B
Wed	18	18	20	15–18 km LSD	18 km LSD	20 km LSD	A
Thurs	8	12	12	8 km easy W	12 km easy W	12 km easy W	A
		8	8	Rest	Fartlek 3 x 2 min hard 5 easy	Hills 2 x 6 x 35 sec jog back	-/C/E
Sat	35	40	40	30–35 km Comrades pace	35–40 km Comrades pace	40 km comrades pace	B/A/A
Sun	12	12	18	10–12 km marathon pace	12 km marathon pace	15–18 km marathon pace	B
Week 7							
Mon				Rest	Rest	Rest W	
Tues	8	10	10	Hills 6–7 x 100 m walk back	6–10 km easy	Track 3 x 800m @ 10-km pace 1 ½ min rec	D/A/B
Wed	18	18	20	15–18 km LSD	18 km LSD	20 km LSD	A
Thurs	8	12	12	8 km easy W	12 km easy W	12 km easy W	A
		8	8	Rest	Fartlek 3 x 2 min hard 5 easy	Hills 2 x 6 x 35 sec jog back	-/C/E
Sat	25	28	28	20–25 km Comrades pace	25–28 km Comrades pace	25–28 km Comrades pace	B/A/A
Sun	12	12	18	10–12 km marathon pace	12 km marathon pace	15–18 km marathon pace	B

APRIL	Dist	Dist B	Dist C	Schedule A	Schedule B	Bill Rowan Schedule	Heart rate
week 8							
Mon				Rest W	Rest W	Rest W	
Tues	10	10	20	8–10 km easy	Hills 5 x 400m walk back rec	a.m. 8 km easy pm Track 5–6 x 1000 @ 15 km race pace rest 1 ½ min	A/D/(
Wed	8	22	25	Fartlek 4 x 1 min hard 2 ½ min easy	18–22 km	21–25 km	D/A/
Thurs	16	8	10	16 km W	8 km easy W	10 km W	B/A/
Fri		8	18	Rest	Fartlek 8 x 30 sec hard 2 min easy	am 8 km easy pm hills 8 x 400 m jog back	-/E/C
Sat	8	10	15	Fartlek 2–4 x 1 min hard 2 min easy	8–10 km easy	12–15 km W	D/A/
Sun	40	40	40	38–40 km Comrades pace. This must be at slow pace or you are likely to overtrain! If using a race then finish should be 1.13 times your best marathon time (I.e. a 3:300 marathoner would take 4 hours for the marathon distance).			A
week 9							
Mon				Rest W	Rest W	Rest	
Tues				If running final qualifying marathon on May 1, then use April 29 and May 2 as rest days and do 5 km fartlek 3 x 1 min hard 4 easy on April 30.			
	289	349	413				
				If running final qualifying marathon on May 1, then use April 29 and May 2 as rest days and do 5 km fartlek 3 x 1 min hard 4 easy on April 30.			
Wed	10	18	18	10 km	15–18 km @ 15-km pace	am 8 km easy pm Track 4–5 x 1 000 rest 1 ½	B/B/(
Thurs	8	8	21	Hills 4–5 x 200 m walk back	Hills 2 x 5 x 35 sec walk back recovery	18–21 km	D/D/
Fri		10	16	Rest	Fartlek 4 x 2 min hard 5 min easy	am 8 km easy pm Hills 7 x 400 m jog back	-/D/D
Sat	25	8	10	22–25 km	8 km easy	10–12 km W	A
Sun	18	30	30	18 km	30–33 km	30–35 km	A

EVERYONE'S GUIDE TO DISTANCE RUNNING

AY	Dist	Dist B	Dist C	Schedule A	Schedule B	Bill Rowan Schedule	Heart Rate
ek 10							
ɔn				Rest W	Rest W	Rest W	
ɪes	10	12	20	8–10 km easy	12 km incl 5-km time trial	am 8 km easy pm Track 5–6 x 1 000 m @ 15-km pace rest 1 ½ min	A/C/C
ɪd	8	8	23	Fartlek 3 x 2 hard 4 min easy	8 km easy	23–25 km LSD	B/A/A
urs	15	17	18	15 km W	15–17 km W	am 8 km easy pm Hills 6 x 400 m jog back	B/A/C
		10	10	Rest	8–10 km easy	10 km easy or rest W	-/A/A
t	30	10	15	30 km Comrades pace	8–10 km easy	am rest pm 15–18 km easy	A
ɪn	25	56	56	20–25 km marathon pace	50–60 km Comrades pace	56 km Comrades pace	A
ek 11							
ɔn				Rest W	Rest W	Rest W	
ɪes	8	10	20	Hills 2 x 5 x 35 sec walk back rec	Hills 6 x 400 m walk back rec	am 8 km easy pm 2 x 2000 @ 10-km pace rest 3 min	D/D/C
ɪd	18	8	16	18 km	8 km easy W	16 km	A
urs	10	15	17	8–10 km easy W	15 km	am 8 km easy pm Hills 2 x 6 x 35 sec jog back	A/B/C
		8	10	Rest	8 km easy W	8–10 km easy or rest W	-/A/A
ɪt	25	30	32	25 km LSD	25–30 km LSD	32–35 km LSD	A
ɪn	25	25	25	22–25 km LSD	20–25 km LSD	25–28 km LSD	A

MAY	Dist	Dist B	Dist C	Schedule A	Schedule B	Bill Rowan Schedule	Heart rate
week 12							
Mon				Rest W	Rest W	Rest W	
Tues	8	8	12	Hills 2 x 6 x 35 sec walk recovery	8 km easy	12 km incl 5-km time trial	D/A/
Wed	20	18	12	18–20 km	18 km	10–12 km easy	A/B/
Thurs	10	8	25	8–10 km easy W	8 km easy W	25 km W	A
Fri		8	17	Rest	Fartlek 8 x 30 sec hard 2 min easy	am 8 km easy pm Hills 2 x 6 x 35 sec jog back	-/D/
Sat	8	12	20	Fartlek 3–4 x 2 min hard 4 min easy	8–12 km easy	20 km LSD	D/A/
Sun	35	38	30	33–35 km Comrades pace or 21.1 @ 80% effort	34–38 km @ Comrades pace or 21.1 race @ 80%	30 km @ Comrades pace or 21.1 race @ 80%	B/B/
week 13							
Mon				Rest	Rest	Rest	
Tues				Commence your taper – drop the distance, keep quality work.			
Wed	8	10	10	Hills 2 x 6 x 35 sec walk recovery	Fartlek 4 x 1 min hard 3 min easy	Track 8 x 400 m @ 10-km pace 1 ½ m recovery	C
Thurs	10	10	18	8–10 km easy W	10 km easy W	15–18 km W	A/A/
Fri	10	10	12	8–10 km easy	10 km easy	12 km with 8 km Time trial	A/A/
Sat	8	8	8	Fartlek 5 x 1 min hard 2 min easy	Hills 3 x 4 x 35 sec with walk back	easy 8 km with 30 sec pick up every 2 km	C/C/
	352	413	521				
Sat	8	8	15	Fartlek 4 x 2 min hard 4 min easy	Fartlek 8 x 30 sec hard 1 min easy	10–15 km easy	C/C/
Sun	21	21	21	21 km at Comrades pace for first 16 km then gradually increase to final km at 10-km race pace.			

EVERYONE'S GUIDE TO DISTANCE RUNNING

NE	Dist	Dist B	Dist C	Schedule A	Schedule B	Bill Rowan Schedule	Heart-rate
ek 14							
n				Rest	Rest	Rest	
s	8	8	10	8 km easy	Hills 2 x 4 x 35 secs walk back	10 km easy	A/D/A
d	15	16	10	12–15 km LSD	16 km LSD	Track 2 x 2000 m @ 10-km pace rest 3 min	A/A/C
urs	8	23	17	Hills 2 x 4 x 35 sec, walk back	23 km Comrades pace	17 km marathon pace	D/A/A
		8	10	Rest	8 km easy	8–10 km easy	-/A/A
t	18	15	23	18 km Comrades pace	15 km Comrades pace	23 km Comrades pace	A
n				Rest	Rest	Rest	
ek 15							
n	6	6	8	Fartlek 4 x 1 min hard 3 min easy	Fartlek 4 x 1 ½ min hard, 4 min easy	4 x 400 m @ 3 000-m pace 3 min rest	D
s	5	8	6	Fartlek 3 x 1 min hard 3 min easy	8 km easy	3 x 400 m @ 3 000-m pace, 3 min rest	D/A/D
d				Rest	Rest	Rest	
urs	4	4	5	Fartlek 3 x 30 sec hard 2 min easy, or rest day	Fartlek 4 x 30 sec hard 2 min easy	Fartlek 4 x 1 min hard 3 min easy or rest	D
				Rest	Rest	Rest	
t				Fartlek 3 x 30 sec hard 2 min easy, or rest day	Fartlek 4 x 30 sec hard 2 min easy	1 x 400 m @ 5-km pace 500 m jog warm up and cool down	
n	90	90	90	**It's Comrades** – IT'S YOUR RACE, enjoy the day and do your best.			
ek 16							
n				Try for 20 minutes of very light exercise such as stationary cycling or swimming/leg kick in water to assist recovery.			
	93	117	125				
EDULE AL	1012	1255	1504	These totals for each schedule are maximums from March to June (excluding Comrades) and hence allow for the occasional problem that interferes with training.			

10 km in 50 minutes

week 1

thur	Day 1	Rest
fri	2	Fartlek 6 km — 3.7 mi → 4 (3 x 45 sec hard, 3 min easy)
Sat	3	3–4 km easy
Sun	4	5–7 km + 5:30 min/km
mon	5	Fartlek 6 km (as above)
tues	6	3–4 km easy
wed	7	6–8 km LSD
		Total 35 km

week 2

thur	Day 1	Rest
fri	2	Fartlek 6–7 km (3 x 1 min hard, 3 min easy)
Sat	3	4–5 km easy — A
Sun	4	5–7 km mod — B
mon	5	Track (5 x 200 60 sec, rest 2 min) — D
tue	6	Rest
wed	7	8–10 LSD
		Total 35 km

week 3

Day 1 Rest
2 Track (3 x 400 1:58, rest 3½, then 2 x 200 in 55, rest 2 min)
3 4–5 km easy
4 6–8 km mod
5 Track (5 x 400 1:58, rest 3½)
6 4–5 km easy
7 8–10 km LSD
Total 38 km

week 4

Day 1 Rest
2 Track (6 x 400 +/- 1:55, rest 3)
3 5 km easy
4 6–8 km mod
5 Track (1 x 400 1:52, rest 2 min. 1 x 200 53, rest 3½, 3 rep)
6 Rest
7 10–12 km LSD
Total 36 km

week 5

Day 1 Rest
2 Track (6 x 400 +/- 1:52, rest 3 min, jog 300)
3 5 km easy
4 6–8 km
5 Track (3 x 800 in 3:50) Rest 4 +/- (jog 500)
6 5 km easy
7 10–12 km LSD
Total 42 km

week 6

Day 1 Rest
2 Fartlek 8 km (4 x 1 min hard, 3 easy)
3 5 km easy (+/- 27–28 min)
4 5–6 km (26–32 min)
5 Rest
6 3–4 km easy (+/- 25 min) stretching
7 10 km easy
Total 33 km

10 km in 45 minutes

week 1

Day 1 Rest
2 Fartlek 6–8 km (3 x 1 min hard, 3 easy)
3 4–5 km easy
4 7–8 km mod 4:45–5:00
5 Fartlek 6–8 km (as above)
6 4–5 km easy
7 8–10 km LSD
Total 44 km

week 2

Day 1 Rest
2 Fartlek 6 km 2 x (1 hard, 2 easy, 1/2 hard, 1 easy)
3 4–5 km easy
4 7–8 km mod 4:45–5:00
5 Fartlek 6-8 km (3 x 1½ hard, 3½ easy)
6 4–5 easy
7 10 km LSD
Total 44 km

week 3

Day 1 Rest
2 Track (4 x 400 in 1:4 rest 2 min)
3 4–5 km
4 7–8 km mod 4:40-4:
5 Track (3 x 800 in 3: rest 4 min)
6 4–5 km easy
7 8–10 km
Total 46 km

week 4

Day 1 Rest
2 Track (5 x 400 in 1:4 rest 2 min)
3 4–5 km easy
4 8 km mod 4:35–4:4
5 Track (3 x 1 000 in rest 5 min)
6 4–5 km easy
7 10–12 km LSD
Total 48 km

week 5

Day 1 Rest
2 Track (3 x 600 in 2:35, rest 3 min)
3 4–5 km easy
4 8 km mod 4:35–4:45
5 4–5 km easy
6 Track (1 x 1 000 in 4:30, rest 2 min, 1 x 800 in 3:30, rest 2, 1 x 600 in 2: rest 2, 2 x 200 in 4 rest 1)
7 8–10 km LSD
Total 47 km

week 6

Day 1 Rest
2 Track (6 x 200 in 48, rest 1:40)
3 4–5 km easy
4 8 km 4:35–4:45
5 4–5 km easy
6 Track (4 x 400 in 1:36, rest 2½ min)
7 11–13 km LSD
Total 47 km

1	Rest
2	Track (6 x 200 in 48, rest 1:50)
3	4–5 km easy
4	6 km mod 4:35
5	Rest
6	Easy 3–4 km
7	Race 10 km in 45 min
	Total 33 km

km in 40 minutes

ek 1

1	Rest
2	Fartlek (5 x 1 min hard, 3 easy)
3	6–8 km easy
4	8–10 km mod 4:20
5	Fartlek (5 x 1 min hard, 3 easy)
6	6–8 km easy
7	10–12 km LSD
	Total 54 km

ek 2

1	Rest
2	Hills 5 x 200, (double effort recovery)
3	6–8 km easy
4	8–10 km mod 4:20
5	6–8 km easy
6	Fartlek (6 x 1 min hard, 3 easy)
7	10–12 km LSD
	Total 55 km

ek 3

1	Rest
2	Hills 6 x 200 (full 2 x effort recovery)
3	6–8 km easy
4	8–10 km mod 4:20
5	6–8 km easy
6	Track (5 x 400 1:30, rest 2 min)
7	12 km LSD
	Total 60 km

week 4

Day 1	Rest
2	Hills 7 x 200 (full 2 x effort recovery)
3	6–8 km easy
4	8–10 km mod 4:15 min/km
5	6–8 km easy
6	+/- 5 km time trial +/- 19 min (NOT FLAT OUT)
7	14 km LSD
	Total 60 km

week 5

Day 1	Rest
2	Track (6 x 200 43, rest 90 sec)
3	6–8 km easy
4	8–10 km mod 4:15 min/km
5	6–8 km easy
6	Track (4 x 400, rest 1 min, 1 x 200, rest 3 min) x 3
7	11 km LSD
	Total 54 km

week 6

Day 1	Rest
2	Track (6 x 200 43, rest 90 sec)
3	6–8 km easy
4	8–10 km mod 4:15 min/km
5	6–8 km easy
6	Track (5 x 400 1:28, rest 2 min)
7	15 km LSD
	Total 58 km

week 7

Day 1	Rest
2	6 km 4:10 min/km
3	Track (2 x 400 1:30, rest 3, 3 x 200 43, rest 1½)
4	Rest
5	4–5 km easy/strides
6	Race 10 km
7	11–13 km LSD
	Total 27 km

Sub-4:15 Marathon

You should be capable of +/- 40 km/week for the last 6–8 weeks.

week 1

Day 1	Rest
2	Fartlek (3–4 x 30 sec hard, 2 easy)
3	4–5 km easy
4	8–10 km mod 6:10 min/km
5	4–5 km easy
6	Rest
7	18–20 km
	Total 45 km

week 2

Day 1	Rest
2	Fartlek (4–6 km x 30 sec hard, 2 easy)
3	4–5 km easy
4	10 km mod
5	Fartlek 4–5 km (2–3 x 1 min)
6	Rest
7	21–25 km
	Total 50 km

week 3

Day 1	Rest
2	Fartlek (4–6 x 30 sec hard, 2 easy)
3	4–5 km easy
4	12–14 km LSD
5	4–5 km easy
6	Rest
7	10 km race +/- 55 min
	Total 40 km

week 4

Day 1	Rest
2	Fartlek (6–8 km min hard, 2 easy)
3	5–6 km easy
4	10 km mod 6:05 min/km
5	5–6 km easy
6	Rest
7	18–21 km
	Total 49 km

A = 55-65% max HR   E = rest
B = 65-85%
C = 85-90%
D = 90+

week 5

Day	1	Rest
	2	Fartlek (3 x 1 min hard, 4 easy, 3 x 30 sec hard, 2 easy)
	3	5–6 km easy – A
	4	8–10 km mod – B
	5	5–6 km easy
	6	Rest
	7	28–30 km LSD

Total 59 km

week 6

Day	1	Rest
	2	5–6 km easy
	3	Fartlek (4–6 x 30 sec hard, 2 easy)
	4	8 km +/- 50–51 min
	5	5–6 km easy
	6	Rest
	7	10 km race +/- 52–53 min

Total 37 km

week 7

Day	1	Rest
	2	Fartlek (3 x 30 sec hard, 2 easy, 3 x 1 min hard, 4 easy)
	3	5–6 km easy
	4	12–15 km moderate +/- 6:00 min/km
	5	5–6 km easy
	6	Rest
	7	25–28 km LSD

Total 59 km

week 8

Day	1	Rest
	2	Fartlek +/- 6 km easy (4 x 30 sec bursts)
	3	6 km easy
	4	5–7 km
	5	Rest
	6	Rest
	7	Race 42 km

Total 60 km

Sub-3:30 Marathon

Should be capable of +50 km/week over the last 6-8 weeks.

week 1

Day	1	Rest
	2	Fartlek (+ 8 km with 3–5 x 1 min hard, 3 easy)
	3	6–8 km easy
	4	Hills 3–4 x 200 (double recovery of effort)
	5	6–8 km easy
	6	15–20 km LSD
	7	12–15 km LSD

Total 64 km

week 2

Day	1	Rest
	2	Fartlek (8–10 km with 3 x 1 min hard, 3 easy, 4 x 30 sec hard, 1 easy)
	3	6–8 km easy
	4	+ 5 km TT
	5	6–8 km easy
	6	18–22 km LSD
	7	10–12 km LSD

Total 63 km

week 3

Day	1	Rest
	2	Fartlek (8–10 km with 4 x 1 min hard, 3 easy. 6 x 30 sec hard, 1 easy)
	3	6–8 km easy
	4	10 km mod + 5:10/km
	5	6–8 km easy
	6	Fartlek (8 km 3 x 90 sec hard, 4½ easy)
	7	20–25 LSD

Total 64 km

week 4

Day	1	Rest
	2	Fartlek (+ 10 km wi... 5 x 1 min hard, 3 e... 6 x 30 sec hard, 1 e...
	3	6–8 km easy
	4	10–12 km mod
	5	6–8 km easy
	6	Fartlek (8 km with 3 x ½ hard, 4½ ea...
	7	20–25 km easy

Total 66 km

week 5

Day	1	Rest
	2	Fartlek (8 x 30 sec h... 2 easy)
	3	5–8 km easy
	4	10 km mod + 5:05
	5	Fartlek (3 x 1 min h...
	6	5–6 km easy
	7	28–32 km

Total 68 km

week 6

Day	1	Rest
	2	Fartlek (1 min hard, 2 easy, 2 min hard, 4 easy, etc – up to 4 min hard, 8 easy)
	3	6–8 km easy
	4	8–10 km mod 5:05
	5	6–8 km easy
	6	Fartlek (8 km 4 x 1 hard, 3 easy)
	7	20–25 km LSD

Total 67 km

week 7

Day	1	Rest
	2	8–10 km TT
	3	5–7 km easy
	4	Fartlek (6–8 km wit... 4 x 1 min hard, 3 e...
	5	5–7 km easy
	6	10–12 km mod +/- 5:00 min/km
	7	Rest

Total 45 km

ay 1   18–20 km
2   5–7 km easy
3   Fartlek easy *(30 sec bursts)*
4   Rest
5   4–5 km easy
6   Rest
7   Race
  Total 70 km

ub-3:00 Marathon

nould be able to do + 60 km/week
r the past 8 weeks.

eek 1

ay 1   Rest
2   Hills 3–5 x 200 *(double recovery as effort)*
3   6–8 km easy
4   12–15 km mod
5   6–8 km easy
6   Fartlek *(8–10 km with 3–5 x 1 min hard, 3 easy)*
7   18–20 km LSD
  Total 69 km

eek 2

ay 1   Rest
2   Hills 4–6 x 200 *(double recovery)*
3   8 km easy
4   5 km TT *(not flat out +/- 98%)*
5   8 km easy
6   Hills 3–4 x 300
7   20–25 km LSD
  Total 67 km

eek 3

ay 1   Rest
2   Track *(3–4 x 1 km in 4:00, rest 5 min)*
3   6–8 km easy
4   12–15 km mod +/- 4:20 min/km
5   6–8 km easy
6   20 km LSD
7   15–20 km LSD
  Total 76 km

week 4

Day 1   Rest
2   Track *(4x 800 in 3:10, rest 4 min)*
3   8 km easy
4   12–15 km mod
5   Hills 4–6 x 200
6   6–8 km easy
7   30–32 km LSD
  Total 80 km

week 5

Day 1   Rest
2   Track *(5 x 800 in 3:10, rest 4)*
3   8 km easy
4   12–15 km mod
5   Track *(3 x 400 1:30 rests, 3 x 200 in 43, rest ½)*
6   20–25 km LSD
  Total 77 km

week 6

Day 1   Rest
2   Track *(6–8 x 400 +/- 1:30 rests)*
3   8 km easy
4   12 km mod 4:15 min/km
5   Track *(3 x 400 1:30, rest 3, 3 x 200, rest ½)*
6   6–8 km easy
7   32–36 km
  Total 72 km

week 7

Day 1   Rest
2   8 or 10 km TT (+/- 98%)
3   6–8 km easy
4   Track *(6–8 x 400 in 1:30, rest 3)*
5   6–8 km easy
6   15 km mod
7   6–8 km LSD
  Total 60 km

week 8

Day 1   Rest
2   6–8 km easy
3   Fartlek +/- 8 km (informal but easy – don't tax yourself)
4   Rest
5   4–5 km easy
6   Rest
7   Race 42 km
  Total 74 km

Symbols used

AM: morning run
PM: evening or afternoon run
W: weight training
TT: time-trial
H/E: hard/easy
R: recovery
LSD: long, slow distance

INDEX

GLOSSARY

The following 'definitions' are a layman's explanation for physiological conditions. For a strict medical definition, consult a medical/sports science dictionary.

aerobic exercise – where oxygen for exercise is provided by the amount of oxygen inhaled

anabolic/catabolic – muscle growth/muscle breakdown

anaerobic exercise – where oxygen requirements of exercise intensity exceeds the oxygen inhaled

ATP (adenosine triphosphate) – the primary chemical used by muscles in the production of energy

bricks – a combination of sessions from 2 or more triathlon disciplines in a continuous training session

bus – a number of runners running in a group in a race

creatine phosphate – the energy system used for short, powerful exercise of 3–45 seconds' duration

DMSO (dimethyl sulphoxide) – an anti-inflammatory agent

fartlek – a Swedish word for a training session with a variety of different speeds continuously mixed

journey race – an ultramarathon race, often from one town or city to another with

lactate threshold – a level of exercise where the amount of lactate produced as a by-product of the exercise equals the rate at which the lactate can be metabolised by the body back to energy

lactate turnpoint pace – research suggests that the production of lactate from muscle exercise is not linear, but sharply increases at a particular intensity of exercise

macro/micro training blocks – training goals are set in short, medium and long term; the objective of a macroblock is achieved through the relevant combination of microblocks

maximum heart rate – the maximum rate at which the heart will beat during all out exercise

negative split – running the second half of an event faster than the second half

pacing schedule – a strategy developed to control the speed of a runner through a race

parluaf cross-country – a cross-country event involving a team of two runners in which each takes alternate times of running over a lap, until the total required number of laps is completed

PB – personal best, also known as PR (personal record) for a particular race distance

peaking – reaching a peak level of fitness ideally at the same time as the goal competition

plyometrics – a series of bounding, hopping, jumping and explosive exercises, used to develop 'elastic strength' in a runner

pronation/supination – the inward roll of the foot (most easily observed at the inner ankle bone)/the outward roll of the foot as the foot moves through its motion on the ground

quality speeds – speeds used to train the quality as opposed to quantity training. These speeds vary depending on the distance of the goal race

quality work – the training done at the quality speeds

race pace – the pace at which a runner can be expected to achieve his best time for a distance

short-term energy systems – those used in flat out efforts in events of up to 1-minute duration

split – the time taken to do a part or portion of a run e.g. in a race a runner may take a time at every km mark – this would provide km splits

taper period – a period used to progressively reduce the training load from the peak training period

training load – this is a measure of the difficulty or work undertaken in training

VO$_2$ Max – this is a measure of the maximum amount of oxygen used by an athlete under maximum effort. It is specific to each person and each sport; typically for runners this is tested on a treadmill where the speed or incline are increased regularly until the runner can run no faster. The amount of oxygen consumed at each pace is recorded and the VO$_2$ Max is expressed as a volume/kg body weight